AUSTRALIAN AUTISM HANDBOOK

Benison O'Reilly and Seana Smith

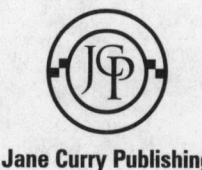

Jane Curry Publishing

DISCLAIMER

The Australian Autism Handbook aims to provide readers with information, but is not intended to be, and is not, a substitute for health and medical advice from a qualified health professional. Jane Curry Publishing does not guarantee or warrant the accuracy, currency, suitability or reliability of any information contained within the book. Diagnosis and treatment of a medical condition should only be undertaken by a qualified health professional and readers should always seek the advice of a qualified health professional before treatment of any condition. In reading this book you accept all risk and responsibility for losses, damages, costs or any other consequences resulting directly or indirectly from relying on information or material contained within it. To the maximum permitted by law, Jane Curry Publishing excludes all liability to any person arising directly or indirectly from using this book and any information or material in it.

First published by Jane Curry Publishing in 2008
(Wentworth Concepts Pty Ltd t/a Jane Curry Publishing)
PO Box 780
Edgecliff NSW 2027

www.janecurrypublishing.com.au

National Library of Australia
Cataloguing in publication data:

Benison O'Reilly and Seana Smith
Australian Autism Handbook

ISBN: 978-0-9804758-1-4
Parenting/Family

Typeset in 11.5/15 Sabon
Cover and internal design by Deborah Parry
Printed in Australia by McPherson's Printing Group

CONTENTS

ABBREVIATIONS

ABA: Applied Behavioural Analysis
ABAS: Adaptive Behaviour Assessment System
ADEC: Autism Detection in Early Childhood
ADHD: attention deficit hyperactivity disorder
ADI-R: Autism Diagnostic Interview–Revised
ADOS: Autism Diagnostic Observation Schedule
AIT: Auditory Integration Therapy
ASD: Autism Spectrum Disorder
CARS: Childhood Autism Rating Scale
CHAT: Checklist for Autism in Toddlers
DISCO: Diagnostic Interview for Social and Communication Disorders
DSM-IV- TR: Diagnostic and Statistical Manual of Mental Disorders 4th edition, Text
Revision
DTT: Discrete Trial Training
GFCF diet: gluten-free, casein-free diet
HFA: high-functioning autism
IBI: intensive behavioural intervention
IEP: individual education plan
IQ: intelligence quotient
LFA: low functioning autism
M-CHAT: Modified Checklist for Autism in Children
NIH: National Institutes of Health
OCD: obsessive compulsive disorder
OT: occupational therapy
PDD: Pervasive developmental disorder.
PDD-NOS: Pervasive developmental disorder — not otherwise specified
PECS: Picture Exchange Communication System
RCT: randomised, controlled trial
RDI®: Relationship Development Intervention
SCERTS®: Social Communication Emotional Regulation Transactional Supports Model
TEACCH: Treatment and Education of Autistic and related Communication-
handicapped CHildren
WISC: Wechsler Intelligence Scale for Children
WPPSI: Wechsler Preschool and Primary Scale of Intelligence

A brief note from the authors

This book is a true collaboration in every sense of the word, but when we started out it made sense to go with our respective strengths. Seana used her journalistic talents to seek out local autism services and experts and the huge Resources Guide is almost exclusively her work. Benison sat down at her desk with a mountain of reports and papers and attempted to translate the science into something parents could understand. We have not announced with loudspeaker who had primary responsibility for writing each chapter (or section therein) but if reference is made to Tom you can probably assume Seana did most of the writing. Conversely, if Joe is mentioned, it is more likely Benison was the main contributor. We hope this is not confusing to readers.

With respect to terminology we have elected to use the phrases: 'child/ren with ASD' and occasionally 'child/ren with autism'. We are not sure about the scientific accuracy of these terms, but both share a personal dislike for the term 'autistic child'. Our children are first and foremost children; autism is just one aspect of who they are and we feel they should not be summed up by that adjective. However some of the other parent contributors to this book have used the word 'autistic' to describe their children. Perhaps these parents are much cooler than we are and we are being a bit oversensitive. We'll leave that for you to judge!

INTRODUCTION

Everyone has worries with their children, dear.
But yours have come early.

A very kind preschool teacher said this to me just at the time my sweet little three-year-old son was being diagnosed with ASD. I burst into tears, of course.

That year of Tom's diagnosis was full of sobbing: a crazy toddler, a new and constantly vomiting baby, a hardworking husband, a new city and no family support. It was all messy enough without adding in a 'lifelong neurological condition'. And the new baby! How could I protect my tiny baby?

I was beside myself. For anguish, despair and desperation, nothing beats your child being diagnosed with an ASD. I thought I had developed some resilience in life, but that hideous year and the diagnosis blew all previous traumas out of the water.

Luckily, time is a great healer as have been early intervention and continuing therapies of various kinds. The baby I worried about so much in 2000 developed normally and is now at school. We went mad and tried for a third; gorgeous baby twins were born in 2006. Oops.

Whilst life in our house is hectic and at times can be hair-raising, overall our family situation is manageable and even, dare I say it, enjoyable? There is some headspace and lots of hindsight, and time to finally write this book — the one I wish someone else had written for me in 2000.

Why this book?

This book aims to be helpful and hopeful. It is written primarily for families whose children are suspected of having an ASD, or who have recently been diagnosed. It is meant first and foremost to be practical.

We hope that there is also valuable information for professionals and even for older 'veteran families' too. Much support and encouragement and some glimpses into possible futures are also offered. There are many voices, most of whom have walked this path before.

We aim to help parents pick a path through the artillery and cannon fire of the awful Autism Wars; has there ever been a disorder which has provoked such dreadful antipathy and argument? Why does no-one seem to want to sit down and find some middle ground? There seems to be no area where there is consensus; from early intervention to genes and the environment, there are ranks of people telling parents that whatever they do is wrong.

Our hope is that by reading this book you can avoid many of the pitfalls we encountered along the way. We set out to write a book which is both positive and realistic; a book that is steeped in science yet at the same time very personal. It was rather an ambitious aim in hindsight but I think we've achieved just that. Of course, we can't cover everything and you will need to do extra reading, but we're optimistic we can point you in the right direction.

Throughout this book you will hear many stories of children and families affected by ASD. As no two children with autism are the same, no two stories can be the same, but you may recognise parts of yourself or your child in some of these tales. Maybe you feel you have made some mistakes along the way. If so, you might be comforted to find out you're not alone. More importantly, if you are struggling with a recent diagnosis we hope these stories will lead you to believe that the future may hold more hope and happiness than you dare to contemplate right now.

This book takes a harmonious approach. We hope that we provide a good balance as co-authors since we took very different paths on our early ASD journeys. With a scientific background, Benison demanded some serious evidence before undertaking any intervention. With her non-scientific background, Seana launched her family straight into the swirling mass of therapies that present themselves to the newly diagnosed.

There is a huge need for more resources and research, and parents will have to fight for their children every step of the way. This is totally unfair, however, we must accept reality and tap into parent power. Parents need to lobby for real change, to demand research be done and research-based treatments be offered. Parents need to encourage doctors, psychologists, teachers and politicians to work together and make some positive changes. The new federal funding announced in 2007 shows clearly that parents do have a voice.

If your child has just been diagnosed, then you will need all your parent power to help your own child for a few years. In the short term it is important to let go of larger concerns and to focus on getting the right interventions for your child. But after that… roll up your sleeves and prepare to fight the good fight!

Tom's story

Tom was born on 9th March 1997, a 4kg boy with Apgar scores of 9 and 9. His birth was easy and I had enjoyed a very relaxed pregnancy.

From the start Tom seemed to have a larger than life personality. He made lots of noise, crawled at seven months and was running around madly by ten months. He was a fearless toddler who climbed constantly. Other babies and toddlers seemed wimpy to me, always hurting themselves and whinging to their mothers.

Tom waved hello and goodbye and he did copy a few words before he was one year old, but his speech just never got going. This really didn't worry me as I thought that he was so quick with gross motor that it would be silly to worry about his other development.

We lived in Karachi, Pakistan for a year from when he was three months. Tom used to vomit a lot and had awful nappies. He was seriously ill once at 12 months, cause unknown. He was a terrible sleeper though I didn't realise how bad until I had other children.

When I look back, I can see that we did have a few early warning signs of ASD. Tom used to gaze out of windows — I turned his highchair away from the window so that he would look at me instead. He didn't crawl normally, but scuttled about like a crab, up on his fingers and toes. He would race away at high speed and never look back. Tom did point but I can see now that it was minimal compared to my subsequent children.

We moved to Australia when he was 18 months old. We had great fun visiting beaches and playgrounds, but I was always having to race to save him from dangerous situations.

If we had known what to look for, we'd have seen ASD clearly by the time Tom was two years old, as that is when the self-stimulatory behaviour started in earnest. Tom fell in love simultaneously with his own reflection and with a plastic Thomas the Tank Engine.

That was an awful year, he faded further and further away, and I became more and more frantic. I was pregnant and suddenly not able to keep up with Tom any more.

At Tom's two-year-old check we were advised to have his hearing tested and we started looking into his speech delay. I look back on this period with great frustration and annoyance: a waiting list to go to a group for parents of late talkers, a waiting list for a speech assessment, a speech assessment where he was really untestable, then a waiting list for speech therapy. That waiting list turned out to be a year long. In my naivety and innocence, I truly thought that if the speech therapists were really worried about Tom they would have made sure he was seen immediately rather than put on a list. Hah! So naive! But the speechies did point me in the direction of an early intervention service and we started going to the playgroup.

Our second son Dexter was born when Tom was two years seven months and thereafter we spiralled towards crisis pretty fast. Tom had no interest at all in his brother, except to try to hit him very hard when he cried. He was a whirling dervish, totally out of our control. He never stayed still, except when he was watching TV and then he was totally still, fixated.

At New Year 1999, a very dear friend did me a huge favour. She sat me down and told me very bluntly that there was something terribly wrong with Tom and I needed to find out what it was and get real help for him. She gave me a piece of paper with the name of a developmental paediatrician and the number of a mother of another child who wasn't talking. 'What's a developmental paediatrician?' I asked, all ignorance and innocence. I made an appointment.

In the midst of trying to deal with my own depression, and my husband's denial, I mentioned to the teacher at the early intervention centre that I was going to see a developmental paediatrician. 'I think Tom might have ADHD,' I said.

'Yes,' she replied, 'or autism spectrum.'

Ting! And that's when our family life changed. Ping! Boom!

That night I looked up autism spectrum on the internet... and knew straight away that Tom had it. Just like that. The process of getting a diagnosis was a mere formality, useful only to have the bits of paper necessary to get the Carer Allowance and a 'special needs' place at preschool.

How bad was he? What did it mean? Would he ever talk? How would we cope? Why did this happen?

Very quickly, I joined Tom as a whirling dervish. We decided to set up a home-based IBI/ABA program. It was an immense relief to do that, to have people come to the house who seemed to know what to do with him. It also seemed as if Tom had simply been waiting for someone to come along who knew how to teach him. He could certainly learn.

For three years we ran the intensive program at home, and then

Tom went to a very small, private school where he was given lots of aide time. We formally stopped the early intervention program at the end of his first year at school.

Tom is eleven now and leads a pretty normal life. He goes to school, he plays rugby and cricket with local teams, he swims and cycles, he fights with his brother.

On the other hand, he has very significant learning issues, especially in maths. His language is delayed and disordered and he is a terribly innocent boy, quite different from his peers. Tom's friendships are genuine, but not the same as those of other boys at eleven. There are occasional dark times too. He can totally lose focus, stim a lot and become obsessive and sometimes aggressive. These times still give us a terrible shock.

But Tom is a very able boy, much more able than disabled. We hope as he enters the teenage years that this can be maintained, and that his life and that of his brothers and sister, and his rapidly-aging parents can be as 'normal' as possible.

In the early days of Tom's diagnosis, I read several books by mothers whose children had largely or completely lost their autistic symptoms and I fiercely hoped that one day I would write a book like that.

Well, this is not it. Tom has not 'recovered' but I think that in many ways our family has recovered and made some peace with it all. On a good day, at least!

Joe's story

When Seana approached me to write this book I was delighted: this book needed to be written. When our son was diagnosed with ASD only a few years ago, there was no definitive, balanced, uniquely-Australian guidebook giving you the basics on diagnosis, treatment, coping and accessing resources. Instead, my husband and I had to make most of our decisions based on scanty pamphlets, the often conflicting advice of professionals and a variety of websites, some of which presented such a gloomy view of autism that I felt like giving up there and then. My background as a medical writer helped, but it's wrong to expect parents to wade through all the scientific literature to get the answers they need.

Joe is the youngest of three boys. His birth was uneventful and as a battle-hardened mum I thought I'd cruise through the newborn period. I was mistaken. Cuddling and human contact seemed to unsettle Joe rather than calm him. He didn't really cry much; he just wouldn't sleep. Of course, I didn't think much of it at the time, just that Joe was a 'difficult' baby. I also noticed he had poor eye contact and rarely smiled and at his six-week check queried this with our paediatrician, who reassured me that all was right. But by the time Joe was eight months old all my previous concerns seemed groundless. He wasn't just a normal baby, he was a charmer, a flirt. His blue-grey eyes sought out the gaze of strangers in the supermarket, only to look away, smiling coquettishly, when he caught their eye. However, even then, my husband, a GP, did wonder that Joe seemed to learn a few words only to lose them.

I think it was about at 12 months that things really started to go wrong. In the photos for his first birthday we couldn't get Joe to raise a smile. I remember him pointing at an aeroplane at 14 months but not after that. People often talk about being too busy to remember their third child's babyhood and so it was with us. During the time Joe was going backwards I was working part-time, organising home renovations, attending to the needs of two other children and doing volunteer work. In the blur of busyness I simply didn't notice.

Joe became a difficult toddler, hyperactive and challenging, but never really socially withdrawn in the way I *thought* people with autism were. I was worried that he didn't talk but friends reassured me that this was just because he was the youngest boy and didn't need to.

It was only when I took Joe to swimming lessons at age two that I realised that he had no idea what the swimming instructor was saying. So off to the paediatrician we went. Joe underwent a barrage of tests — genetic screenings, lead levels, hearing tests and an EEG, the latter to exclude epilepsy. All came back normal. Autism was briefly discussed but dismissed (at least in my mind) and Joe was given a diagnosis of receptive and expressive speech delay.

For the next year, as Joe got worse, I clung to that diagnosis like a lifeline. He babbled but barely spoke, he couldn't do the simplest puzzles, he lined up toys but didn't play with them. Then he started looking at things out of the corner of his eyes. I was later to discover this was a self-stimulatory behaviour common to many people with autism. But at that time I didn't want to think about autism — that happened to 'other people', not to us.

Of course there were days of despair during that year when I wondered just what was wrong with my beautiful little boy. But ironically, at the time of diagnosis I was more upbeat: Joe had been given some educational videos for Christmas and had learnt his ABCs, numbers and shapes by watching these. I now know that this language was echolalia (the echoing of words and phrases, a common symptom of autism) but at the time I thought his emerging speech was a sign that things might finally be coming right.

February 27th 2004 was the day Joe was diagnosed with an ASD. He was just three. But if I said it was the worst day of my life that wouldn't be true. That came two days later when we hosted a third birthday party for him. As I compared him with the happy, talkative preschoolers the stark reality of his autism hit me. I shed tears for the future I thought he would never have.

Once the blinkers came off, and I started reading about ASD all Joe's symptoms became blindingly obvious. Then I went too far the other way. I cried and railed against my fate. I resented all other mothers and their 'normal' children. And for a short time, Joe ceased to be my little boy and became a diagnosis. I saw all his behaviour through the prism of autism. My husband James, grieving also, was much wiser. One day, when Joe had a particularly bad tantrum and I blamed it on autism, James pointed out that a typical four-year-old girl had had a much worse tantrum in his consulting rooms that day.

Gradually these feelings started to recede and I came to realise that this child was still my beautiful boy and, what's more, he needed my help. I got up, dusted myself off and started looking at therapy options. After wading through all the possibilities, James and I decided that the best option for Joe was a home-based intensive ABA program.

We employed six bright, young university students who came to our house every day, to slowly and painstakingly teach Joe how to sit at a table and attend, complete simple tasks, imitate actions, understand and speak words, play and generally make sense of the world. Joe made wonderful gains but we got greedy for more, so after a year or so of intensive ABA we added another therapy called Relationship Development Intervention®. This parent-run program specifically targets the differences in thinking, emotion and communication which can make relationships hard for people with autism. Joe's response to this program has delighted us all.

Joe is now seven years old. He attends a private special-education school and loves it. He shows a particular aptitude for maths and to my delight is reading the same school readers that his older brothers read. Much more importantly, he is developing into a happy little boy who loves playing with his dad and brothers and is making his first tentative steps toward friendship with his school friends. He has a winning smile and a cheeky sense of humour. Of course, he still has an ASD diagnosis and lots of other challenges such as attention deficit disorder, speech delay and some curious obsessions and whims. But the sunny little baby who smiled at strangers in the supermarket never really left us and has emerged from the worst bonds of autism to charm us all again.

Of course Joe is only seven years old. We are under no illusions that there won't be difficult times ahead but we are going to keep working with our little boy until he becomes a big boy and then a man. Hopefully we'll prove those pessimists wrong and he will go on to lead a happy and productive life. But, whatever challenges lie ahead we know that there will be lots of good times, too.

Finally, before you embark on this book, I'd like to let you on a couple of secrets. Firstly, you may find that having a child with a disability uncovers strengths and abilities in you that you never knew you had. Having Joe has made me a kinder and wiser person. I no longer sweat on the small stuff, and, if anything, my main fault is that I've become intolerant of people who fuss about trivialities. It's now my belief that if you and your children are healthy and reasonably happy, and you have enough money to live on, anything else is just a bonus.

Secondly, in a society that seems to expect all our children to be high achievers it's easy to imagine that a disabled child might be harder to love. Instead I've found the reverse to be true. Watching our little fellow struggle and overcome all the challenges thrown his way has made him so much more precious in our eyes. We despair at his occasional setbacks and triumph at his successes. I expect you will find the same and will come to love your little person more than you could ever have imagined. Good luck on your journey.

1

I wish someone had told me that everything will be alright. You will pass through stages — deny it, fight it, grieve about it, then you will find peace and joy in your little person.

Kelly Hargreaves, mother of Daniel

AUTISM SPECTRUM DISORDERS AND YOUR CHILD

He ran around on his tippy toes, constantly in motion. He wasn't talking and he didn't play with toys properly, only ever rolling cars back and forth in front of his eyes. He was obsessed with his own reflection in the mirror. He loved music and loved to dance staring at his reflection. Why didn't he ever want to dance with me?

When my son was 18 months old, a friend brought her nine-month-old baby round to our house. I had so much fun with the baby; there was constant interaction between us. I realised that this was completely absent with my own little boy.

She was so distant from us we found it hard to engage her. We would have to say her name at least six times before she would acknowledge us, often staring into space as if in a trance. We put this down to a hearing problem but test results showed otherwise.

He was my first child so I didn't know what to look for although I knew he was different. I was a full-time mum and was involved in

*every kids' group around, trying to be incredibly social, but I had
this baby and then toddler, who wasn't. He constantly cried, wasn't
interested in anything the others were, wouldn't take instructions
and he was often obsessed with one toy or the sand-pit.*

*I thought that maybe he was just incredibly smart as he would
remember everyone's name, the alphabet/numbers, mimic
newsreaders and kids' characters. He spoke like an adult and was
reading signs at shopping centres when he was only two. Perhaps
he didn't want to mix with other children because they weren't at
his intellectual level? He loved to sit and talk to the mums rather
than go and play.*

*He didn't respond to his own name; he didn't understand a word
we said to him; he had no speech whatsoever — in fact he was
pretty silent. He walked in circles and pushed chairs; he hand-
flapped; he had poor eye contact and he ran away from people.
He treated people like objects, walking over the top of them and
climbing them. He had a thing about switches.*

*Any outing became a nightmare and she could not take pleasure in
things that other children loved like going to the park, the beach,
indoor play centres or friends' houses; she did not know how...
She never showed excitement for anything except the TV.*

*He was fine on his own at home — I thought I was in heaven
because he'd sit for up to two hours doing the same thing...
compared to all the other kids who were up and down and all
over the place... But then as soon as we went out or had other
kids around — he was a biting monster if they jostled him. Or he
would get angry and frustrated with their random actions and
yell and hit and kick and push.*

These are the voices of people whose lives have been turned upside
down by an autism diagnosis for a beloved child. These people speak
for the growing number of Australian families affected by autism

spectrum disorders (ASDs). A recent prevalence study of ASDs in Australia found an estimated one child in 160 with an ASD in the 6–12 year old age group, which translates to 10,000 6–12 year olds. If we extrapolate the data further, to other age groups, there could be as many as 125,000 people with an ASD in Australia and half a million Australians living in families affected by ASD.[1]

This estimated prevalence is very similar to that reported in the USA and other countries and confirms that ASDs are much more common than originally thought.

If you are reading this book there is a good chance that you have joined, or are about to join, this not-so-exclusive club. Perhaps your child or the child of someone close to you has just been diagnosed with an ASD. Or maybe you don't even have an official diagnosis yet but are worried that your child is affected. Whatever the case, we hope it's some comfort to know that there are many people out there who understand exactly what you are going through. They may be just statistics now but one day some of these people will be your friends.

In this chapter we describe autism and some of its symptoms, explain the different diagnoses which all fall under the ASD umbrella, and touch briefly on the emotional impact of an ASD diagnosis. In the next we will go through the steps involved in diagnosing and assessing children. This information is not meant to be a substitute for thoughtful discussions with the people who assess your child, but at such an emotional time it's going to be difficult to take in everything they say. Hopefully we will be able to fill in a few of the gaps.

Some technical terms are necessary. However, they will be in *italics*, followed by explanations in simpler terms; there is also a glossary. A lot of this terminology may seem intimidating at first but before long it will become very familiar.

What is autism? What is an ASD?

Autism is a neurological disorder which disrupts normal child development in the first few years of life. Symptoms are typically present by the age of three, although sometimes these will be very subtle and diagnosis may not occur till some years later.

Autism is characterised by differences and delays in:

- **Communication** — both verbal (understanding and using spoken language) and non-verbal (such as pointing and smiling). Children with autism may have no speech, delayed speech, or rote and repetitive speech. They might be able to recite whole scripts from videos but be unable to have a two-way conversation.
- **Social Interactions** — relating to other people and sharing emotions. Young children with autism don't share their experiences with you: they don't yell out 'Look at me, Mum' like typical kids. They usually play alone even when other children are around and often appear to lack awareness of others.
- **Routines and repetitive (or stereotyped) behaviours** — such as repeating words (*echolalia*) or body movements (hand flapping, toe walking). Kids with autism often having a liking for sameness and will rigidly follow routines. They may play in an unusual way (lining toy cars up in a perfect line rather than playing imaginatively with them). Older children may talk obsessively about one topic.

Children with autism usually don't look physically different from other children and there is no blood test to tell if they have autism; it is diagnosed only by observing behaviour. In recent times we've also recognised that people with autism often display an under- or oversensitivity to sensory stimuli — for example, they may block their ears at the sound of the vacuum cleaner and refuse to wear certain clothes, but then, paradoxically, not seem to notice pain — but these sensitivities are not part of the diagnostic criteria for ASD.

The word autism comes from the Greek word *autos*, which means *self*. Like schizophrenia, autism has probably existed throughout history, but neither condition was actually recognised until relatively recently. In 1943, American psychiatrist Leo Kanner published a report on 11 young children who had similar symptoms, including social aloofness and unusual restricted interests. He called this 'early infantile autism'. Coincidentally, a year later, an Austrian, Hans Asperger, published a report on a similar group of children. Amongst the children in Asperger's study were some with superficially normal language development and IQ. However, because his work was not published in English, Asperger's contribution was not widely recognised until 1981, when psychiatrist Lorna Wing coined the term Asperger's syndrome to describe the 'high-functioning' children he had talked about almost 40 years earlier.

There was a bleak period around the 1960s when autism was believed to be a psychological disorder, caused by bad parenting. The term 'refrigerator mother' was used to describe cold, uncaring mothers who apparently 'failed' to bond with their child. Thus parents not only had to deal with this devastating diagnosis, they were also unfairly blamed for the condition! Fortunately we live in more enlightened times. Autism is now recognised as a disorder of brain development with a strong genetic component, which, if not exactly 'curable' in the strict sense of the word, can respond, sometimes dramatically, to the educational and medical interventions of today.

The more severely affected children Kanner described in 1943 would probably be diagnosed with autistic disorder today. This is the best known of a group of pervasive developmental disorders (PDD) currently outlined in the American Psychiatric Association's *Diagnostic and Statistical Manual of Mental Disorders IV (DSM-IV)*, the official manual used by most professionals for diagnosis. Other types of PDD include Asperger's disorder, childhood disintegrative disorder, and Rett's disorder.

PDD is a not a very parent-friendly term so doctors more commonly talk about ASD. This term is used to describe three of these PDD — autistic disorder, Asperger's disorder and pervasive developmental disorder not otherwise specified (PDD-NOS).

These disorders all share three common areas of concern: qualitative impairments in social skills, qualitative impairments in communication skills and restricted and repetitive interests and behaviours. However, as the name implies, ASD represents a *spectrum* of severity and children with ASD can vary widely in abilities, intelligence and behaviour. Some children will avoid eye contact and seem totally aloof whereas others will look at you and sometimes smile and hug. Some children will have learning difficulties whereas others will be of superior intelligence. Some will be nonverbal, whereas others will display impressive vocabularies. Some children will have obvious stereotypic behaviours (commonly known as *self-stimulatory* behaviours or '*stims*') such as finger-flicking and hand flapping whereas others will blend into school without any outward sign of their condition. But what all these children have in common is a different way of thinking — a way which makes the everyday tasks of socialising and communication very, very difficult.

Explaining the official diagnostic criteria

Autistic disorder is also sometimes known as 'classical' autism. For a diagnosis of autistic disorder a child must meet a specified number of the 12 criteria in the DSM-IV covering: impairment in social interactions, impairment in communication and repetitive behaviours and stereotyped behaviour patterns (see Table 1, below). However, just *how* these impairments and behaviours manifest themselves will vary greatly from one child to the next.

Some (but not all) children with autistic disorder also have an *intellectual disability* — usually defined as below average intelligence (IQ less than 70) associated with significant difficulties with everyday living and self-care skills.

Table 1. Diagnostic criteria for Autistic Disorder

A. A total of six (or more) items from (1), (2), and (3), with at least two from (1), and one each from (2) and (3):

(1) qualitative impairment in social interaction, as manifested by at least two of the following:

✓ (a) marked impairment in the use of multiple nonverbal behaviours such as eye-to-eye gaze, facial expression, body postures, and gestures to regulate social interaction

✓ (b) failure to develop peer relationships appropriate to developmental level

✓ (c) a lack of spontaneous seeking to share enjoyment, interests, or achievements with other people (eg by a lack of showing, bringing, or pointing out objects of interest)

✓ (d) lack of social or emotional reciprocity

(2) qualitative impairments in communication as manifested by at least one of the following:

✓ (a) delay in, or total lack of, the development of spoken language (not accompanied by an attempt to compensate through alternative modes of communication such as gesture or mime)

(b) in individuals with adequate speech, marked impairment in the ability to initiate or sustain a conversation with others

✓ (c) stereotyped and repetitive use of language or idiosyncratic language

✓ (d) lack of varied, spontaneous make-believe play or social imitative play appropriate to developmental level

(3) restricted repetitive and stereotyped patterns of behaviour, interests, and activities, as manifested by at least one of the following:

(a) encompassing preoccupation with one or more stereotyped and restricted patterns of interest that is abnormal either in intensity or focus

(b) apparently inflexible adherence to specific, non-functional routines or rituals

✓ (c) stereotyped and repetitive motor mannerisms (eg hand or finger flapping or twisting, or complex whole-body movements)

✓ (d) persistent preoccupation with parts of objects

B. Delays or abnormal functioning in at least one of the following areas, with onset prior to age 3 years: (1) social interaction, (2) language as used in social communication, or (3) symbolic or imaginative play.

C. The disturbance is not better accounted for by Rett's Disorder or Childhood Disintegrative Disorder.

Reprinted with permission from the Diagnostic and Statistical Manual of Mental Disorders, Fourth Edition, Text Revision, (Copyright 2000). American Psychiatric Association.

The DSM-IV diagnostic criteria for *Asperger's disorder* (commonly known as Asperger's syndrome) are very similar to those of autistic disorder, except that children diagnosed with Asperger's have, by definition, at least an average IQ and superficially normal early language development (defined as single words by the age of two years and communicative phrases by three). We say *superficially*, because while they may develop speech at an appropriate age their manner of speaking is often unusual. For example, they may use words more appropriate for a 'college professor' and talk only about a very narrow range of interests.

The diagnosis of *pervasive developmental disorder – not otherwise specified (PDD-NOS)* is usually given when a child presents with impairments in social interaction, communication and behaviour but their symptoms are not severe enough or of sufficient number to qualify for a diagnosis of autistic disorder. PDD-NOS is also sometimes referred to as 'atypical autism.'

Much has been made of the 'explosion' in ASD diagnoses in recent years but most of this growth has been in cases of Asperger's syndrome or PDD-NOS and these conditions are probably more common now than classic autistic disorder. Also, you will notice that you tend to see more boys than girls diagnosed with ASD; overall the ratio is about 4:1.

The terms *high-functioning* and *low-functioning* are also sometimes used to describe people on the autism spectrum. These terms aren't clearly defined, but low-functioning autism (LFA) is generally used to describe individuals who also have a significant intellectual disability (low IQ) whereas high-functioning autism (HFA) describes those with a normal or near-normal IQ.

Children with LFA tend to have more severe symptoms, struggle with speech and learning and generally have a more difficult path to independence. The worst affected may never develop functional speech and will need support into adulthood.

However, children with HFA, and those with Asperger's syndrome in particular, have their own challenges. The term 'high-functioning' can be misleading: a child with a high IQ may still have significant social difficulties. Unfortunately, because they don't look different from other kids, their social problems are often met with little understanding, causing considerable anxiety and stress. As leading UK autism expert Patricia Howlin puts it, 'Seemingly so close to 'normality' there is constant pressure for them to 'fit in' in ways that would never be demanded of a less able autistic child'.[2]

The bottom line is that no matter where a child sits on the autism spectrum they are going to need more help and support to succeed than a typical child.

'Normal' versus 'typical'

Throughout this book we will refer to average people (*that is those without an ASD diagnoses*) as *'typical'* not *'normal'*. Normal is a subjective term and not widely accepted in the autism world. In many autism publications people without ASD are described by the more politically correct term *neurotypical* or NT for short. However, we've chosen to just use typical.

EARLY SIGNS OF AUTISM

Most children with Autistic Disorder/PDD-NOS receive their diagnosis somewhere between their second and fourth birthdays but, in retrospect, their parents often realise that subtle symptoms of autism were present much earlier. Studies of home videos suggest that many children who subsequently go on to develop an ASD may display signs around, and even before, the age of 12 months. Current international research is focusing on the early signs of autism, which should eventually lead to earlier diagnosis, earlier treatments and hopefully better outcomes for children with ASD. One of the foremost researchers in this area in Australia is Robyn Young.

Dr Young is an Associate Professor in the School of Psychology and Director of the Early Intervention Research Program at Flinders University, South Australia. She and her colleagues have developed **Autism Detection in Early Childhood (ADEC)**, an effective, validated screening tool for identifying autism and autistic tendencies in children as young as 12 months. Dr Young has kindly agreed to summarise the research on the early signs of autism:

Although we now recognise early intervention is essential for children with autism, such intervention depends upon us recognising the early signs of this disorder and subsequent diagnosis. At present, our understanding of autism tends to focus on behaviours that are not apparent until later in childhood, including delays in language, a lack of social skills and the presence of stereotypic and ritualistic behaviours. These behaviours remain the focus of most of the autism diagnostic tools currently available and largely dictate how we think about the disorder.

Few people are aware of the behavioural differences or abnormalities that may precede and perhaps even lead to these difficulties. As a result, recent research has begun to focus on these early behavioural characteristics, most of which relate to joint attention behaviours, the absence of which might be noted from as early as six months of age and continuing throughout early infancy. Specific examples include:

- not turning when one's name is called
- a lack of gaze switching from an interesting object to another person's face
- a lack of interest in others
- poor eye contact
- avoiding the gaze of others
- a reduced ability to follow the point and gaze of others
- a lack of showing or pointing.

Young children with autism have also been found to not respond typically to emotional displays of others, suggesting a lack of empathy. This may present as:

- reduced emotion
- appearing overly placid
- failing to demonstrate a typical range of facial expressions
- a lack of response to the social cues of others (eg responding to a smile).

Researchers have also noted unusual development of play behaviours in infants who later develop autism. Such indicators include:

- repetitive and non functional use of objects (eg lining up toys or spinning wheels)
- attachments to particular objects (ie constantly carrying around a particular toy).

Although sensory abnormalities do not form part of the diagnostic criteria for autism, there is evidence that most children with autism also present very early on in their development with sensory abnormalities. These include:

- abnormal responses to sound or appearing deaf
- excessive mouthing of objects
- oversensitivity to tastes, smells and touch
- watching hand or finger movements

- • showing interest in minor details
- • visual staring and fixation on objects
- • looking at objects from unusual angles
- • insensitivity to pain, heat or cold.

If intervention programs commence when children are older, they typically focus on addressing the secondary deficits such as language delays and social problems. If we are able to diagnose autism earlier we may be able, through early intervention, to prevent some of these secondary deficits developing and give these children a better start on life. By identifying autism at a young age, families can also start to come to terms with the diagnosis and gain support at an earlier age.

Facing your fears

Could my child have an ASD?

All of the mums and dads who you will hear from in this book have, at some stage, had to ask themselves this most-difficult question. And of course, in their case, the answer was always 'yes'. We expect that most people reading this book will be some way along the path to the same conclusion, but perhaps some will be finding that journey a little bumpier than others. It is thus important to touch on the emotional consequences of accepting your child has an ASD.

In Uta Frith's book, *Autism, Explaining the Enigma*, she quotes autism mother, Anne Lovell:

It is to my mind one of the most exquisitely cruel aspects of early childhood autism that it only becomes apparent to parents very slowly that there is anything wrong with their child.[3]

Like any other, the parent of an ASD child celebrates the arrival of an apparently typical baby and starts to make the usual plans and dreams for their future. But then slowly, ever so slowly, the realisation strikes them that something is just not right. It can be unspeakably hard to face up to this and let go of those cherished hopes and dreams.

Complicating this is the fact that children with ASD rarely fit the image most of us have ever had in our minds of autism — that is, if we ever thought of it at all.

I wish I had known that autism looks different in every child. A friend's little boy was diagnosed with autism but he was very different from my son. Her boy had no language and lost all eye contact with others. Although I knew something was wrong with my son, I didn't think it could be autism because not only did he have some words, but he looked at me and smiled.

When people are confronted with this situation they can respond very differently. Some mothers 'diagnose' their own children and then go to the professionals to have it confirmed. Others try to shut out these scary thoughts until someone helps them to face their fears. Still other parents are informed by a professional that their child has an ASD but refuse to believe it, seeking second and even third opinions. Sometimes one spouse will be accepting whilst the other will remain in denial. There are no rules.

No, sorry, there is a rule...

Almost universally, parents agree that if they have to learn that their child has an ASD, then it is better to learn about it as soon as possible. In later chapters you will read further about why it is important to diagnose children and start early intervention as soon as possible. But for the moment, here are some parents' thoughts, reflections and wishes as they look back on those months around diagnosis.

I wish I hadn't gone into denial and blamed his lack of speech on his dummy. I was too frightened to think that there might be something wrong with this beloved baby we had waited so long and tried so hard for. I should have thought more about why three different people had looked at my son and mentioned autism (I was highly offended at the time). If only I had known what the symptoms of autism were — for when I did see them after his diagnosis, I knew without a doubt that they described my son.

I visited our community health centre many times in an exhausted state. He was labelled as 'badly behaved' and a parenting course was suggested. I regret he was ever labelled as naughty, because that's how he was treated until he was diagnosed when he was four years old. I accidentally came across an article on Asperger's in a weekend paper at the same time a new teacher at his preschool suggested speech therapy. It was the best day of my life, and my son's.

I regret wasting a year listening to doctors who kept telling me that my son was 'delayed' but would 'catch up'. I should have arranged a full assessment as soon as I realised something was wrong.

As our son got to around 20 months with absolutely no language, we started to become concerned about his development. My biggest regret is that we didn't follow-up on these concerns sooner. So many people kept saying things like 'I know so-and-so who didn't talk until they were five, and he's perfectly alright'; or 'He's developing at his own pace, let him be'. The message I took out of all this was that I was at fault for being a pushy and neurotic older mother when my concerns were actually right on-the-money.

Denial is a dangerous place to live when your child has been diagnosed with autism. You need to work through the initial shock and despair and get moving to have any real chance of improving their future.

Of course, no-one expects you to be happy and comfortable with this diagnosis. You still have a lot of grieving to do.

As the parent of the ASD child, give yourself two years to come to terms emotionally with your child's diagnosis, go through the phases of grief at the 'loss' of what your 'hopes and dreams' were for your child, and to embrace who they really are. Be gentle with yourself, and find a support group or person with whom you can feel safe.

So acknowledge these feelings but recognise that an ASD won't go away if you ignore it; unfortunately, things will probably get worse. The sooner you accept your child has a problem the sooner you can commence interventions which will help — perhaps even transform — your child and, importantly, allow your family to regain some hope and equilibrium.

1. Australian Advisory Board on Autism Spectrum Disorders. (2007). The prevalence of autism in Australia. Can it be established from existing data? Overview and Report. www.autismaus.com.au/aca/pdfs/PrevalenceReport.pdf
2. Howlin, P. (1998). Practitioner review: psychological and educational treatments for autism. *Journal of Child Psychology and Psychiatry*, 39, 3, 307–322.
3. Frith, Uta. (2003) *Autism. Explaining the Enigma* 2nd edn, Malden, MA, Blackwell Publishing.

Additional references:
4. Dover, CJ, Le Couteur, A. (2007). How to diagnose autism. *Archives of Diseases in Childhood*, 92, 540–545
5. Wing L. (1996). Autism spectrum disorders. *BMJ*, 312, 327–328
6. Wing L. (1981). Asperger's syndrome: a clinical account. *Psychological Medicine*, 11, 115–129.
7. American Academy of Pediatrics Committee on Children with Disabilities. (2001). The Pediatrician's Role in the Diagnosis and Management of Autistic Spectrum Disorder in Children. *Pediatrics* 107, 5 www.pediatrics.org/cgi/content/full/107/5e85
8. American Psychiatric Association. (2000). *Diagnostic and Statistical Manual of Mental Disorders*, Fourth Edition, Text Revision (DSM-IV-TR®), Washington DC: American Psychiatric Association.
9. Perry, A. and Condillac, R. (2003). Evidence-Based Practices for Children and Adolescents with Autism Spectrum Disorders: Review of the Literature and Practice Guide. Children's Mental Health Ontario. Toronto, Ontario, Canada.
10. Wray, J, Silove, N, Knot, H. (2005). Language disorders and autism. *Medical Journal of Australia*, 182(7), 354–360.
11. National Initiative for Autism: Screening and Assessment. (2003). *National Autism Plan for Children (NAPC)*. The National Autistic Society, London.

2

Autism is not a disease, it is a pattern of brain development that causes a recognisable collection of behavioural and developmental traits, many of which may be partially familial. As such, every child is a unique individual and yours has some additional needs to help achieve his/her potential. Education and behaviour management are the cornerstones to improvement and this process needs to be involved daily to some degree. Medication, diets and other suggestions sometimes help to improve particular symptoms and make the child more able to learn, but without early intervention and teaching little is learnt. When choosing treatments remember that anecdotes are no more reliable than the average news report or advertisement. It has been said that it doesn't matter as much what you do, so long as you do it early enough and often enough. Your child needs to be a part of your family and so his/her needs do have to be balanced with the ongoing needs of all the family including yourself — martydom is no substitute for motherhood (or fatherhood).

Dr David Starte, Service Director at the Chatswood Assessment Centre, Clinical Associate Lecturer in the Department of Paediatrics and Child Health, University of Sydney, School of Medicine and member of the Board of Directors of Aspect.

THE DIAGNOSTIC PROCESS

This diagnosis does not change who he is. He is the same child you loved when you walked in this door.
Dr Robyn Young

If you've got any message from our parents' stories it's that ASDs can present themselves in many different ways — chapter 1 contained a list of early indicators. This chapter aims to move further along the path to diagnosis of an ASD, especially in older children and explain some of the specifics of diagnosis and assessment. While we recognise that many of you may have already been through at least part of this process we think you may still find it helpful to understand the rationale behind the barrage of tests and assessments your child has been, or is about to be, subjected to.

The following signs are **red flags** for a possible ASD:

- lack of babbling or pointing by 12 months
- no sharing of interest in objects or activities with another person

- • no single words by 16 months, or no two-word (non-echoed) phrases by 24 months
- • any loss of language or social skills at any age.

If any of these signs describe your child — and you haven't already done so — you should go to your doctor and seek referral for a developmental assessment immediately. Even if your child doesn't end up having an ASD they may well have another problem with their development (such as a general learning disability or a language disorder) which needs investigating.

In the first year of baby's life there are often no obvious pointers to an ASD. It's at about 18 months that most parents have their first concerns, usually because speech isn't developing. However, as Robyn Young explained in the previous chapter; deficits in *joint attention* may actually be present much earlier. A typical one-year-old will be able to follow their parents' gaze or point (for example, if their parent shows them an aeroplane in the sky) and will show enjoyment in sharing an object of interest with another person by looking back and forth between the two. These behaviours tend to be missing or at least reduced in a young child with an ASD. Of course, you have to be actually *looking* for these things to notice that they are missing. If it's your first baby you might well not pick these up if your child seems to be doing everything else (sitting up, walking etc) at the right time.

There is also a group of children with ASD (estimated to be up to one-third) whose parents report apparently typical development up to the age of 18 months or two years before their children start to lose words and regress. However, it now appears that word loss occurs most commonly at the very early 10-word stage and that these words may never have actually been used in a communicative way.

Children with autistic disorder and PDD-NOS can also present with developmental delays in areas other than language and social development: they may not be able to draw, do puzzles, or feed and dress themselves independently. Some children may have an intellectual disability as well, but in other cases it's actually the autism which is stopping them from learning things. These children often don't pick up new skills by observation and imitation, the way typical kids do.

There are now a number of autism-specific screening checklists, which, although not 100% perfect, can aid us in detecting ASDs and help distinguish them from other causes of developmental delay.

We've already mentioned the **Autism Detection in Early Childhood (ADEC)** screening tool in chapter 1. Another is the **Checklist for Autism in Toddlers (CHAT)** which was developed in the United Kingdom and can be administered by doctors when children are approximately 18 months of age. Imitation, pretend play and joint attention are assessed through a series of parent questions and direct observation of the child. If a child fails more than a few items in the CHAT it is recommended they be referred for further assessment, as their chances of having an ASD are quite high. However, the CHAT does not pick up all children who subsequently go on to be diagnosed with an ASD.

The **Modified Checklist for Autism in Children (M-CHAT)** is an expanded American version of the CHAT. It contains 23 questions which require a yes/no answer. You can access the M-CHAT and scoring system yourself at the First Signs website. Not all children who fail the M-CHAT checklist will go on to be diagnosed with an ASD but a failure certainly indicates that your child needs further assessment.

First Signs is a really helpful website: www.firstsigns.org. The website is dedicated to the early detection of and intervention for children with developmental delays and disorders.

In most cases a diagnosis of autistic disorder can reliably be made between the ages of two and three years. In the case of children with PDD-NOS or Asperger's syndrome diagnosis at this age may be less clear cut (although with better diagnostic and early screening tools now available this situation is likely to improve in coming years). In particular, *stereotypies* such as finger flicking and peripheral eye gazing may not appear until a child is three years or older so very young children may not display all the behaviours described in the

DSM-IV criteria (certainly our own boys had many more of these symptoms at three years than they did at two).

If there's any doubt about the diagnosis your paediatrician may refer you for further specialist testing, perhaps give a preliminary diagnosis of PDD-NOS or occasionally recommend a period of 'watchful waiting'. If the last course is recommended don't assume you're in the clear — make sure you get your child reassessed *regularly* (every three months) and keep a close eye out for new symptoms to report. Your paediatrician may recommend you start your child in early intervention anyway, as in the event they turn out not to have an ASD, they are very unlikely to be harmed by (and more likely to benefit from) this therapy.

In the case of children with HFA and Asperger's syndrome, concerns often don't develop until they are exposed to the greater social demands of school. Some children with Asperger's are even thought to be 'advanced' because of their special interests or sophisticated vocabulary. With this in mind the British National Autism Plan for Children has developed a list of features which may discriminate 'high functioning' children with ASD once they reach school-age (Table 1). They developed this list mainly for teachers and health care workers but it is also useful for parents. As you can see, many of these signs are quite subtle and could easily just be attributed to 'bad behaviour'. If some of these features remind you of your child please investigate further. At the very least, an official diagnosis may lead them to receiving more help and understanding at school.

Table 1: Alerting features of ASD in primary school age children

1. Communication impairments
- Abnormalities in language development, including muteness and odd or inappropriate intonation*
- Persistent echolalia
- Reference to self as 'you,' 'she,' or 'he' beyond 3 years
- Unusual vocabulary for child's age or social group
- Limited use of language for communication or tendency to talk freely only about specific topics

2. Social impairments
- Inability to join in with the play of other children or inappropriate attempts at joint play (may manifest as aggressive or disruptive behaviour)
- Lack of awareness of classroom 'norms' (criticising teachers; overt unwillingness to cooperate in classroom activities; inability to appreciate or follow current trends—for example, with regard to other children's dress, style of speech, or interests)
- Easily overwhelmed by social and other stimulation
- Failure to relate normally to adults (too intense or no relationship)
- Showing extreme reactions to invasion of personal space and extreme resistance to being 'hurried'

3. Impairment of interests, activities and behaviours
- Lack of flexible, co-operative, imaginative play/creativity although certain imaginary scenarios (eg copied from videos and cartoons) may be frequently enacted alone.
- Difficulty in organising self in relation to unstructured space (eg hugging the perimeter of playground and halls)
- Inability to cope with change or unstructured situations, even ones that other children enjoy (such as school trips, teachers being away etc)

Other factors: Unusual profile of skills and deficits (for example social and motor skills very poorly developed, whilst general knowledge, reading or vocabulary well above chronological/mental age). Any other evidence of odd behaviours (including unusual responses to sensory stimuli); unusual responses to movement and any significant history of loss of skills.

National Initiative for Autism: Screening and Assessment. (2003). National Autism Plan for Children (NAPC). Reproduced with permission from The National Autistic Society, London.

*for example, speaking in a flat expressionless voice

Diagnosis and assessment — what's involved

We can only talk in general terms in this section, as the diagnostic process does vary between, and even within, states and territories. Please refer to the chapter at the back of this book for the specific agencies involved in diagnosis and assessment in your area.

In Australia, diagnosis and assessment for ASD is provided by a range of agencies, including specialised assessment services (funded by state governments), state-based autism associations and paediatricians and psychologists working in the private sector.

Government-funded diagnostic assessment is usually performed by a multi-disciplinary team, which may include a psychologist, a doctor (paediatrician or child psychiatrist) and a speech pathologist and, in some cases, an occupational therapist and/or social worker. These multi-disciplinary assessments may take place over several appointments on several days.

If your child is suspected of having an ASD you should arrange for an assessment as soon as possible, because there can be very long waiting times, especially for the some government-funded services.

If you find that waiting times in your area are unacceptably long (anything more than a few months) we'd strongly recommend you consider having your child privately assessed. There will probably be some out-of-pocket costs involved but the sooner you have a diagnosis the sooner you can start getting the right help for your child, in the form of early intervention. Also, once your child has an official diagnosis, you may find you are eligible for some government financial assistance, such as the Carer Allowance/Payment.

From 1 July 2008, new Medicare items for ASD diagnosis are available. These include:

- new specialist Medicare Benefits Schedule (MBS) items for paediatricians and child psychiatrists for diagnosis and the development of treatment plans for children aged up to 12 years;
- new Medicare items for developmental psychologists and speech pathologists to assist with aspects of the assessment.

This is a very positive development and hopefully should lead to a more timely and less expensive diagnostic process for many families but we are obviously unable to assess the full impact of these changes at this time.

A diagnostic assessment may include some or all of these assessments:

PAEDIATRIC MEDICAL ASSESSMENT

Your child will be seen by a paediatrician who will assess your child and probably recommend or organise further medical tests. They may give you a diagnosis at this stage or possibly refer your child for further specialist assessment and diagnosis. Some medical tests are recommended to make sure your child does not have any other conditions which could explain their symptoms (see Table over).

DEVELOPMENTAL AND FAMILY HISTORY

A professional will interview you and document your family history and the developmental history of your child, including their early developmental milestones, language, social development and play. Ideally both parents should participate in this interview. In some cases the interviewer may use a semi-structured interview tool such as the *Autism Diagnostic Interview–Revised (ADI-R)* or the *Diagnostic Interview for Social and Communication Disorders (DISCO)*.

It might sound obvious, but it's best to be absolutely honest when answering questions about your child's skills and development. Whilst it might be tempting to 'talk up' your child's abilities, the assessment team must have an accurate picture of your child in order to recommend an appropriate intervention program.

BEHAVIOURAL OBSERVATIONS

A health professional will observe and interact with your child to assess communication, social and play skills. Ideally these observations should take place in more than one setting as familiarity with the environment may influence behaviour: for example, children may cope reasonably well at home but do less well in a noisy, busy

TEST	WHAT'S INVOLVED	WHY IT MAY BE NECESSARY
Physical examination and history.	The doctor will measure your child's height, weight and head circumference and conduct a neurological examination. They may ask questions about diet, bowel and bladder function and sleeping habits and possible fits.	To look for physical signs of other conditions which may explain your child's symptoms, such as tuberous sclerosis or fragile X syndrome, and to identify any other medical problems which may need investigation and treatment.
Hearing test	Routine testing followed up with further audiological investigations if any doubts remain.	To exclude hearing loss as cause of language delay. Even mild to moderate hearing loss in young children can cause problems with language development.
Genetic testing (chromosomal analysis and DNA testing)	Blood test	To test for possible genetic disorders, such as fragile X and/or Rett syndrome.
Full blood count; iron, folate (folic acid) and vitamin B12 levels	Blood test	To check for deficiencies, especially if your child's diet is limited.
Lead testing	Blood test	To test for lead toxicity, especially if your child eats or mouths non-food items such as dirt or chalk or you live in a house where there may be lead-based paint.
Electroencephalogram or EEG	A test to measure brain waves to look for signs of seizures. Your child will probably need to attend hospital for this test.	This test is not routinely recommended, but may be indicated if epilepsy is suspected (eg if you report a history of seizures or regression in your child.)
Thyroid function test; creatine kinase level; urine metabolic screen.	Blood and urine tests.	These tests are also not routinely recommended, but may be performed to exclude conditions such as an under-active thyroid or metabolic condition as a cause of your child's symptoms.

childcare centre or preschool. Primary school-aged children should be observed at school.

Some professionals may use standardised observation tools such as the *Autism Diagnostic Observation Schedule (ADOS)*, a 30–45 minute assessment which sets different tasks for children of different ages and language ability, for example, a younger child may have to pretend they're at a birthday party.

Although not strictly a diagnostic tool, another commonly used instrument is *Childhood Autism Rating Scale (CARS)*, which rates your child based on how their behaviour compares with that of a typical child. Children who score above a given point may go on to be diagnosed with autism.

You may find these assessments very confronting. Most people do. It's no fun having someone tell you all the things your child can't do — all the things that typical children just pick up naturally. Look at this assessment as a benchmark, against which you can measure your child's progress once they start in an intervention program.

COGNITIVE ASSESSMENT

A psychologist may assess your child's *cognitive* (learning) abilities. Intelligence (or IQ) tests are traditionally used to assess cognitive abilities, but these can sometimes be difficult to perform in children with ASD because:

- some tests require a level of verbal understanding and/or verbal responses which are beyond the capabilities of many children with an ASD (Therefore your child should have a speech and language assessment beforehand so that the tester knows to use a test which is appropriate for their language skills).
- children with ASD are not usually motivated to 'perform' so compliance can be a problem. (It is therefore essential that the person conducting the test has experience in ASD.)

Even if these factors are taken into account, the first time a young child undergoes one of these assessments they may still perform relatively poorly, simply because they don't really understand what's expected of them. So it's also good to think of your child's first cognitive assessment as a benchmark — the *minimum* they're likely to be capable of. As they grow and learn this may well change.

This was certainly the case with Joe. He didn't have too many skills at the time of his first assessment, but those he did have he decided not to demonstrate during the test. He was subsequently assessed as being very developmentally delayed. When he was reassessed after 20 months of early intervention he understood more and was a lot more co-operative. Thus the psychologists were able to get a much more accurate picture of his real abilities.

Some of the better known IQ tests include the **Wechsler Preschool and Primary Scale of Intelligence (WPPSI)**, and, for those who are school-aged, the **Wechsler Intelligence Scale for Children (WISC)**.

These IQ tests are not appropriate for younger children (under four years of age). **The Griffiths Scales of Mental Development** and **Bayley Scales of Infant Development** are developmental tests which can help identify cognitive and other delays in younger children.

Some people believe that measures of *adaptive behaviour* (everyday living or self-help skills) may be a better predictor of a child's development than IQ tests. Assessment tools commonly used by psychologists to assess your child's daily living, motor and social skills include the **Vineland Adaptive Behaviour Scales** and the **Adaptive Behaviour Assessment System (ABAS)**.

COMMUNICATION ASSESSMENT

A speech pathologist trained in ASD will conduct some tests to assess your child's *expressive* and *receptive communication* skills — ability to express and understand language. Children may also have their pragmatic language skills assessed. *Pragmatic language skills* refer to how effectively a child uses words and gestures to communicate, and are best observed in informal situations, such as during play.

OTHER ASSESSMENTS

Sometimes occupational therapy assessment may be recommended, to see if your child has any sensory issues (see page 83) or problems with muscle tone and co-ordination. If you are fortunate, you may also be offered a meeting with a social worker to discuss your individual family situation.

At the end of this process you should be given a comprehensive report on your child's abilities and needs. Depending on the results, this report should give you access to government support and services, as well as provide valuable information which can be used by early intervention services. At this time you should also receive information and advice on further assessment and interventions.

We hope the professionals you are dealing with during the diagnostic process will be sympathetic and understanding. But even so, diagnosis can still be a harrowing time:

The diagnosis dragged me from that warm and fuzzy place called denial which I retreated back to when the scary thoughts (like maybe there is something wrong with my son?) became too real.

Some diagnostic teams did not possess the art of giving bad news in a way that motivates people to want to do something about it... I wanted to develop an action plan to do something... I wanted the 90:10 rule; to spend 10% of the time on the problem and 90% on what could be done about it.

My husband was quite matter of fact about D-day. But even though I knew exactly what was coming, I was still distraught on the day. Afterwards I went off for a swim and a cry. That's the day I learned that you can cry doing breaststroke or backstroke but it's almost impossible to cry doing the crawl.

If you are like most parents, you will feel terrible grief at this time. You will probably feel that your child's future has been snatched away from you. But an ASD diagnosis does not have to define your child or their future.

What an official diagnosis will do is give your child access to financial, educational and social support they might otherwise be denied. Diagnosis is the first step towards getting help.

As we waited for that first diagnosis, a couple of people tut-tutted saying that three years old was far too early to 'label' a child. Oh that attitude makes me want to scream. I couldn't disagree more! If we don't understand exactly what a child's issues are, how can we get going with treatment? And a diagnosis is not a label. My son may have a diagnosis, and we tell people about it when we need to. But we absolutely do not label him.

A diagnosis helps prove to other people (and yourself) that something is wrong, something is different, allowances have to be made. It can open doors to support including financial. It helped get us the right kind of help and support for our son... Having the diagnosis also helped me seek out like-minded parents for sharing emotions and successful procedures.

We spent most of the time working out a plan of treatments. The doctor told us to start on the implementation plan and 'see where we would end up'... I walked out 10 feet above the ground. I did have a diagnosis but I also had a direction to follow.

1. Wray, J, Silove, N, Knot, H. (2005). Language disorders and autism. *Medical Journal of Australia*, 182, 7, 354–360.
2. Baird, G, Cass, H, Slonins, V. (2003). Diagnosis of autism. *BMJ*, 327, 488–493.
3. American Academy of Pediatrics Committee on Children with Disabilities. (2001). The Pediatrician's Role in the Diagnosis and Management of Autistic Spectrum Disorder in Children. *Pediatrics* 107, 5. www.pediatrics.org/cgi/content/full/107/5e85
4. National Initiative for Autism: Screening and Assessment. (2003). *National Autism Plan for Children (NAPC)*. The National Autistic Society, London.
5. Robins, DL, Fein, MA, Barton, ML, Green, JA. (2001). Modified checklist for autism in toddlers (M-CHAT). www.firstsigns.org
6. American Academy of Pediatrics Council on Children with Disabilities. (2007). Identification and evaluation of children with autism spectrum disorders. *Pediatrics* 120, 5, 1183–1215.
7. Dover, CJ, Le Couteur, A. (2007). How to diagnose autism. *Archives of Diseases in Childhood*, 92, 540–545.
8. Caronna, EB, Augustyn, M, Zuckerman, B. (2007). Revisiting Parental Concerns in the Age of Autism Spectrum Disorders: The Need to Help Parents in the Face of Uncertainty *Archives of Pediatric and Adolescent Medicine*, 161, 406–408.
9. Australian Advisory Board on Autism Spectrum Disorders. (2007). The prevalence of autism in Australia. Can it be established from existing data? Overview and Report. www.autismaus.com.au/aca/pdfs/PrevalenceReport.pdf
10. New Zealand Ministries of Health and Education. (2006). Draft Evidence-based Guideline for Autism Spectrum Disorder. Wellington: Ministry of Health. www.moh.govt.nz/moh.nsf/pagesmh/5597/$File/draft-asd-guideline-jan07.pdf

3

I don't think we can underestimate the importance of valuing the child as a unique person. I have met some amazing little personalities, children who shine through their autism, even better when they are part of a family where they are loved and accepted for themselves. I'm not sure that obsessively chasing a cure for the autism might not result in the loss of the child.

Dr Jacqui Roberts, Research Associate in the Disability Studies Initiative in the Faculty of Health Sciences, Sydney University

HOW DID THIS HAPPEN?

It's natural to ask: 'How did this happen to my child?' Unfortunately it's not an easy question to answer. Indeed, the answer may well differ from one child to the next. There is growing consensus amongst scientists that autism is not a single disorder but a *group* of disorders with many different causes ('autisms' rather than autism), which would explain why symptoms and severity can vary so much.

The *Autism Phenome Project*, a large study at the University of California, Davis, M.I.N.D. Institute, is hoping to shed some more light on this question. This study will enrol 1,800 children aged 2–4 years (most will have autism but there will be two comparison groups of typical and developmentally delayed kids) and follow them for several years. Each child will undergo a thorough medical examination, testing of their immune systems, brain structures and functions, genetics, environmental exposures and blood proteins. Researchers are hoping to be able to identify different subgroups, or *phenotypes* of autism, so that treatment and prevention strategies can be specifically targeted.[1]

Unfortunately it will be some years before the main results of this research are known. In the meantime, here is what we know about the causes of autism *right now*.

ASDs ARE NOT CAUSED BY BAD PARENTING

We've already discussed this. The myth of the 'refrigerator mother' has well and truly been debunked.

GENETICS PLAY A BIG ROLE

There is a lot of evidence to support the idea that our genes play a big role in the development of ASDs:

- ASDs are more common in boys than girls.
- Families with one child with autism have a greater chance (2–8%) of having another child with autism when compared with the general population.
- Family members of a person with an ASD (including extended family) tend to have higher rates of ASD-like language delays and social difficulties.
- Twin studies have found that when identical (*monozygotic*) twins (who have the same genetic makeup) have autism, *both* will have some form of autism up to 90% of the time. When non-identical (fraternal or *dizygotic*) twins have autism, both will have autism in only around 10% of cases. If genes were not involved in autism you'd expect the rate of autism to be the same for both types of twins.
- Autism is associated with a number of recognised genetic disorders, such as fragile X and tuberous sclerosis.

However, after many years of investigating the genetic basis of autism there is still not a known mode of *inheritance* (the manner in which genes and traits are passed from parent to child) suggesting that the genetics are complex. It appears that multiple genes (possibly more than 10) contribute to autism and ASD susceptibility, but how particular genes interact to produce the very different picture of autism from one person to the next remains unclear.

Genetics are a major area of international autism research. If you are interested in reading more on autism and genes the US National Institute of Child Health and Human Development has produced a comprehensive booklet on the topic. Go to: www.nichd.nih.gov/health/topics/asd.cfm

BETTER RECOGNITION HAS LED TO AN INCREASE IN ASD DIAGNOSES

If you compare prevalence rates of autism 30 years ago to those of today it would be easy to conclude that all the talk of an 'autism epidemic' — or even better, 'autism tsunami' — is correct. However, experts believe this increase is mostly due to us getting better at recognising the disorder, combined with a broadening of the diagnostic criteria of ASD (Asperger's disorder wasn't even included in the DSM until 1994). It's easy to imagine how people with Asperger's could have just been thought 'eccentric' or 'unsociable' 20 years ago and thus slipped through the diagnostic net. At the other end of the spectrum, there is research suggesting that many 'lower-functioning' children with autism and intellectual disability were simply classified as 'mentally retarded' in the past.

However, we can't completely rule out the possibility that environmental factors are triggering a genetic predisposition in selected children, resulting in a real increase in ASD prevalence.

BRAIN RESEARCH IS HELPING US TO UNDERSTAND AUTISM BETTER

Another major area of research is focussed on the brain. Doctors are using imaging technologies such as magnetic resonance imaging (MRI) to look at how the structure of brains of people with autism differ from those of typical people. They are also using this sort of technology to see how the brain works: for example, they will set the same task (such as observing facial emotions) for a group of autistic people and a group of typical people and see which areas of their brains 'light up' in response.

One popular theory is that autism could be a result of faulty neurological circuitry — the fibres of nervous system tissue that interconnect the individual parts of the brain. Deprived of effective connections, the different brain areas must work independently. This could explain why some people with an ASD may have superior abilities at spelling or maths but be poor at multi-tasking and social skills, areas which require a more 'co-ordinated' brain.

How this disruption to the circuitry occurs is still unclear but there is research showing that in some young children with autism the brain develops too quickly. It may be because this accelerated growth occurs at the 'wrong' time that the brain wiring becomes faulty. This research has implications for treatment, too. If this theory proves correct, experts such as Nancy Minshew believe that therapies which stimulate brain areas to work together — by exercising problem-solving skills and creative thinking — may prove effective.[2,3]

IS PARENTAL AGE A RISK FACTOR?

Results haven't been consistent, but some studies have found that older fathers and mothers (defined as being over 35 years) may be at increased risk of having a child with an ASD.[4,5] Older parents, as a rule, are more likely to have children with a range of developmental and other disorders, probably because of genetic factors. However, older mothers also have a higher risk of pregnancy and birth complications — premature delivery, low-birth weight babies and 'difficult' births — all of which have been associated with ASDs (although once again not consistently).[4] In scientific publications, factors that raise the risk of ASDs are often called *risk factors*.

Raising the risk means an increase in the chance of developing a disease or condition. There are, however, very few things that we do that will increase our risk in such a way as to lead us to inevitably develop a disease or problem. For example, smoking increases the risk of developing heart disease and cancer, but not *every* smoker develops heart disease or cancer and some non-smokers do. So, if you happen to be an older parent this doesn't mean that it was inevitable that you would have a child with an ASD and your age is not enough to explain why your child has an ASD. On the other hand, the general trend to delay parenting in our society may turn out to be a small piece in the puzzle of why the number of children being diagnosed with autism has risen in recent years. More research is needed.

OR SOMETHING IN THE ENVIRONMENT?

There are theories that environmental factors may contribute to some cases of ASD. Research is being conducted to identify possible environmental factors and the ways in which these could trigger the expression of autism in a child who is genetically predisposed.

An environmental factor that increases the risk of ASD could be anything that affects development from the time of fertilisation. We've already mentioned birth complications, but other pregnancy-related factors which have been implicated include: viral infections, autoimmune disorders, use of some epilepsy medicines, an underactive thyroid, smoking and heavy alcohol use.

Research groups, such as the M.I.N.D. Institute, are also investigating whether exposure to environmental pollutants such as heavy metals (lead and mercury) and organic solvents might increase the risk in children who are genetically predisposed. However, as yet, none of these suggested environmental factors has been *proven* to increase the risk of autism.

THE VACCINE CONTROVERSY

The environmental factor most often accused of contributing to the rise in ASD diagnoses is our childhood immunisation program. Two potential 'culprits' have been proposed.

Thiomersal, the mercury-based preservative used in some vaccines. Because of concerns about mercury toxicity and its effects on the central nervous system, it was theorised that the use of thiomersol-preserved childhood vaccines might be contributing to some cases of autism. However, to date, studies have not found any consistent association between the use of thiomersal-containing vaccines and the prevalence of ASD. A 2004 review of 12 of these studies concluded 'Studies do not demonstrate a link between thiomersal-containing vaccines and ASD'.[6] More research is continuing, especially in the US.

In Australia, thiomersal has been removed from all routine childhood vaccines since 2000, with the exception of one type of hepatitis B vaccine (Engerix®-B paediatric formulation) which may contain trace amounts left over from the manufacturing process. Therefore, if you have a young child who has recently been diagnosed with an ASD it's very unlikely they have been exposed to thiomersal through their immunisation program.

Measles, Mumps, Rubella (MMR) vaccine is a combination vaccine given to children at 12 months and again at four years of age. Because the signs of autism often become apparent around the same time children receive their first MMR vaccine, some parents worry that the vaccine has caused their child's autism.

In 1998, a small British study raised the question of a connection between MMR vaccine and developmental disorders, including autism.[7] The researchers suggested that MMR vaccination caused inflammatory bowel disease (IBD) in the children, which then led on to autism. However the study design and conclusions have been widely criticised: for example, the study included only 12 children and there was no control (comparison) group of typical children. Also, in at least four of the children studied, symptoms of autism appeared before symptoms of IBD. In 2004, 10 of the 13 original authors of the 1998 study retracted the study's interpretation.

Since that time, several large European and American studies have failed to find a link between MMR and ASD. A 2005 study from Japan found that ASD rates continued to rise after the MMR vaccine was discontinued and replaced with single vaccines.[8] Groups of experts, including the World Health Organisation and American Academy of Pediatrics, believe there is no convincing evidence that the MMR vaccine is associated with autism or IBD.

In summary, based on current research, the mainstream medical community does not believe there is a link between ASD and either thiomersal or the MMR vaccine. However, many parents and a smaller group of health professionals (several of whom have a very active presence on the Internet) continue to dispute these conclusions.

The MMR research is summarised in a fact sheet produced by the National Centre for Immunisation Research and Surveillance (NCIRS), based at The Children's Hospital at Westmead (Sydney). There is also a fact sheet about thiomersal. If you're interested go to: www.ncirs.usyd.edu.au and follow the links.

The Australian Government has also produced fact sheets on thiomersal and MMR through their *Immunisation: Myths and Realities* supplements: www.immunise.health.gov.au/internet/immunise/publishing.nsf/Content/uci-myths

For further information on current research in Australia see the appendix by Dr Deb Keen.

We'll finish with a cautionary note. It is natural for you to want answers to why your much loved child has developed this seemingly crippling disorder and we know it's frustrating that no simple explanations are forthcoming. But please don't get bogged down thinking about the past at the expense of the here and now. Right now you need to stay focussed on getting the best treatments for your child. By concentrating your energies on the present you have the best chance of creating a better future for you and your child.

1. UC Davis M.I.N.D. Institute. (2006). *UC Davis M.I.N.D. Institute Research The Autism Phenome Project.* www.ucdmc.ucdavis.edu/newsroom/releases/archives/mind/2006/Autism%20Phenome%20Project%20Facts.pdf

2. Just, MA, Cherkassky, VL, Keller, TA, Minshew, NJ. (2004). Cortical activation and synchronization during sentence comprehension in high-functioning autism: evidence of underconnectivity. *Brain* 127, 8, 1811–1821.

3. National Institute of Child Health and Development. (2004). Brains of people with autism recall letters of the alphabet in brain areas dealing with shapes. Finding supports theory that autism results from failure of brain areas to work together (Press Release). www.nichd.nih.gov/news/releases/final_autism.cfm

4. Kolevzon, A, Gross, R, Reichenberg, A. (2007). Prenatal and perinatal risk factors for autism. *Archives of Pediatric and Adolescent Medicine*, 161, 326–333.

5. Croen, LA, Najjar, DV, Fireman, B, Gether, JK. (2007). Maternal and paternal age and risk of autism spectrum disorders. *Archives of Pediatric and Adolescent Medicine*, 161, 334–340.

6. Parker, SK, Schwartz, B, Todd, J, Pickering, LK. (2004). Thimerosal-Containing Vaccines and Autistic Spectrum Disorder: A Critical Review of Published Original Data. *Pediatrics*, 114, 793–804.

7. Wakefield, AJ, Murch, SH, Anthony, A, et al. (1998). Ileal-lymphoid-nodular hyperplasia, non-specific colitis, and pervasive developmental disorder in children. *Lancet*, 351, 637–641.

8. Honda, H, Shimizu, Y, Rutter, M. (2005). No effect of MMR withdrawal on the incidence of autism: a total population study. *Journal of Child Psychology and Psychiatry*, 46, 6, 572–579.

Additional references:

9. American Academy of Pediatrics Council on Children with Disabilities. (2007). Identification and evaluation of children with autism spectrum disorders. *Pediatrics* 120, 5, 1183–1215

10. Wray, J, Silove, N, Knot, H. (2005). Language disorders and autism. *Medical Journal of Australia*, 182, 7, 354–360

11. Frith, Uta. (2003). *Autism. Explaining the Enigma* 2nd edn, Malden, MA, Blackwell Publishing

12. Coleman, M. Ed. (2005). *The Neurology of Autism*, New York, Oxford University Press.

13. Windham, GC, Zhang, L, Gunier, R, Croen, LA, Gether, JK. (2006). Autism spectrum disorders in relation to distribution of hazardous air pollutants in the San Francisco Bay Area. *Environmental Health Perspectives*, 114, 9, 1438–1444

14. National Centre for Immunisation Research and Surveillance of Vaccine Preventable Diseases. *Thiomersal Fact Sheet* www.ncirs.usyd.edu.au/facts/thiomersal.pdf

15. MacIntyre, CR, McIntyre, PB. (2001). MMR, autism and inflammatory bowel disease: responding to patient concerns using an evidence-based framework. *Medical Journal of Australia*, 175, 127–128.

4

You may seek the help of many other professionals but always remember that voice inside of you. A mother's intuition is so important. When looking at the interventions available for your child ask yourself does this make sense? How does this feel? Does this professional take time to explain and ask what I think? Every child with ASD is different and they all have their own personality outside the ASD.

Edwina Scerri, Kaleidoscope Network

EARLY INTERVENTION

If you have a child with an ASD who is not yet at school the single most important thing you must do is get them enrolled in an early educational intervention program. Although there is no magic pill or potion which can cure autism, a good, intensive, early intervention program can hugely improve symptoms and give your child the opportunity to learn and become independent. With the right early intervention, some children with ASD can grow up to lead normal, or near-normal, lives. According to the American Academy of Pediatrics: 'early diagnosis resulting in early, appropriate and consistent intervention has... been shown to be associated with improved long-term outcomes'.[1]

However, even if your child is already at school many of the intervention options discussed below are still relevant for primary school age children and beyond.

This is not meant to be a comprehensive guide (the reference list at the end of this chapter includes some more detailed reviews) but will hopefully point you in the right direction.

What to look for in a good early intervention program

What should you look for in an early intervention program? This is a difficult question for parents struggling to come to terms with an ASD diagnosis. There are lots of different options out there and nearly everyone you speak to will offer a different opinion. This can be a confusing and, frankly, quite frustrating time.

We are fortunate therefore that, in recent years, a number of expert committees in the English-speaking world — boasting qualifications in paediatrics, psychology, psychiatry, education and related disciplines — have reviewed the research on early intervention in ASD.[2-8] The conclusions of these expert groups have been remarkably similar. Following is a list of characteristics *they* agree are important in an early intervention program.

STARTING AS EARLY AS POSSIBLE

You should aim to start your child's educational intervention as soon as possible after diagnosis, or even before you have an official diagnosis if an ASD is strongly suspected. We know that this may seem daunting when you are still adjusting to the reality of having a child with autism. However, doing something positive should help to lift your mood and, once you witness your child making progress, the worst feelings of grief can hopefully recede.

So why is earlier better?

Early intervention can prevent or reduce challenging behaviours such as tantrums or self-injury, which often result from communication problems. Can you imagine how frustrating it must be for these young children unable to express their needs? If we equip our children with the skills and ability to communicate at an early age many of the worst behaviours can simply be avoided.

Also, there is some evidence that children who start intensive intervention before the age of three respond faster than children who begin after the age of five. Stroke and brain injury research has shown that previously damaged and underused parts of the brain can be strengthened with 'exercise'. That's what early intervention aims to do — 'rewire the brain'. The theory is that very young children's brains are more *plastic* (able to be re-shaped) and that new neural connections can be made more easily than in the brains of older children.

However, this is not a hard and fast rule. The latest research suggests that remodelling and rewiring of the brain continues throughout childhood, adolescence and even beyond. Older children can definitely still benefit from these interventions, although in some cases their progress may be a bit slower.

HAVING A PROGRAM OF SUFFICIENT INTENSITY

Experts now agree that early intervention for ASD should be intensive, although there is no strict consensus on the exact number of hours. Some recommend a *minimum* of 15 hours a week; others suggest it should be 20–25 hours a week.

If anyone remains unconvinced, we now have Australian Government-sponsored guidelines which specify: 'a minimum of 20 hours a week over two or more years is essential for young children to make major gains'.[9] You can access these guidelines yourself at: www.health.gov.au/internet/wcms/publishing.nsf/content/mental-child-autbro

If you choose intensive behavioural intervention (page 47) your service provider will probably recommend even more hours — 30 or even 40 hours a week. In Joe's case, he ended up doing about 30 hours a week of therapy in his first year. He coped with this remarkably well, although it must be said that much of the 30 hours was spent learning through play and he had lots of short breaks in his schedule.

However, it is not just the number of hours that you have to consider. The quality of those hours is as least as important. For intervention hours to be effective your child has to be more than just physically present — *their mind must be meaningfully engaged*. Initially at least, this means that your child will probably need lots of individual attention (see below), as it's easy for ASD children to 'zone out' when they are involved in group activities.

If this all sounds scary remember that not all learning need take place in the confines of a classroom. Intervention hours may include play sessions, where the goal is co-operative play; or time at preschool where children work towards defined goals, such as eating morning tea independently and sitting quietly for story time. Even household chores can provide learning opportunities if you deliberately set out to involve your child and engage them in the activity. For example, you could help your child count fruit into a bag at the supermarket and teach them important social goals such as staying close and waiting patiently in line.

AUTISM SPECIFIC CURRICULUM

Children with an ASD have unique social and communication challenges so the curriculum content of any intervention program should be *autism specific*.

There are five important skills your child should be working towards in their program:

- to focus and pay attention
- to imitate others
- to understand and use language
- to play appropriately with toys
- to socially interact with others.

Of course no two children with an ASD are exactly alike, so your child's program should be *individualised* to their relative strengths and weaknesses. Some children pick up language relatively easily; others find it more difficult and may need visual supports such as the *Picture Exchange Communication System (PECS)* (discussed on page 78). Some children will need extra help with motor skills: jumping, kicking balls, writing and drawing. Self-help skills can also be taught through an intervention program. These can include getting dressed, making a snack or independent toileting, all skills necessary for future self-sufficiency.

A POSITIVE APPROACH TO CHALLENGING BEHAVIOURS

Most children with ASD will develop challenging behaviours, such as 'stimming' and tantrums, from time to time. A good intervention program will have pro-active strategies in place to prevent challenging behaviours: making learning fun and motivating, carefully structuring the environment (see below) and providing lots of positive reinforcement, such as verbal praise or a favourite toy, for good behaviour.

Of course, even with the best intervention programs some problem behaviours are unavoidable. If so, the teacher/therapy providers should conduct a *functional analysis* to establish the reasons behind that behaviour, introduce changes to reduce that behaviour and provide more acceptable alternatives. For example, if they find that a child usually tantrums during a particular language program the most logical conclusion might be that he is trying to escape that task by 'playing up'. In this case the response might be to reduce the difficulty of the work for a time, ignore the tantrums (difficult but possible) and reinforce on-task work with lavish praise and a favoured activity afterwards. You might see an increase in tantrums in the short term, but down the track you would expect to see the problem diminish.

STRUCTURED AND SUPPORTIVE ENVIRONMENT

All children respond well to predictability and routine, but for children with ASD this is especially important. Particularly if your child is in a preschool setting, the school day should be as structured as possible and follow a predictable timetable. Some children will need extra help with *transitions* between activities, especially if there are unexpected changes to the routine. Providing them with a visual schedule of the day's activities can help reduce anxiety.

The physical teaching environment should also be well-organised and free of distractions. Many children with ASD have sensory sensitivities and can be disturbed by things we wouldn't notice, such as fluorescent lights. Some children cannot work around particular noises such as lawn mowers, vacuum cleaners or drills.

Predictability and routine are especially important in the early months of learning, but as your child progresses, it is important to gradually introduce changes to the routine. This helps in developing independence and skills for coping with the realities of the outside world. It could mean moving from 1:1 instruction to group lessons and learning in more natural settings, such as preschool.

FAMILY INVOLVEMENT

Family involvement is essential for the success of any intervention program. There is no point in having the best intervention program that money can buy, if the lessons learnt are not followed through in the family home. Your family should be actively involved in goal-setting and planning. You should also receive training in how best to communicate with your child and to apply, or *generalise*, the skills they have learnt. As your child moves through the program you should expect regular feedback on their progress.

Some parents choose an even more active role and become therapists themselves. This can be a good way to save money, although it will not suit all people. For some intervention programs, such as RDI (discussed on page 57), the parents are actually required to implement the program.

INDIVIDUALISED ATTENTION

Your child should be given an individualised education plan, specifically tailored to their strengths and needs. This plan should take into consideration your family situation and priorities. For example, a priority for you might be to teach them how to request drinks and snacks, to make your home life a little easier.

It is essential that your child receive sufficient individualised attention on a daily basis for their education goals to be realistically met. As your child progresses they should become able to learn as part of a group but in the early stages of treatment at least some 1:1 attention is recommended.

SYSTEMATIC TEACHING

The teaching goals for your child should be carefully planned, and include strategies to generalise these skills in the home and community settings.

Progress should be carefully monitored and the education plan adjusted accordingly. Be very wary of any program which doesn't offer ways to measure its effectiveness. It is also not helpful to have vague goals such as 'increase in spoken language' or 'improved behaviour'. To properly assess progress you need to record data on behaviours which can be measured, such as the number of spontaneous spoken requests in a day or the number of tantrum episodes over the week.

TRANSITION SUPPORT

Children with autism usually need a lot of support when it's time to start school. Good early intervention programs will include a formal *transition to school* program, which will teach school skills to help them to function independently, and ideally include a formal *integration program* so that they can gradually adjust to their new environment.

CONTACT WITH TYPICALLY DEVELOPING CHILDREN

There is evidence that, in the right setting, children with autism can pick up valuable social skills from typical children. Ideally, your child's intervention should include some opportunity to mix with *typically developing peers* (ordinary children about their age). However, if you plan to send your child to a mainstream preschool remember that these can be noisy and chaotic places and your child is likely to need lots of support to succeed. They will probably need an integration plan, visual supports such as an activity schedule and perhaps even a personal aide or *shadow* to encourage play with the other children.

That's it from the professionals. However, we'd like to add one more recommendation from the other 'experts': mums and dads who have negotiated the early intervention path before you.

TEACHERS/ THERAPISTS WHO CAN ENGAGE YOUR CHILD

It is probably stating the obvious to say that good intervention programs should employ teachers and supervising therapists with appropriate qualifications, be it in special education, psychology, speech pathology or occupational therapy. They should also be specifically trained in working with children with ASD. Junior staff can be less qualified, but should receive ongoing training and close supervision from more qualified personnel.

However, the most important quality that teachers and therapists should have, which transcends academic qualifications, is the ability to engage your child. The best therapists can look past the autism symptoms and see the child within; they will know how to laugh and play and have fun, but also how to impose discipline in a kind and consistent manner. Your child will really enjoy being with these people and will learn best with them. If you come across one you should try to hold onto her (or him) for as long as possible. Fortunately they are more common than you might think.

If a therapist comes for a job interview and doesn't even ask to meet my son, I now know not to give them a job. The people I employ are the ones who get down on the floor and say hello to my son, even before they speak to me.

Some different intervention models

Unfortunately, like almost everything to do with ASD, early intervention can be a controversial topic. There is certainly no controversy about the fact that early intervention is extremely important for your child's learning and progress, but there are arguments about which are the most effective programs.

The problem is that it is difficult and expensive to conduct good quality studies of early intervention in ASD and as a result much of the published research isn't very good. Some well-established intervention models, particularly ABA, have a lot of evidence behind them, but others have less independent research.

It is even *more* difficult to conduct studies comparing two different intervention programs. And, unfortunately, you can't just compare the results of two separate studies of intervention models, because the children in the individual studies might be quite different from one another in terms of age, IQ and severity of symptoms (and this would influence response to treatment). Also, the *outcome measures* (that is the signs the researchers are looking for as measures of progress, such as change in IQ, school placement or autism symptoms) often differ from one study to another. In summary, you would be comparing apples with oranges.

In the end you will have to make a judgement based on the evidence available, feedback from professionals and other parents, your own personal philosophies and — regrettably — on availability and economics: some of these interventions can be difficult to access and very expensive.

Warning: Each of these intervention models has its own unique terminology which can be a bit intimidating if you are not familiar with it. We have tried to avoid scientific jargon as much as possible but the occasional technical phrase has slipped through.

INTENSIVE BEHAVIOURAL INTERVENTION (INTENSIVE APPLIED BEHAVIOURAL ANALYSIS OR ABA)

On one of those dark days following Joe's diagnosis, our paediatrician sat us down to discuss early intervention options. He mentioned ABA but said that to run an intensive home program would cost $40,000 per year and would involve one of us having to give up work. I immediately thought, 'Well we won't be doing that'. Then I went away and did the research and a few months later resigned my job and committed our family to spending tens of thousands of dollars on Joe's intervention over the next few years. What changed my mind?
One thing really – evidence.

So what is ABA?

Applied behavioural analysis, or ABA, is a treatment methodology based on BF Skinner's theory of *operant conditioning*, which in summary is, consequences have an effect on behaviour. According to this theory, a child is more likely to learn and retain behaviours for which there are positive consequences (positive reinforcement) and less likely to learn or maintain behaviours for which there are negative or neutral consequences.

Many behavioural interventions use a variety of different ABA methods (for example, the functional approach to managing challenging behaviours, discussed on page 43, has its foundations in ABA). However, the best known ABA technique, and the one that still forms the basis of most in-home intensive behavioural programs, is *Discrete Trial Training (DTT)*. In DTT learning is broken down into small, discrete steps, which the children can master more easily. Rewards (or *reinforcers*) are offered to motivate the children while they are learning these new behaviours and skills. For example, a therapist might give the instruction 'Come here' and if the child responds correctly (ie comes to the therapist) they are rewarded with praise ('very good!') and some bubble blowing or a tickle. If the child does not respond with the correct behaviour the reward is simply withheld. However, early in any program, the child receives reinforcement just for trying, so the whole experience remains a successful and positive one. These discrete trials are repeated several times over, until the child masters the skill.

For children with ASD, DTT and other ABA methods can be used to:

- teach play, academics, social skills, communication and *adaptive living skills* (fine and gross motor skills, eating, toileting, dressing etc)
- encourage desirable behaviours, such as attending to the teacher and completing set tasks
- reduce undesirable behaviours, such as self-injury or 'stims'
- generalise desired behaviours to different settings (home, school etc)

People use the terms intensive behavioural intervention and ABA interchangeably, but this is not strictly correct. Behavioural teaching, based on ABA methods, need not necessarily be intensive and 1:1. Many early intervention programs will use behavioural methods to teach skills (especially living skills, such as toilet training) and to manage problem behaviours, but will not use these techniques exclusively. *Intensive behavioural intervention (IBI)* is an individualised intervention program which involves the systematic use of ABA techniques, delivered on a 1:1 basis (usually) for at least 20 hours a week. The evidence discussed below relates to IBI or *intensive* ABA programs.

The evidence for intensive behavioural intervention

In 1987, Dr Lovaas and colleagues at the University of California, Los Angeles, published a groundbreaking study of intensive behavioural intervention in young children with autism.[10] They compared three groups of children — one group of 19 children received 40 hours of 1:1 behavioural intervention a week over 2–3 years; the other or control groups (with 19 and 21 children respectively) received less than 10 hours a week of therapy over this time. At the end of the study they found that 47% of the children in the intensive intervention group passed normal first grade, had average or above average IQ scores and, according to their teachers, were 'indistinguishable' from their school friends. In the control groups only one child succeeded in normal first grade placement and had a normal IQ on testing.

In subsequent years there has been much criticism of the Lovaas study and its methods and especially the claim that some children in the IBI group had actually 'recovered.' A major sticking point was that no researchers had been able to reproduce the striking results of this study. However, this criticism has recently been countered by the work of the Wisconsin Early Autism Project (WEAP).[11] The WEAP was a randomised study which followed 23 young children, who received an average of 32 or 40 hours a week of IBI for four years. At the end of the study, 48% had normal IQ and language scores and were succeeding in regular schools, although about a third of these still had mild social difficulties. The remaining children also improved but their gains were more modest.

It must be remembered that both the Lovaas and WEAP studies represent absolutely best practice and therefore the best possible outcome. They were conducted in the university departments with the highest quality teaching, supervision and monitoring. Such programs don't currently exist locally and it's probably unrealistic to expect a parent-run home IBI program to meet such standards. The characteristics of the child can also affect response to treatment — research indicates that children over five and those with lower IQs may not respond as dramatically, although they are still able to learn using behavioural methods.

Thomas Insel, Director of the (US) National Institute of Mental Health has suggested a figure of about 20–25% for the best outcome children. In the words of Dr Insel, children who respond to intensive intervention 'may not be exactly free of rituals and social deficits but they will be subtle. These will be kids who can attend regular school and achieve things and be very successful. The key here is getting to them at an early stage'.[12]

Whatever the controversy, there is no doubt that ABA is a very effective teaching method for children with ASD. What's more, most but not all studies have found IBI to be more effective, in terms of raising IQ, language and skill levels, than 'eclectic' special education programs (a mixture of DTT, *sensory integration* and TEACCH [see page 62]) with a similar number of teaching hours.

So why isn't every child doing intensive behavioural intervention? Are there any downsides?

The number one negative is the cost. This is certainly not because the local ABA providers* are in the business of making big profits; it's simply that paying the wages of therapists for 30–40 hours a week costs a lot. Some parents take on some of the therapy themselves to reduce costs; others become very inventive at raising money. However, the fact remains that intensive ABA programs are beyond the financial reach of many Australian families.

---

*Just to confuse you IBI providers generally call themselves ABA providers!

Also, if you chose to go down this path, please be prepared for some negative comments, as IBI has many detractors. Some critics complain that it is 'just like training monkeys' and it's true that the learning theories which underpin ABA are based on animal behaviour studies. However, we all know that rewarding good behaviour works for people, too. As autism author, Karen Siff Exorn points out, why would businesses offer corporate bonuses to their employees if not to motivate them to perform? [13]

Nonetheless, there has been a move in recent years to what are referred to as *contemporary ABA programs*, which have a reduced emphasis on DTT and greater emphasis on spontaneity, incidental learning, teaching in real-life settings and allowing the child to choose games and activities. Contemporary ABA programs encourage the use of 'naturally occurring reinforcers' (for example, rewarding a request for a food or activity with that food or activity) and there is some evidence that this approach may be more effective than relying on 'artificial' reinforcers such as toys. One of the best known examples of contemporary ABA is *Pivotal Response Training*, a program developed by Dr Robert and Lynn Koegel.[14]

Joe's program included many contemporary ABA elements. He spent just as much time playing with toys and goofing around with his therapists, as he did at DTT, and I was pleased about that.

Finally, there are the logistic issues. You can't approach a home-based IBI program half-heartedly. You need to be intimately involved — recruiting therapists, attending clinics, developing learning materials and the like — and will be expected to generalise the skills your child is working on outside therapy hours. This can be especially hard if you have other young children at home. However, since we've already identified parent involvement as an important characteristic of successful intervention programs, you could actually consider this an upside of home ABA programs.

If you are interested in intensive behavioural intervention we list ABA service providers in the state by state chapters at the end of this book.

Alistair was diagnosed with ASD just before his third birthday...
Though we have investigated and 'dabbled' in other approaches,
ABA has been the cornerstone of Alistair's intervention program,
around 30 hours a week. From day one he took off, almost
exponentially in the first 18 months. Our life revolved around his
schedule, but we turned out to be one of those lucky families that
is rewarded with dramatic improvement. His original diagnosis of
intellectual impairment proved to be incorrect and the little boy
that was considered moderate to severely autistic now ranks as
mild.

Alistair is currently in year 1 at a local mainstream school, his
initial full-time support (funded by us) now minimal. He keeps up
academically, has friends, a girlfriend, plays in the soccer team and
loves annoying his big brother. He still has weaknesses in
expressive language and social interaction... but his intervention is
now something that we fit into our family life, rather than revolve
around.

ABA is extremely hard going and expensive, not always delivering
the results our son has achieved. The most important thing it has
done for us and I believe it can do for the majority of families, is
to give back some sort of family lifestyle. We now have the
knowledge and tools to tackle problem behaviours and the ability
to help our child deal with a world that often overwhelms him.
We can eat in restaurants, visit friends, take holidays, go to the
supermarket, movies, amusement parks, bowling alleys, beaches,
ride buses, get haircuts... we have a quality of life.

Though every parent who begins an ABA program hopes for
'recovery', you accept that it is rare. Alistair is not and may never
be 'indistinguishable', but he continues to grow, improve and
amaze us. Most parents only celebrate when their child achieves
the extraordinary. For us, achieving the ordinary is extraordinary
and we get to celebrate every day.
BARBARA MORROW, MOTHER OF ALISTAIR.

DEVELOPMENTAL INTERVENTIONS

Developmental or relationship-based interventions are based on research into typical child development and focus on the child's ability to form positive, meaningful relationships with other people. We are going to discuss two — DIR®/Floortime™ and the RDI® Program — which are currently available in Australia.

DIR®/Floortime™

DIR®/Floortime™ is the brainchild of Dr Stanley Greenspan and Dr Serena Wieder. DIR® stands for *Developmental Individual-Difference Relationship-Based Model,* but is commonly referred to as 'Floortime', for reasons we'll explain later.

Developmental interventions such as DIR®/Floortime are based on developmental psychology research from the last few decades. Fundamental to this has been the discovery that children learn *cognition* (the ability to think, reason, and remember), language, emotional and socials skills through their interactions with other people, firstly and most importantly their primary caregivers.

However, according to the Floortime model, children with autism have unique *biological challenges,* such as difficulties with sensory modulation and motor planning (see page 83), which interfere with learning and cause these important relationships to go awry. DIR®/Floortime therefore aims to help a child work around these difficulties and re-establish an emotional relationship with their primary caregivers.

Greenspan and Wieder have identified six developmental milestones they believe are necessary for a child to master in order for them to learn and succeed in the world. The DIR®/Floortime intervention is designed to guide a child through these milestones.

1. *Self-regulation and interest in the world*: the dual ability to take an interest in the sights, sounds and sensations of the world and to calm oneself down.
2. *Intimacy*: the ability to engage in relationships.
3. *Two-way communication*: the ability to engage in two-way communication with gestures. For example, a baby learns to reach out for her daddy so that he will pick her up.

4. *Complex communication*: When a child can string a series of gestures together in order to express their intentions and is able to read the gestures of others as well.
5. *Emotional ideas*: the ability to create ideas. The ability to form ideas develops first in pretend play, for example when a boy learns to race and crash toy cars, rather than just spin their wheels.
6. *Emotional thinking*: the ability to build bridges between ideas to make them reality-based and logical. When a child can link ideas together into logical sequences and play, and can describe their feelings instead of acting them out: 'I am mad because you took my toy.'

Each child is first assessed and provided with an individually-tailored intervention program. Several hours a day (up to 6–10 sessions of 20–30 minutes) are then spent in child-directed play sessions. These sessions are referred to as 'floortime' as the adult (parent, therapist or other helper) and child often play together on the floor. According to Greenspan, interactive play, in which the adult follows the child's lead, will encourage the child to 'want' to relate to the outside world.[6]

Once a child has made sufficient progress, play dates with typically developing children are introduced. To address the child's biological challenges (referred to earlier), regular occupational therapy, physiotherapy and/or speech therapy sessions are also recommended.

For many children, the Floortime home-program is combined with an educational intervention. The preference is for a supportive preschool with opportunity to interact with typically developing peers, but in the USA at least, DIR®/Floortime is often incorporated into home-based ABA programs.

Whilst DIR®/Floortime appears to be in its fledgling stages in Australia there are therapists operating in some capital cities. We've listed their details in the back of this book. Indications are that Floortime is a relatively lower-cost intervention model and therefore might be more financially accessible for some families.

How effective is DIR®/Floortime™?

As with most early intervention models in autism, this is a difficult question to answer at present.

In 1997 Greenspan and Wieder published a detailed case review of 200 children who had participated in the DIR®/Floortime model for two or more years. In measures of social-emotional functioning, 58% were reported to have had 'good to out-standing' outcomes.[7] An in-depth study of 20 of the highest functioning children found that they were indistinguishable from age-matched typical peers on assessments of emotional functioning using the *Functional Emotional Assessment Scale (FEAS)* and the *Vineland Adaptive Scales* (see page 26). A recent follow-up of 16 of these children, 10–15 years after they'd started Floortime, found all to be functioning well in mainstream schooling and enjoying friendships.[15]

Whilst this all sounds very promising, it is difficult to really compare these outcomes with those of other interventions because the main instrument used to measure progress (FEAS) was specifically developed for the DIR®/Floortime model. Also, to date, Greenspan and Wieder have published all their outcome research in a journal they founded themselves and therefore have been criticised for not subjecting their research to independent scrutiny.

Fortunately, we should know more in a few years. A research study is currently underway in Canada, comparing the progress of two groups of randomly-assigned preschool age children. One group will receive intensive DIR®/Floortime for two years; the other will receive the same intervention but delayed by 12 months.[16] Presumably we will expect to see a faster rate of progress in the children who start Floortime straightway. Standard assessments such as IQ and the *Autism Diagnostic Observation Schedule (ADOS)* (see page 25) will be used, as well as measures of social emotional functioning. Excitingly, this study is also monitoring brain function, in the hope of picking up changes to suggestive of brain remodelling (see page 41).

In summary, DIR®/Floortime has some important qualities of effective intervention programs — in particular it is individualised and requires (indeed demands) lots of family involvement.

More information on DIR®/Floortime™ is available at
www.floortime.org or www.icdl.com.

*Our son Will was diagnosed with autism when he was just 28
months old. Will regressed from a very happy but placid baby to a
toddler who would lie on the floor all day and stare at the
ceiling... He tolerated us in his world but didn't show any response
to affection, laughter or play.*

*Floortime looks at the level of communication your child is
capable of and comes up with strategies to increase the quantity
and quality of communication... whilst incorporating the sensory
needs of the child.*

*We would spend hours every day following Will's lead,
encouraging him to make the first contact and then extending each
play piece until he was able to sustain an interaction for 15
minutes. Floortime is not just about play, it is also used in
everyday life situations — turning routines such as dinner/bath etc
into opportunities to encourage communication and fun.*

*Three years later we still attend a Floortime session every week...
Will is a very happy, well-regulated boy who can transition
between many environments without getting anxious or being
fixated on a particular interest. Although he can only say a few
words he understands the importance of needing to communicate
with a person and through gestures, a few words and PECS is able
to do this.*

*Floortime can be complemented with many other therapies
including school, speech and motor activities. It is not just for
children with special needs – try it with your other children and
watch their confidence grow!*

SUE BROCKHOFF, MOTHER OF WILL.

Our son was diagnosed with ASD at the age of 18 months... One of the first referrals we received was to an occupational therapist, trained in the DIR®/Floortime model. This proved to be the best referral we could ever hope for... The DIR®/Floortime principles of 'follow the child's lead' and 'enter the child's world' were able to be applied during active and movement-based play sessions, using our son's ability to swing, climb and balance with a skill beyond his years... He has always enjoyed these sessions and they have been the foundation of a comprehensive early intervention program.

The DIR®/Floortime model comprises six developmental levels or stages and we have found these very helpful in showing our son's steady progress... Having commenced this therapy with barely Level I capabilities, our son, now five, has progressed to Level V. This therapy can be intense and at times exhausting, but once you are familiar with it, the rewards are many. Our son now enjoys many activities that he once found bewildering, frustrating and exhausting. A trip to the beach is now a delight: endless sand to sift through exploring fingers, rock pools and waves to paddle in and rocks to climb on — no longer a cause for sensory overload. The quality of family outings has greatly improved: our son can now sit and enjoy a dinner out, or watch his older sister perform in the school band or her ballet concert, quite calmly.

Our son has become an endearing, happy, loving little boy with a very cheeky sense of humour and we feel DIR®/Floortime is greatly responsible for this.

GREG AND CARINA WALKER, PARENTS OF JOHN.

The RDI® Program

RDI® or *Relationship Development Intervention®* is a developmental intervention, based on research which has found that children typically learn through interaction with parents and other caregivers. RDI was founded by Dr Steven Gutstein and Dr Rachelle Sheely in 1996. Its base is in Houston, Texas, but there are now RDI Certified Consultants practising throughout much of the world, including an increasing number in Australia.

According to the research that underpins the RDI® Program, the universal deficit of people with ASD, no matter how 'high-functioning', is a failure to develop *dynamic intelligence*: the abilities required to succeed in a dynamic and changing world. It is this lack of dynamic intelligence, Gutstein argues, which explains why many adults on the autism spectrum struggle to form friendships, marry and hold down satisfying jobs.[17]

Dynamic intelligence is described as being composed of the following abilities, things most of us take for granted:

1. *Experience-sharing*: To be able to use language and non-verbal communication to express curiosity, invite others to interact, share our perceptions and feelings and co-ordinate our actions with others.
2. *Dynamic analysis*: To be able to monitor and continually *regulate* our behaviour in order to participate in collaborative relationships (for example, adjusting to rapidly changing topics in a typical conversation).
3. *Flexible and creative problem-solving*: The ability to see the 'big picture', to solve problems that have no 'right' or 'wrong' answer, and to 'go with the flow'.
4. *Episodic memory and self-awareness (foresight and hindsight)*: The ability to reflect on past experiences and anticipate potential future scenarios; to be able to consider, prepare, evaluate and dream.
5. *Resilience*: The ability to cope with a 'messy' unpredictable world, where setbacks and mistakes are unavoidable.

The RDI® Program is therefore designed with the specific and ambitious aim of developing dynamic intelligence in children with ASD. For this, parents are required to be the primary therapists, or *guides*.

Parents of typical children instinctively act as guides in interactions with their children. They challenge their child (*the apprentice*) to take more responsibility for *co-regulation* (maintaining the connection), all the time making sure they are not pushing too hard and the encounter remains an enjoyable one. This process is called *guided participation*. Then, as their sense of competence grows, typical infants and toddlers start to actively seek out new information and challenges. This is how they grow and learn.

However, because of their communication challenges, guided participation never really gets started with ASD children. And then, children with ASDs start avoiding encounters characterised by change or novelty, missing out on dynamic learning opportunities.

RDI aims to re-establish this important relationship between parent and child. The goal is for the child to regulate their actions and thoughts with their parent or caregiver, which allows dynamic intelligence to gradually develop.

In guided participation activities (several of which are conducted throughout the day) parents are instructed to slow down and carefully pace their demands for co-regulation, so that their child can begin to feel competent and have the desire to take on more responsibility. Challenges are added in small manageable amounts, so the child has opportunity to assimilate the added complexity.[18] For example, on one day a child might hand his mum the washing for her to put in the machine; the next day the roles might be reversed and she will pass the washing to him. It's crucial that these interactions remain enjoyable, so that the children realise that parents (and later other people) are fun to be around.

RDI also requires that parents talk less and change their communication style — reducing the amount of *imperative* language they use (language that places a demand on someone else, such as a request, 'Come here' or a question 'What is this?') and increasing their *emotion-sharing language* (inviting another to share some aspect of their experience, 'Wow, that's great' or 'Eww, that's yucky').

RDI requires a serious and long-term family commitment: it is not something you can fit in 'here and there' around other therapies. RDI is continually evolving but the current version has over 1100 developmentally-staged objectives. Parents are advised to attend RDI workshops (introductory two-day and/or intensive four-day training) and work under the supervision of a Certified Consultant, who will assess the child and devise an individualised treatment plan. Training workshops are held in Australia occasionally, but some parents have had to travel to the US. In addition, many children will need other therapies such as occupational or speech therapy to deal with co-occurring disorders not specifically targeted by RDI.

Late in 2007 the RDIos was established. This subscription-only, web-based operating system facilitates online communication between clients and their consultants and offers other support such as a video library, webinars, e-learning and chat groups.

The evidence for the RDI® Program

Two RDI studies have been accepted for publication. The first, which at the time of writing is still *in press*, is a retrospective study of 31 children (2–9 years old); 17 who participated in the RDI® Program and 14 who received other interventions (ABA or special education).[18] After 16 months, 70% of children in the RDI group had improved at least one diagnostic category in their *Autism Diagnostic Observation Schedule (ADOS)* — there are three diagnostic categories: 'autism', 'autism spectrum' and 'non-autism' — compared with none in the control group. Also, prior to treatment, only one child in each group was in mainstream schooling but by the end of the assessment period 13 of the RDI® group were 'mainstreamed', whereas there was no change in the comparison group.

Once again, these results are impressive, but the study methods have been criticised, especially with respect to selection of the control group. The study was not randomised and the children in the RDI group were younger, received therapy for longer and had higher IQs than those in the control group, all of which may have influenced the outcome.[6]

The second study reviewed progress of 16 young children enrolled in RDI programs for at least two and a half years.[19] Prior to treatment, ten were classified as having 'autism' and three as 'autism spectrum' on ADOS testing (there was no data for the remaining three). At the end of the study period there were no children in the 'autism' group, six in the 'autism spectrum' group and ten in the 'non-autism' group, with corresponding improvements in the ADI-R (see page 23), parent-rated measures of flexibility and mainstream school placement. However, there was no control group in this study and all children were classed as 'intellectually high-functioning' (IQ ≥ 70), so results cannot necessarily be generalised to all children on the autism spectrum.

Also, Gutstein and Sheely are cautious to remind us that ADOS categories are not the same as the diagnostic categories used by clinicians, so a 'non-autism' ADOS result alone does not mean a child has 'recovered' and is no longer on the autism spectrum.

Our experience with RDI has been very encouraging — we have noticed big improvements in Joe's experience-sharing, *social referencing* (looking to our reactions to guide his behaviour if faced with uncertainty) and resilience when faced with life's little setbacks. He talks a lot more too, especially to share his impressions with us, and we believe (although we cannot be sure) that this is largely because of RDI. However, the ultimate aim of RDI® is to improve the quality of life of adults on the spectrum and obviously it will be some years before we know whether it can deliver on that score.

For more information on the RDI® Program, including a list of Certified Consultants, visit www.rdiconnect.com

Our youngest of two children was diagnosed with autism just before his third birthday... We were a family crippled, unable to leave the home because our son couldn't cope with the outside world. From all the information we received we just kept reading about the impairment in relationships which was the main concern for autism sufferers, rendering them into an isolated and depressed life. So in our search for intervention for our son we chose to remediate as much as we humanly could his relationship impairment.

We 'Googled' relationship intervention and RDI came up;

everything that RDI had to offer was what we felt we were looking for to help our son have a quality of life... We started RDI as our main intervention immediately and we haven't looked back since; we now have our family life back, where we can go out and enjoy outings together and simple trip to the supermarket is a fun experience instead of an embarrassing and exhausting one. RDI is an intensive home-based program and it's not for everyone but for us it was what we needed to get us and our son through to a better place...

We experienced in the first few months of RDI our son placing his arms around our necks for the very first time and saying 'I love you!' He started looking in our eyes in anticipation trying to figure out what we might do next; we had laughter back in the home instead of screaming meltdowns. RDI and autism have shown us the better side to our life, a slow motion view of how to go about enjoying every moment, something that we didn't appreciate with our first son.

RDI is a journey that assists us and our son to achieve our goals of quality of life... The autism road is still a challenging one at times but we have comfort in knowing that now we have the proper road map to deal with detours and anything else that may come along.
ANTHONY AND LEARNE BRISCHETTO, PARENTS OF PATRICK.

COMBINED INTERVENTIONS
These interventions combine elements of behavioural and developmental models.

TEACCH and structured teaching
TEACCH or *Treatment and Education of Autistic and related Communication-handicapped CHildren* was founded by the University of North Carolina in 1972. TEACCH is a structured teaching approach which does not rely on one specific technique, but provides a comprehensive range of services to children, adolescents and adults with autism.

Perhaps to distinguish their intervention from ABA, the proponents of TEACCH do not claim to 'cure' autism but rather to help people with ASD to reach their potential, so they can function more independently in the home, at school and the wider community.[8]

Gary Mesibov, the Director of Division TEACCH, explains this further:

> We emphasize individualized assessment to understand the individual better and also 'the culture of autism,' suggesting that people with autism are part of a distinctive group with common characteristics that are different, but not necessarily inferior, to the rest of us... This is different from espousing a model of 'normal' behaviour for everyone and requiring people with autism to fit into that mould, whether that is comfortable for them or not.[20]

A major emphasis of the TEACCH program is the use of *structured teaching.* They recommend minimising visual 'clutter' in the classroom, which can be distracting to children with autism, and organising the learning environment so that children can understand what they are meant to do in each different area. For example, in a preschool there might be separate areas designated for play, schoolwork and eating, with colourful visual cues to remind the children what happens where. The TEACCH approach also stresses the importance of providing predictable routines throughout the day to help reduce anxiety, a major barrier to learning. As children with autism tend to be visual learners, picture schedules and other visual cues are used extensively. By providing this structure and support children are able to function more independently and rely less on adult prompting. However, the longer term plan is a gradual reduction of these supports, so the child is eventually able to succeed in less structured surroundings.

TEACCH specialised school-based programs use a variety of teaching methods, from traditional special education to structured behavioural teaching: 'Structured teaching says nothing about where people with autism should be educated; this is a decision based on the skills and needs of each individual student. Some can work effectively and benefit from regular educational programs, while others will need special classrooms for part or all of the day...'[20]

According to their website[21] TEACCH early childhood programs emphasise 'individual instruction based on on-going assessment, close collaboration with families and the development of the child's motivation and skills' in a variety of curriculum areas including:

- building attention, organisation, generalisation and independence
- functional expressive and receptive communication skills
- play and social skills
- developmentally appropriate cognitive, motor and self-help skills.

For more information on TEACCH visit www.teacch.com

So is TEACCH effective?

To date there isn't much research looking at the longer-term outcomes of young children who have been through TEACCH programs. Research from the 1990s found that children who were non-verbal and had IQ scores in the 30–50 range at age three reported a quite substantial increase of just over 20 IQ points by age seven. Unfortunately there was no control group in these studies so it is not possible to say with certainty that all the gains reported in these children resulted from the TEACCH program.[8]

However, the Division TEACCH academics are extremely well-respected and have published widely on the nature of autism, structured teaching, language and communication and many other aspects of their program. The TEACCH program also includes many of the characteristics that experts agree are important in an early intervention program, such as an autism-specific curriculum, a structured environment, systematic teaching and individualised attention. As a result TEACCH is one of the most widely used approaches for ASD worldwide.

Division TEACCH does not operate any centres in Australia. What you will find, however, is that many local programs will adopt its structured teaching methods as part of wider or eclectic programs and you may come across these in your search for an early intervention program for your child.

For example, the Queensland-based AEIOU Centres use visual supports to promote independence, but as a component of an intensive centre-based program that primarily emphasises play skills and social skills development.

Our son Riley was diagnosed with autism eight days before Christmas in 2003 at the age of two and a half...

During Riley's first year at AEIOU the progress that he made was amazing, it exceeded our expectations. The intense early intervention program with 25 hours a week of speech therapy, occupational therapy as well as the early education teachers and teacher's aides brought about incredible changes in Riley. He started talking, dressing himself, following directions, waiting, turn-taking and instead of playing by himself in his room he started seeking out his brothers to play with. We could even take him out to the shops and to restaurants. Sometimes the smallest things are taken for granted but when you have a child with autism these small things all add up to great things.

Riley now attends his mainstream Prep class and enjoys every minute of it. We will be forever inspired by Riley who has taught us so many things and worked so hard through tears and tantrums to get where he is today — we are all very proud of him.

We will be forever indebted to all of the therapists, teachers and staff for giving Riley the chance to be the best that he can be... we only hope that many more children with autism can have the same chance.

LYNDA AND STEVE FOULIS, PARENTS OF RILEY

The SCERTS® Model

The SCERTS® model is a relatively new intervention, but one that is likely to be adopted more widely in Australia in forthcoming years. Like TEACCH, SCERTS is a teaching philosophy rather than a method, and draws on developmental and contemporary ABA methods as required, based on an assessment of an individual child's strengths and needs.

Developed in the US by autism experts Barry Prizant, Amy Wetherby, Emily Rubin, Amy Laurent and Patrick Rydell, SCERTS is a comprehensive education program with three interdependent treatment goals: [22]

1. *Social Communication*: Developing spontaneous, functional communication and secure, trusting relationships with children and adults.

Using *social-pragmatic* language methods (which encourage spontaneity in communication and teaching in natural settings) the SCERTS® model targets two core challenges in social communication:

Joint attention, (see page 11), which is a predictor of language development and to a varying degree is impaired in all children with autism.

Symbol use, or learning to use and understand gestures (such as pointing or nodding) and words appropriately. It also involves *symbolic* or imaginative play. SCERTS encourages the use of signing or picture communication systems (see page 77) to support verbal communication.

2. *Emotional Regulation*: Enhancing the ability to maintain a well-regulated emotional state for learning and interacting.

Children with autism tend to find it harder to regulate their internal emotional state and ignore distracting sights and sounds in the environment. If they are not in a well-regulated state they find it hard to learn. SCERTS therefore aims to give children the skills to self-regulate and/or request someone else to help them. A good example of this was at a mainstream primary school, where a young girl with ASD who suffered from anxiety was allowed to use a visual anxiety barometer to tell the teacher when she needed to retreat from the classroom and jump on a mini-tramp to calm herself down.

3. *Transactional Support*: Supporting children, their families, and professionals to maximise positive social experiences across home, school and community settings.

To support generalisation of learning, SCERTS emphasises the importance of providing *transactional support*. This could include *interpersonal support* (training parents, teachers and carers in the best way to communicate with the child), *educational support* such as visual aids and activity schedules, and support for the family so they are better educated and able to cope with the challenges of raising a child with ASD.

There are no certified SCERTS practitioners as such, but the SCERTS training manuals are available for purchase. These include a detailed description of the model as well as a curriculum-based assessment, data collection and program planning forms. The manuals have primarily been designed for children in the preschool and early primary school years but its authors claim the model can be adapted to suit older children as well as accommodating the needs of children with a wide range of abilities , whether 'high' or 'low functioning', verbal or non-verbal.

The SCERTS® model is new — the authors even claim it be a 'next generation' intervention model — and as yet there is no outcome research evaluating the entire model. However, the authors claim that the model draws from a variety of evidence-based treatment methods and also includes all the characteristics of effective intervention programs, as outlined in first part of this chapter.

The SCERTS® manuals and other information on the program are available at www.scerts.com

So that's it in a nutshell for education interventions (or at least some of the better-known ones). Of course your child may require supplementary interventions such as speech and occupational therapy but these will be discussed later.

Some of you may prefer the skills and language focus of ABA whereas others will lean towards the relationship-based developmental interventions. Some of you may like the idea of a home-based program whereas for others still a preschool program might be the ideal. Sometimes other realities will intrude, such as cost or availability (especially if you live in a rural and regional area). To help you in your search we have provided the following table, which includes a list of questions you might wish to ask intervention providers.

Some questions you might wish to ask early intervention providers.

- What kinds of intervention, therapy, and services do you provide?
- Do you have a particular philosophy on working with children with autism spectrum disorder?
- How many hours per week do these services require, and how much of this is one-on-one time with the child?
- Please describe a typical day or session.
- What experience do the teachers and/or therapists have in working with children with autism?
- What experience does the person who supervises the program have? How closely does the program supervisor work with the therapists, teachers, and parents?
- What kinds of ongoing training do your full- and part-time staff participate in?
- Are parents involved with planning as part of the intervention team?
- Do you provide a parent training program?
- How much and what kinds of involvement are expected of parents and family members?
- Are parents welcome to participate in or observe therapy and/or group sessions?
- What techniques do you use to manage difficult behaviours?
- Please describe your program for communication and language development. Do you use a picture communication system, sign language, other kinds of communication systems, or all of these?

- Are there opportunities for integration with typical and/or higher functioning children?
- How do you evaluate the child's progress, and how often?
- How do you keep parents informed of the child's progress?

Reprinted from the Clinical Practice Guideline Report of the Recommendations, Autism/ Pervasive Developmental Disorders, Assessment and Intervention for Young Children (Ages 0–3 Years), 1999, with permission of the New York State Department of Health.

Finally there is the vexed issue of cost. At the time of writing, public funding for early intervention in autism, and support for people with disabilities in general, remains inadequate. We have tried to include all the avenues you can call on for federal and state government support in the back of this book, but if you don't have much money to spare you may still find yourself on long waiting lists for publicly-funded intervention services.

Fortunately, thanks to the energetic efforts of parents and professionals in the autism community, awareness is rising and governments are finally taking more notice. In July 2008 we welcomed the federal government's *Helping Children with Autism* (HWCA) package to support ASD diagnostic and intervention services but at this stage it's too early to say how much impact this package will have at grassroots level.

A 2007 study, which found that the estimated annual cost of ASD to the community was between $4.5 and $7 billion stated:

Whilst this is beyond the scope of the current study, it is evident that there is an ongoing need for community and policy dialogue, in areas such as… investment in strategies that could potentially alter the outcomes for at least some children with ASD, such as early intervention. In particular, if this improves educational and employment outcomes for even a small number of people, the benefits (via reductions in costs and improvements in quality of life outcomes) will be sizeable.[23]

And so the fight for more funding and services will continue. We hope that the continued activism of parents will lead governments to recognise that providing early intervention for children with ASD is not only morally necessary, but makes good economic sense, too.

1. American Academy of Pediatrics Committee on Children with Disabilities. (2001). The Pediatrician's Role in the Diagnosis and Management of Autistic Spectrum Disorder in Children. *Pediatrics*, 107, 5, 1221–1226.
2. New York State Department of Health. (1999). 'Intervention Methods for Young Children with Autism' in *Clinical Practice Guideline Report of the Recommendations, Autism/Pervasive Developmental Disorders, Assessment and Intervention for Young Children (Ages 0–3 Years)*. www.health.state.ny.us/community/infants_children/early_intervention/autism/ch4_pt1.htm
3. New Zealand Ministries of Health and Education. (2006). Draft Evidence-based Guideline for Autism Spectrum Disorder. Wellington: Ministry of Health www.moh.govt.nz/moh.nsf/pagesmh/5597/$File/draft-asd-guideline-jan07.pdf
4. Perry, A. & Condillac, R. (2003). *Evidence-Based Practices for Children and Adolescents with Autism Spectrum Disorders: Review of the Literature and Practice Guide*. Children's Mental Health Ontario. Toronto, Ontario, Canada.
5. National Initiative for Autism: Screening and Assessment. (2003). *National Autism Plan for Children (NAPC)*. The National Autistic Society, London.
6. Roberts, JMA & Prior, M. (2006). *A Review of the Research to Identify the Most Effective Models of Practice in Early Intervention for Children with Autism Spectrum Disorders*. Australian Government Department of Health and Ageing, Australia.
7. National Research Council. (2001). *Educating Children with Autism*. National Academy Press, Washington.
8. MADSEC. (2000). *Report of the MADSEC Autism Task Force*: Maine Administrators of Services for Children with Disabilities.
9. Prior, M and Roberts, J. (2006). *Early Intervention for Children with Autism Spectrum Disorders*. Australian Government Department of Health and Ageing, Australia www.health.gov.au/internet/wcms/publishing.nsf/content/D9F44B55D7698467CA257280007A98BD/$File/autbro.pdf
10. Lovaas, OI. (1987). Behavioral treatment and normal educational and intellectual functioning in young autistic children. *Journal of Consulting and Clinical Psychology*, 55, 1, 3–9.
11. Sallows, GO and Graupner, TD. (2005). Intensive behavioral treatment for children with autism: four-year outcome and predictors. *American Journal on Mental Retardation*, 110, 6, 417–438
12. Vastag, B. (2004). Autism interventions come of age. *JAMA*, 291, 23, 2807–2808.
13. Siff Exkorn, K. (2005). *The Autism Sourcebook*, Regan Books (Harper Collins), New York.
14. Koegel, LK and Le Zebnik, C. (2004). *Overcoming Autism*, Viking (Penguin Group), New York.
15. Weider, S, Greenspan, S. (2005). Can children with autism master the core deficits and become empathetic, creative and reflective? A ten to fifteen year follow-up of a subgroup of children with Autism Spectrum Disorders (ASD) who received a comprehensive Developmental, individual-Difference, Relationship-Based (DIR) approach. *The Journal of Developmental and Learning Disorders*, 9, 39–61.
16. Caseinhiser, DM, Stieben, J, Shanker, SG. Assessing behavioral and neurophysiological outcomes of intensive DIR® Intervention for children with autism. [poster] www.icdl.com/staging/dirFloortime/research/index.shtml
17. The Connections Center. What is the RDI® Program? www.rdiconnect.com/default.asp
18. Gutstein, SE. (2005). Relationship Development Intervention. Developing a treatment program to address the unique social and emotional deficits in autism spectrum disorders. *Autism Spectrum Quarterly*. Winter issue.
19. Gutstein, SE, Burges, A, Montfort, K. (2007). Evaluation of the Relationship Development Intervention Program *Autism*, 11, 5, 397–411
20. Mesibov, G. What is TEACCH? www.teacch.com/whatis.html
21. Division TEACCH Early Childhood Services Program. www.teacch.com/intervention.html

22. Prizant, BM, Wetherby, AM, Rubin, E, Laurent, AC. (2003). The SCERTS Model. A transactional, family-centered approach to enhancing communication and socioemotional abilities of children with autism spectrum disorder. *Infants and Young Children*, 16, 4, 296–316.
23. Synergies Economic Consulting for the Autism Early Intervention Outcomes Unit (AEIOU). (2007). Economic Costs of Autism Spectrum Disorder — Executive Summary. www.aeiou.org. au/files/Exec%20summary_FINAL_May07.pdf

Additional references:
24. Howard, JS, Sparkman, CR, Cohen, HG, et al. (2005). A comparison of intensive behavior analytic and eclectic treatments for young children with autism. *Research in Developmental Disabilities*, 26, 4, 359–383.
25. Eikeseth, S. (2005). Intensive Behavioural Intervention for children with autism. A reply to Prior. *Journal of Paediatrics and Child Health*, 41, 7, 391–392.
26. Magiata, I, Charman, T, Howlin, P. (2007). A two-year prospective follow-up study of community-based early intensive behavioural intervention and specialist nursery provision for children with autism spectrum disorders. *Journal of Child Psychology and Psychiatry*, 48, 8, 803–812.
27. The Floortime Foundation. Our approach. www.floortime.org/ft.php?page=Our%20Approach
28. The SCERTS® Model. www.scerts.com

5

All of my four beautiful children are a gift to us, but Cooper has changed me. He has taught me so much more than I ever could have expected or will ever be able to teach him. He has opened my eyes to true human spirit, whether it be genuine and kind or selfish and cruel. He has taught me to fight, to stand up for what I believe in and to have an opinion. I have so much grief for what he will never experience, but I have so much joy from his words, his love. I will fight for him, and all other children with autism, and together we can give these children the opportunity to live to their true potential and inspire us all.

Holly Priddis, mother of Cooper

OTHER HELPFUL INTERVENTIONS FOR YOUR ASD CHILD

If you are fortunate enough to get your child enrolled in a good quality early intervention program this should go along way towards addressing the big hurdles that stand in the way of their development. But some children require a bit more help.

I always understood the need for speech therapy — after all it was pretty obvious Joe needed to talk more — but at the start I was less clear on the benefits of other interventions, in particular occupational therapy. I have subsequently discovered just how important some of these apparently peripheral therapies can be to a child's progress.

In this chapter we will therefore review other helpful interventions in ASD, focussing on three major problem areas: communication, motor skills and senses, and social skills. For most of these interventions you will need the expert guidance of a professional but others, with the right skills and training, you will be able to implement by yourself at home.

We do not claim to discuss every therapy promoted for ASD, just the more established ones. Down the track you may discover that your child really benefits from art or music or horse riding or whatever but at this early stage it is important to get the basics right.

Interventions for communication

SPEECH AND LANGUAGE THERAPY

A common theme amongst parents is an overwhelming desire to get their child to talk. Of course, teaching a child to speak doesn't mean their problems are over — just ask any parent of a child with Asperger's syndrome — but being able to communicate is a basic human need. We can trace many of the behavioural problems of people with ASD back to communication difficulties.

The good news is that, with intervention, the majority of children with ASD do learn to talk. However, communication is much more than just speech. Communication is a complex process involving the following elements, all of which can be impaired:

Receptive communication — receiving and understanding the messages from others.

> Children with ASD may have problems attaching meanings to words and not understand facial expressions, body-language and other forms of non-verbal communication. They may also have problems concentrating and get distracted by other elements in their environment (noise, movement, people), which can make it very difficult to get and keep their attention.

Expressive communication — sending information or messages to other people.

> People with ASD may have difficulties getting another person's attention (for example, pointing); knowing the correct word or symbol for what they want; using language, pictures or other non-verbal communication strategies to get what they want and/or being able to understand the social and *pragmatic* rules of communication. Some may actually have verbal *dyspraxia*, making it physically difficult for them to articulate sounds and speech.

Pragmatic language skills involve the social conventions of language.

Children with ASD may have problems adjusting their voice volume to the situation, interpreting body language, asking and answering questions, commenting, making jokes and understanding the rules of language. They often do not understand the rules of conversation such as turn-taking, staying on topic, rephrasing something when it's misunderstood and giving background information to an unfamiliar listener. Their conversations tend to be repetitive and one-sided — talking 'at' people, instead of with them. In essence they are likely to have little interest in or ability to use communication to establish and maintain contact with others.

Speech and language therapy should therefore ideally address all these problems, not just focus on getting your child to speak. Speech and language therapy is provided by a speech pathologist (formerly known as a speech therapist). Speech pathologists complete a degree at university which covers all aspects of communication including speech, writing, reading, signs, symbols and gestures.[1]

The first thing a speech pathologist should do is assess your child's existing language and communication skills, using a variety of formal (standardised) and informal assessments. Once they've established exactly what your child's communication skills are they can set about developing an individualised intervention program. For children who already have some language the focus of this intervention program may be on improving comprehension, increasing the complexity of speech, or correcting problems with articulation or *intonation* (children with ASD may have a flat, monotone or high pitched voice). Usually the focus is on teaching through play, making the sessions enjoyable for teacher, pupil and anxious parent!

For children for whom language is a bigger hurdle, behavioural methods can be used to encourage communication. Behavioural techniques are most effective if they are taught in natural settings, using natural routines and natural consequences. An example of this might be restricting your child's access to the fridge, so that they have to use words, sounds or picture symbols to request food or drinks.

It's important to realise that one hour a week of speech therapy is not going to solve your child's communication problems, but a speech pathologist can help ensure that you, and all those living and working with your child, use effective and consistent strategies to encourage speech and improve understanding. It's this day-to-day consistency of approach that will make the most difference in the long term.

Some speech pathologists are employed by state government health and disability services (refer to the rear section of this book for more information). You may be eligible to receive some government-funded speech therapy for free. Unfortunately there can be waiting lists for these free services and because of the demand you may be only allocated a short time block of services. Other speech pathologists may be employed by early intervention programs or in schools to provide general support to all children with communication difficulties.

Many more speech pathologists work in private practice, which means you probably will have to pay to see them, although you may be able to claim at least some of the expense back if you have private health insurance 'extras' cover and families can claim a rebate for up to five speech pathology services per year through the Medicare Enhanced Primary Care plan (see page 222). From July 2008, some parents may also be able to access ASD-specific speech pathology services through the federally-funded *Helping Children with Autism* initiative (see page 219).

It's essential you look for a speech pathologist with interest and experience in ASD. While there are lots of paediatric speech pathologists out there, many of them have experience mainly with children who just have language disorders or articulation problems; it is whole different kettle of fish working with a child with ASD, largely because of their problems with attention and concentration. Hopefully your child will learn to pay attention through their early intervention program and speech lessons will take off, but in the interim an ASD-trained speech pathologist will be able to help you with visual supports or other forms of augmentative communication (discussed below).

Even if you do locate a number of ASD-trained speech therapists in your area you might still need to shop around to find one you like. Some will be very busy and not have any vacancies in their schedule and others still may not 'click' with you or your child. However, we don't mean to imply that speech pathologists are a particularly troublesome bunch! This piece of advice could refer to any therapist or professional working with your child.

The Speech Pathology Australia website includes private speech pathologist directories for some of the larger Australian states. Click on the Public Information link at: www.speechpathologyaustralia.org.au

AUGMENTATIVE COMMUNICATION

Augmentative communication might sound a bit intimidating but it merely means the use of sign language, photographs, picture communication symbols or mechanical devices (such as speech generating devices) to replace or *augment* speech.

Augmentative communication interventions can support both expressive and receptive communication. The most commonly used are those with visual symbols — photos, pictures and written words.

Visual symbols such as flash cards, timetables and choice-making boards are used to aid receptive communication even in children who are able to talk. With time you will learn how to make these visuals yourself, but in the beginning your speech pathologist (or early intervention provider) should be able to advise you. Some people prefer to purchase commercially produced visual aids (see back of the book for some stockists) or software such as Boardmaker® (for a free trial see www.mayer-johnson.com) but you can also use digital photos that you take yourself.

Joe had a visual choice board at preschool, with symbolic representations of painting, puzzles, dress-ups and so on to help him choose activities. Even now he has a not-100%-successful visual reminder to wash his hands after using the toilet (though I think the cavalier attitude to personal hygiene is as much a 'boy thing' as an 'ASD thing')!

For pre-verbal children visual supports are even more important. Picture symbols can be used as a substitute for speech, allowing these children to request and communicate in a functional way.

Probably the best known visual augmentative communication system is the *Picture Exchange System* or *PECS*. PECS was developed in 1985 by Dr Andrew Bondy and Lori Frost. PECS begins with teaching a student to exchange a picture of a desired item with a teacher, who immediately provides that item as *reinforcement* or reward. As they progress through the program, children can be taught to construct simple 'sentences', comment and answer questions. The *Picture Exchange Communication System Training Manual (2nd ed)* provides information on how to implement PECS effectively. PECS is considered a useful and effective approach for children with ASD and can complement many educational programs.

For more information about PECS, including Australian training workshops visit www.pecsaustralia.com

There are other types of augmentative communication systems. The first of these is *manual (hand) signing*, which appears to be particularly popular in Britain. Supporters of manual signing argue that it makes communication 'visual' for children with autism and this may augment and promote the development of speech.[2]

Probably the best known of the manual signing systems is *Makaton*®. Makaton® is a vocabulary of key word signs and natural gestures, which was first introduced into Australia in the 1980s. It borrows some features from Auslan, the sign language of the deaf community in Australia, but is specifically designed for children and adults who can hear but have difficulty speaking. Makaton® uses speech together with a sign (gesture) and/or a symbol (picture). Symbols are used when a child has problems with hand movements (some children with ASD have fine motor challenges), making signing difficult, and to develop reading and language skills.

It is very important that speech is used together with signs and symbols. Research indicates that manual signing can speed up a child's acquisition of receptive and expressive language, although it appears that some children will do better with signing than others.[3] Your speech pathologist can advise you if signing is suitable for your child.

Makaton® Australia is based at the University of Newcastle. For more information, including details about Australian workshops go to: www.newcastle.edu.au/centre/sed/makaton/

Speech generating devices (also known as *voice output communication aids*) are being used increasingly. The simplest of these devices stores a single pre-recorded message, which is produced in the form of digitised speech when the child presses a button marked with a picture or symbol. The more elaborate speech generating devices have software that allows users to create and combine words and produce sentences in the form of computerised synthetic speech.

Many children with autism are motivated to communicate by speech generating devices and research has shown that these devices can support comprehension and request-making and increase interaction with adults and peers.[2]

Of course these devices are not suitable or indeed necessary for many children with ASD and you would only consider using one if recommended to by a speech pathologist.

Many parents are understandably upset when a speech pathologist suggests using augmentative communication to support expressive communication in their child. They feel that they are 'giving up' on the goal of speech. However, this is not the case. Research shows that, rather than delaying the acquisition of speech, augmentative communication such as PECS or Makaton® may actually stimulate speech development. At very least, if your child is one of the few who does not develop functional speech, they will have an effective means of communicating with you.

THE HANEN PROGRAM® *MORE THAN WORDS*™

The Hanen Centre is a charitable organisation based in Toronto, Canada, committed to helping children communicate effectively by supporting their parents, teachers and caregivers. *More Than Words*™ is a family-centred program specifically designed for parents of preschool age children with ASD. It was adapted from Hanen's *It Takes Two to Talk*™ program for families of young children with expressive and/or receptive language disorders and shares many features in common with this program.

More Than Words is based on the *social-pragmatic* theory of language development, which argues that communication develops in the context of interactions between the child and the important adults in their life.

The goal of *More Than Words* is to 'empower parents to become the primary facilitators of their child's communication and language development'.[4] Parents are therefore encouraged to use their child's everyday activities as learning opportunities.

Through *More Than Words* training, parents learn to be more responsive to their child's attempts at communication and to structure the environment to increase the motivation to communicate and interact. However, *More Than Words* does not stick strictly to a 'follow the child's lead' approach, as favoured by Floortime™ (see page 53) — parents are sometimes encouraged to take the lead with a child who is difficult to engage. They learn to prompt their child to interact using a variety of explicit (verbal) or natural (for example, an expectant look) cues, depending their child's level of competence. Parents are also instructed in a language-modelling strategy called the Four S's — 'Say less and Stress, go Slow and Show' (use visual supports).[4]

Parents meet for 8–10 group classes and also receive three individualised in-home videotaping and coaching sessions, all overseen by a Hanen certified speech pathologist. Program materials include an illustrated guidebook of the course content. Parent education and social support are important features of the program. The speech pathologist takes on the formal role as educator and counsellor, but the group sessions allow parents opportunities to share experiences with people in similar situations.

There is limited research to date on the *More Than Words* program. British researchers found that children of parents who had been through the program had a larger vocabulary at seven months follow-up than a group of children whose parents had delayed their participation in the program. Whilst researchers were unable to detect a difference between the two children's groups in social communication skills, the parents in the active treatment group scored higher in the delightfully named *Joy and Fun Assessment*, which looked at their use of fun words ('wheee!'), pretend games, simplified language and imitations.[4]

The *More Than Words* program is not intended to replace other intensive interventions for children with ASD but is designed to give parents skills to support other treatments that their child may receive throughout their life.

The Hanen Program® is offered by a number of providers throughout Australia. Even if there are no Hanen courses in your area you can still purchase their *More Than Words Parent Guidebook*, an excellent resource to help foster communication between you and your child. Program development is also underway in Canada for a new Hanen Program called *TalkAbility*™ — The Hanen Program for Parents of Verbal Children on the Autism Spectrum. *TalkAbility* is designed for families with children aged three to seven who can talk, but find conversation-making and friendships more challenging.

More information on the Hanen® Program and resources can be obtained at: www.hanen.org

Our youngest son Dallin was diagnosed with ASD when he was three years old... He had no speech, no communication skills and very little receptive language... When we were offered a chance to participate in the 'More Than Words™' course, we jumped at the chance to better communicate with our little boy.

The course helped us realise that there was more to communicating than just words. We were able to identify the stage of communication Dallin was at, and how his preferences and

actions determine how he senses the world. It taught us to also use methods such as visuals, signing and cues. It taught us different strategies that involved observing, waiting, listening, repetition and providing fun opportunities for him to communicate.

It has been over three years since we did the 'More Than Words' course and Dallin's communication skills have increased immensely. Yet we still use the same principles and strategies we learnt from the course to help in his developing language. The beauty about 'More Than Words' was that it enabled us to help open up Dallin's world of communication, as well as our understanding of that world.

'More Than Words' is a detailed, intelligent and practical course that gave us hope and encouragement, so that every little milestone in Dallin's communication — from pointing to a picture of a drink, to his first attempt to sign the word 'more' and eventually, to his utterance of a 2-word phrase — was seen as a great achievement and brought waves of happiness to our family.
LILIETA LINDBERG, MOTHER OF DALLIN

I signed my son Connor (ASD, then aged 33 months), and myself, up for the 'It Takes Two to Talk' Hanen program being run by Lifestart (in Sydney). He had severe expressive and receptive language disorder and had only six words (none of which was 'Mum').

The Hanen program was life changing for all the family... My son had no desire to talk, and he found it very confronting when people spoke to him; he hated it all. After this stark discovery, the Hanen program helped us to motivate him to interact with us and eventually to talk. Basically we made it worth his while — to reward him saying 'I WANT' as in 'I want ice cream' we gave him ice-cream at 7am in the morning.

The first time he said 'train' and pointed to one we screamed, stopped the car and got on the train for one stop. He rewarded us by saying 'car' and 'bird' looking out the window of the train, accompanied by the all-important pointing.

Hanen helped us to develop the pre-language skills first, to build strong foundations, to take a few steps back, then move forward steadily in tiny increments, instead of constantly trying to make the giant leap to speech. It took us down to his level, to look at the world through his eyes, and try to make it more interesting, more exciting...We learned how to connect and communicate with our child and to make each other laugh.

Hanen gave us homework every week for six weeks, and came to the house three times and filmed us at play... At the group sessions, we looked at all our tapes and learned from each other and each other's children. ..The last week the topic was reading books, and we learned simple tricks to involve our children, such as getting them to turn the pages, which helped give them some control over what was happening. I still use this to this day, helping with reading groups at my son's mainstream school.

CAROLE JAPP, MOTHER OF CONNOR

Interventions for motor skills and senses

OCCUPATIONAL THERAPY

Occupational therapists (OTs) work with children with autism and their families to improve the child's ability to participate in activities of daily living, play and school.

Although motor skills are generally less affected than language and social skills in children with Autistic Disorder/PDD-NOS, some children can have significant problems in this area.

- *Gross motor skills* are the abilities required to control the large muscles of the body for walking, running, sitting and other activities.
- *Fine motor skills* generally refer to the small movements of the hands, wrists, fingers, feet, toes, lips, and tongue.

Both these may be delayed in ASD, affecting things like ball skills, balance, imitation, handwriting, cutting with scissors and sense of rhythm. Some children may have low muscle tone, oral motor problems (affecting speech) and motor planning (the ability to plan and execute a series of movements) problems, also called *dyspraxia*.

For children with Asperger's syndrome (often known for their clumsiness) motor skills often lag behind cognitive and language abilities.

If your child does turn out to have gross and/or fine motor delay an occupational therapist could work with them to improve their:

> *Everyday living skills* — using cutlery, putting on shoes and socks and drinking from a cup.
>
> *Hand skills* — picking up small things, writing and drawing, using scissors and pasting.
>
> *Play skills* — using toys, catching a ball or participating in sports.

However, modern OTs have expanded their repertoire and may now work to improve attention and concentration, social skills and more. During a typical session an OT may use equipment such as exercise balls, climbing gyms and obstacle courses to help a child build muscle strength and co-ordination, as well as address fine motor skills such as writing and drawing. OTs will also consult with schools and other intervention providers and can advise on modifications, such as a specially-designed computer mouse for a child with fine motor difficulties. Many OTs have become experts in managing sensory processing issues (see below) and a few have also branched out into offering Floortime™ therapy (see page 53). OTs teach as much as possible through play so sessions should be enjoyable for your child.

If you decide to consult an OT, it's important to look for one with experience in ASD; someone who understands sensory issues and how communication difficulties can impact on behaviour. The initial assessment should focus on motor and self-help skills and *sensory profile*. This information will be used to develop an individualised program for your child.

There are OTs employed by government services and you may be eligible for some free consultations; however, demand for free services is usually fierce. Private OTs charge for their services but you may be able to recoup some of the cost through the Medicare's *Enhanced Primary Care* plan or private health insurance. Refer also to the federal government *Helping Children with Autism* funding initiatives (page 219) for information on Medicare rebated ASD-specific OT services for eligible children aged fifteen years and under.

A *limited* range of mental health-related OT services may be accessed through the Medicare's *Better Access to Mental Health Care* program. More information on this program can be found on the OT Australia website. This website also provides a link to state by state directories of private occupational therapists working throughout Australia. www.ausot.com.au/

Joe has low muscle tone and motor planning difficulties. For a time we thought this wasn't such a big deal compared with all his other issues, until someone wise pointed out that these deficits might actually be impacting on his ability to play. It's pretty hard to build sand castles or play with trains if you are struggling just to sit upright and move your limbs in the direction they are meant to go.

At age four he was diagnosed with moderate gross motor delay, which means he was about two years behind in his gross motor milestones. Through the efforts of a wonderful paediatric physiotherapist we stumbled across he has caught up much of this delay. Paediatric physiotherapists are less common in Australia than OTs and are rarely consulted by parents of children with ASD. However, in the US they often work with ASD kids. Our son's physio has worked with him on exercise balls, balance beams, scooter boards etc to increase his core stability, balance and co-ordination. We are now working on skipping, bike riding and soccer skills and he is now only about six months behind in his milestones. Swimming lessons are also on the agenda. (Some of the larger swimming pools offer Special Needs swimming classes, so if you feel your child will need specialised tuition keep an eye out for these).

We also consulted an excellent OT about Joe's fine motor skills, as he refused to draw or colour in for a long time and I really thought he would never learn to write. To our amazement, through the efforts of his OT and school teachers he is now forming most of his letters correctly and writing and drawing messily, but very enthusiastically. He may still need a keyboard to write assignments in the future but he can at least write enough now to get by.

MANAGING SENSORY PROCESSING ISSUES

Many children with ASD display unusual responses to sensory stimuli or 'sensory issues', although like all symptoms associated with ASD the severity will vary from one child to the next and can even change in an individual child over time. Joe used not to notice any bumps or bruises at age three but now he certainly does and cries and whinges accordingly.

Sensory processing has been defined as 'the way our brain takes in and organises sensory information from our body and the environment'.[5]

Sensory processing difficulties in ASD can manifest as either an under- or over-responsiveness to sensory stimuli and can affect any of the common senses as well as balance and movement (the *vestibular* system) and/or information from muscles and joints (referred to as *proprioception*). Some examples are listed in Table 1. At first glance some of these examples may appear contradictory but what they are illustrating is that sensory processing difficulties will vary from one child to the next. These patterns can even be uneven within an individual child: a child may be over-sensitive to some sounds but under-sensitive to touch.

Table 1. Examples of unusual sensory processing in children with ASD

SENSORY SYSTEM	BEHAVIOURS YOU MIGHT SEE IN YOUR CHILD
Visual (sight)	May shade eyes or squint in strong sunlight or under fluorescent lights.
	May look at items from unusual angles (eg out of the corner of their eyes). *looks up when touching*
	May enjoying flickering objects such as fingers, computer screens.
	May show minute attention to visual details in books etc
Auditory (hearing)	May become upset at loud noises eg vacuum cleaners, lawn mowers.
	May be distracted by sounds other people don't hear (eg computers, fans) or hum to screen out unwanted noise.
	May appear to be selectively deaf.
Tactile (touch)	May avoid other people's touch, especially light touch, and be irritated by certain clothes or foods.
	May refuse to have hair brushed or cut.
	May avoid messy play.
	May not react to pain, heat or cold.
Vestibular (movement of body in space)	May get car sick.
	May avoid climbing equipment and sports and be uncomfortable on stairs. *Hard to climb stairs*
	May enjoy spinning and show no signs of dizziness.
	May be constantly on the move.
Proprioceptive (where a certain body part is and how it is moving)	May hold items either too loosely or too tightly.
	May enjoy firm touch or massage.
	May like rough-and-tumble play.
	May have difficulty dressing.
Olfactory (smell and taste)	May dislike strong smells or tastes
	May eat a very restricted diet or only bland foods.
	May crave strong smells or tastes.
	May eat non-food items

Sensory processing issues can have a big impact on behaviour, learning and even social relating. It's easy to imagine how an over-responsive child might have trouble concentrating if distracted by the sound of chairs scraping and lights humming and the glare of fluorescent lights. There are also children whose need to seek sensory input means that they are on the move *all* the time; it's hard to keep them still long enough for them to learn anything. In contrast a child who is under-responsive to sensory stimuli may come across as tired, lazy or distracted. The challenge is to find an optimal level of arousal (or alertness) for these kids so that they can pay attention and learn.

Sensory integration therapy aims to help a child respond appropriately to sensory information and targets the vestibular, tactile and proprioceptive senses. Generally delivered by OTs, this treatment may involve: swinging in a hammock, playing in a ball pit, balancing on beams, and brushing or stroking. Therapists select activities for each child based on his or her particular 'sensory profile.'

Despite its widespread use and acceptance, there is not much good quality research to show that sensory integration therapy can improve behaviour and learning in children with autism. This doesn't necessarily mean that sensory integration is ineffective — it's just that the research performed to date has not looked at this question in a systematic way.[2] Thus experts recommend that you don't use sensory integration therapy as your child's *primary* intervention, but it (and occupational therapy in general) may be important as part of a more comprehensive intervention program. If nothing else, sensory integration therapy sessions are likely to be enjoyable and relaxing for your child.

It is also important to make the distinction between sensory integration therapy and day-to-day management of sensory difficulties associated with ASD. A good OT will be able to advise you (and your child's teachers) on how to alleviate any sensory problems limiting your child in daily life. For example, if your child is upset by loud classroom noise at the end of a school day they could be allowed to get ready for home before everyone else.

Alternatively, if they are bothered by woollen clothing they could be permitted to wear a different fabric. To help with learning, an OT could also recommend some calming (such as wearing a weighted vest) or alerting activities ('movement' breaks) that could be built into your child's day. Often quite small environmental changes will help your child cope better at school or preschool, thereby reducing the chance of problem behaviours.

> If you feel sensory processing is a significant problem with your child we'd recommend you seek out an OT with experience in this area. Refer to the OT Australia website. Also, there are some good books in this area. *The Out-of Sync Child* by Carol Stock Kranowitz and Lucy Jane Miller is a favourite.

AUDITORY INTEGRATION TRAINING

Auditory Integration Training (AIT) was developed by Guy Berard as a technique for improving abnormal sound sensitivity in individuals with learning disorders including autism. These hypersensitivities are believed to interfere with a child's attention, comprehension, and ability to learn. Other similar sound therapies include the Tomatis Method and Samonas Sound Therapy.

AIT typically involves a child attending two 30-minute sessions per day for ten days. During a session, a child wears specialised earphones to listen to music with selected frequencies filtered out. Proponents claim that AIT and similar sound therapies can improve auditory processing and concentration of children with ASD.

Whilst many parents will testify to the benefits of AIT, this is another ASD therapy where the research is quite patchy. A recent Cochrane review (see page 109) of the evidence of effectiveness of AIT and other sound therapies for children with autism concluded:

No clear evidence yet for auditory integration therapy's effect on autism... Six relatively small studies met the inclusion criteria for AIT... These largely measured different outcomes and reported mixed results. Suggestion of benefit in two outcomes requires corroboration by further research using well-designed trials with long-term follow-up.[6]

There are AIT (sometimes called Berard Method) practitioners operating throughout various regions of Australia.

For Tomatis visit: www.tomatis.com.au/

For Samonas Sound Therapy: www.samonasaustralia.com/

Interventions for social skills

One of the defining characteristics of ASD is a 'qualitative impairment in social interaction'. Social difficulties affect all children on the spectrum, regardless of their IQ and overall level of functioning.

The popular image of someone with autism is Dustin Hoffman's 'Rainman' — a person locked in his own world and indifferent to approaches of others — but the reality is a bit more complex than that. Researchers have actually identified three distinct social groups amongst children with ASD:

- *Aloof* children will try to avoid other kids completely.
- Another *passive* group will rarely initiate social contact but will accept it happily enough when it's offered.
- A third group of children actually like being with people but because they appear *odd* (use odd language, obsess on obscure topics, and miss the social cues) they often have problems making and keeping friends.

These groups, whilst distinct, aren't necessarily fixed and many children tend to move from the aloof to the passive or odd group as they get older.

Children with ASD have problems in many areas which are the foundation of successful relationships: joint attention, sharing and co-operating, using and understanding body language, imitation and imaginative play. In addition they are often unable to understand and empathise with the feelings or perspectives of others; you will sometimes hear this referred to as a deficit in *theory of mind*. In a typical child an ability to 'read' the mind of others develops remarkably early — around the age of five. Theory of mind is not necessarily absent in people with ASD but their ability to 'mind read' tends to develop much later and perhaps be less sophisticated than that of their typical peers.

Because of all these problems it's not surprising that many of the interventions for ASD target problems in social relating: the developmental interventions Floortime™ and RDI® focus first and foremost on social relationships, but there are other interventions that may help.

SOCIAL SKILLS TRAINING

Social skills training is an umbrella term used to describe such techniques as one-to-one social skills therapy, social skills groups, peer modelling and video modelling (more on the last one later). Training may be facilitated by a psychologist, a behavioural therapist, a speech pathologist or special education teacher.

Social skills training is always going to be an inexact science, because social encounters never follow a pre-determined script. However, it is possible to teach your child many social conventions that will help them to fit in: how to greet another person, the need to stand in line at the supermarket, the importance of not touching other people's belongings etc.

Teaching social skills using *naturalistic* behavioural techniques such as pivotal response training (see page 51) has been shown to be effective. Indeed, evidence suggests that social skills training is most effective if it takes place in natural settings and within regular routines and activities. This might mean you need to teach your child a whole different set of social skills for the home, school, shops and peer-group.

In one-on-one training the child and therapist will work on a specific skill, for example, greeting a person or joining in a classroom routine. Generally the skill is taught, role-played, discussed, then feedback is given and the skill is practised again. For younger children, social skills training may also revolve around play skills, such as turn-taking and sharing or participating in simple interactive games like 'duck, duck, goose.'

For older children with good language social skills groups may be useful. Through discussions, games and activities these children can learn about body language, recognising emotions, conversation skills and theory of mind. Research has found that participants generally enjoy these group sessions and they may even boost self-esteem, but some programs have been less successful at producing long term social gains.[7] Once again, the key to success of these strategies is *generalisation*; your child is going to need to use their newly-acquired skills in real-life situations to produce any lasting change.

Peer-modelling is probably the best studied of the social skills techniques. This involves a trained adult facilitating a play session where a typical child acts as a role-model for the child with ASD, taking the lead in sharing, helping and conversation; for young children 'play-dates' may involve playing simple board games, building block towers and listening to stories together. In the most successful programs the peers undergo specific training in how to encourage play and social interactions. Peer-modelling has also been used in schools, at least overseas, to help the child with ASD learn school rules and routines.

> If you're interested keep an eye out for social skills programs (a few are listed at the back of this book), although many programs tend to be targeted at older children and teenagers. Your state autism association may also be able to refer you to local social skills training programs.

SOCIAL STORIES™
Developed by Carol Gray in the early 1990s, *Social Stories*™ are short narratives which help children learn how to respond appropriately to specific social situations. Written in the first person, a basic social story consists of *descriptive* sentences (which explain the 'who, what, when, where and why' of a situation), *perspective* sentences that explain how the situation affects other people, and *directive* sentences, which suggest a socially appropriate response. Stories are often accompanied by pictures and photographs. The beauty of Social Stories is that they can be written by almost anyone (once the technique is understood) and customised to the individual

needs of the child.

We have used Social Stories often with Joe. For example, we have written stories to explain toilet training and why he wasn't allowed to play outside at pre-school on rainy days. We've found them particularly useful to help him comprehend anxiety-producing situations, such as the time mummy and daddy had to go overseas without him for a week.

To date there is limited research on the effectiveness of Social Stories, but what there is has produced positive results, at least in school-aged children.[2] More research is needed to assess their effectiveness in preschool-age children, who may have less language comprehension.

For more information on Social Stories™ go to: www.thegraycenter.org

VIDEO MODELLING

I am a great fan of video modelling. My enthusiasm is two-fold: in my days as a showbiz showoff, I worked as a TV producer for the BBC and Channel 9, and from the age of one, Tom was a total TV addict.

Simply put, *video modelling* is the use of video to teach children specific skills.

International researchers have studied the efficacy of video modelling for children with ASD, with positive results. A study in 2000 found that video modelling was more effective than live modelling in teaching a variety of skills to children with autism. Importantly, video modelling promoted generalisation of these tasks across different persons, settings, and stimuli, whereas live modelling did not.[8]

The message seems to be that it is sometimes easier for children with ASD to learn from a video than from a live model (a teacher or a peer). This may be because the child finds it easier to focus on a small screen with no other sensory or social distractions.

Research has shown that video modelling is an efficient way to teach language, social skills, self-help skills and play skills. It is also used to help prepare children for new situations or activities.

Following are some examples of how parents and teachers can use video modelling:

- video a new preschool or school and show it to your child as part of the transition process
- video a sibling or friend having a haircut, or visiting the dentist; video the route to the doctor or therapist's office, so that your child understands where they are going
- video short play scripts using your child's own toys and a much-loved friend or family member playing
- video other children playing party games
- video simple language concepts at the appropriate level for your child (eg 'I **caught** the ball', or **in front** and **behind**).

The video models do not need to be of good quality, children don't seem to mind wobbly filming and messy close-ups. The idea is to film short segments (1–2 minutes) and then show them several times.

Video self-modelling involves videoing your child doing something, editing out the parts which were not successful, and then showing them the rest. It can be used to improve social skills, sports skills, play skills and even gross motor activities.

Many children with ASD are visual learners. If your child loves to watch TV and seems to pay better attention to the screen than to people, then it is worth attempting some video modelling. If your child is already copying things they see on television, then video modelling is definitely for you.

There are some pre-made video modelling DVDs available which have been made specifically for children with an ASD. Although the effectiveness of these has not been studied there are anecdotal reports of them working very well with some children

During Tom's years of early intervention we made lots of video models. These worked really well for him, and I met many other families who found that video models were a quick and efficient way of teaching skills to their children.

Recently, I made a video self model of Tom saying the nine times table (he was reading it from a piece of paper under the camera) and it helped him to learn. I also video Tom playing with other children and playing sport then show him all the good bits.

So dust off that video camera and zoom out to buy some new tapes. Also pester your early intervention professionals; if they don't already use video modelling, tell them they need to get started!

The 2006 book, *Video Modelling and Behaviour Analysis* by Christos Nikopolous and Mickey Keenan, is an academic examination of the use of video modelling. While it is not as parent-friendly as would be ideal we would recommend it for families as well as teachers and other professionals.

Unfortunately, video technology can have its downside, too. ASD kids often develop a passion for TV, computers, DVDs and electronic games. It's okay to allow children some 'screen-time' (parents often use it as a reward for desirable behaviour) but it's a good idea to put some sensible limits on this. The more time they spend in front of an electronic box, the less time they will have to develop any competency in the more challenging but ultimately more rewarding world of people.

Managing the social problems of autism is the hardest part of being an ASD parent, so please seek as much help as you can. If it's just after diagnosis, you might be tempted to cocoon yourself away from family and friends and their irritatingly 'normal' kids. But, remember, family and friends can also provide you and your child with valuable social contact. Find your most kind and tolerant friends and mix with them and their kids. You may find that their young children are very tolerant of your child's little eccentricities.

Hopefully you'll find some sympathetic professionals to guide you through the social minefield, but look out for books and publications which can provide you with tips on how to successfully negotiate holidays, trips to the shops and eating out at restaurants with your child (Karen Siff Exkorn's, *The Autism Sourcebook* is great for this, as is the British National Autistic Society website www.nas.org.uk). Having an ASD child does not necessarily mean the end of *your* social life, but it will take a bit more preparation and planning if it's to be successful.

1. Speech Pathology Australia. *Fact Sheet.* What is a speech pathologist? www.speechpathologyaustralia.org.au/library/Fact%20Sheet%201.1%20What%20is%20 a%20SP.pdf

2. Roberts, JMA & Prior, M. (2006). *A Review of the Research to Identify the Most Effective Models of Practice in Early Intervention for Children with Autism Spectrum Disorders.* Australian Government Department of Health and Ageing, Australia.

3. Howlin, P. (1998). Practitioner review: psychological and educational treatments for autism. *Journal of Child Psychology and Psychiatry* 39, 3, 307–322.

4. The Hanen Centre®. (2007). *Research Summary: More Than Words™*. The Hanen Program® for Parents of Children with Autism Spectrum Disorder. www.hanen.org/web/Portals/0/ HostedFiles/MTWResearchSummary2007.pdf

5. Mora, L. *Sensory processing in daily life. Presentation at Child and Adolescent High-Functioning Autism and Asperger's Syndrome Seminar for Parents and Carers*, The Children's Hospital Westmead, 10th September, 2007.

6. Sinha, Y, Silove, N, Wheeler, D, Williams, K. Auditory integration training and other sound therapies for autism spectrum disorders. *Cochrane Database of Systematic Reviews* 2004, Issue 1. Art. No.: CD003681. DOI: 10.1002/14651858.CD003681.pub2.

7. New Zealand Ministries of Health and Education. 2006. Draft Evidence-based Guideline for Autism Spectrum Disorder. Wellington: Ministry of Health. www.moh.govt.nz/moh.nsf/ pagesmh/5597/$File/draft-asd-guideline-jan07.pdf

8. Charlop-Christy, MH, Loc Le, and Freeman, KA. (2000). A comparison of video modeling with in vivo modeling for teaching children with autism. *Journal of Autism and Developmental Disorders*, 30, 6, 537–552.

Additional references:
9. Hart, C. (2006). The role of the speech pathologist and communication problems in the autism spectrum disorders, in *The Clinician (Volume 3) — Acceptance and the Autistic Disorders*, Child and Adolescent Mental Health Statewide Network (CAMHSNET), 206–209.

10. Perry, A and Condillac, R. (2003). *Evidence-Based Practices for Children and Adolescents with Autism Spectrum Disorders: Review of the Literature and Practice Guide.* Children's Mental Health Ontario. Toronto, Ontario, Canada.

11. Pyramid Educational Consultants. What is PECS? www.pecs.com/WhatsPECS.htm

12. Makaton Vocabulary Development Project. *About Makaton®* www.makaton.org/about/about.htm

13. Frith, U. (2003). *Autism: Explaining the enigma* 2nd edn, Blackwell Publishing, Malden MA, USA

14. Wong, M. (2006). Teaching social skills and anxiety management in children with autistic spectrum disorders in *The Clinician (Volume 3) — Acceptance and the Autistic Disorders*, Child and Adolescent Mental Health Statewide Network (CAMHSNET), 127–133.

15. Siff Exkorn, K. (2005). *The Autism Sourcebook*, Regan Books (Harper Collins), New York.

16. Law, M. (2006). Autism *Spectrum Disorders and Occupational Therapy — Briefing to the Senate Standing Committee on Social Affairs, Science and Technology*, Ottawa, Canada.

6

Work backwards — look for other people who have already achieved good results with a certain intervention, and ask them exactly how they did it.

Don't just try something new because it sounds hopeful, stick to definite successes. Surround yourself with supportive, positive, enthusiastic people. Don't waste energy on the mediocre or the harbingers of doom, you know the ones who say: 'Oh you poor things'.

Carole Japp, mother of Connor

THE
MEDICAL MAZE

Picture this scenario. You walk out of the paediatrician's rooms in a daze, after hearing that your child has an ASD. You go home, log onto the Internet and look up the 'official' websites, which all say something like this: 'Autism is a life-long disability. There is currently no known cure'. But then you start searching further and discover seemingly dozens of websites offering treatments which they claim can 'cure' or 'reverse' autism. What's going on? Are these claims to be believed? Who's right?

Unfortunately the official view is much closer to the truth. There is no 'miracle cure' for autism. The very fact that there are so many and varied therapies is testimony to that. As Joe's paediatrician succinctly put it, 'if there was a cure for autism, there would only be one cure'. This quote probably sums up the current situation best:

When you have many medical therapies, often contradictory, two possibilities exist. One is that the correct therapy for that disease has yet to be identified. The history of medicine is replete with incidents in which multiple, unsatisfactory therapies are offered until the single effective treatment for a single disease is discovered. The second possibility is that there is no such thing as one medical treatment because autism is not one disease after all, but a syndrome, a final common pathway of many, many different diseases, each of which may require its own medical therapy. In such cases accurate diagnosis must precede therapy.[1]

But let's not be too pessimistic. Researchers throughout the world are strenuously working to improve our understanding of autism and to search for more effective treatments for this perplexing condition. The future of a child diagnosed today is much more promising than that of a child diagnosed only 10–15 years ago. And while there may be no quick fix there is certainly a lot you can do to help your child right now.

Remember that ASD is a spectrum — a spectrum which ranges from people with a significant disability (low functioning autism) to very high functioning people who can cope pretty well in the world with little or no support. There are many examples of able people with ASD going on to lead successful adult lives and, whilst autism may remain a life-long condition, for these people at least, it is not much of a 'disability'.

Current interventions aim to reduce your child's symptoms and equip them with new abilities, *at very least* to reduce the level of their disability and at best to give them the opportunity to live a near normal life. This is not something that can be achieved overnight. It will probably be a long and difficult journey which may require a multi-pronged approach of early intervention, speech and/or occupational therapy, medication and, for some people dietary changes and complementary medicines.

With this sort of approach a very few lucky children will improve so much that their symptoms will all but disappear. These children are sometimes referred to as 'recovered.' Maybe your child will be one of the fortunate few, but the majority will not. Whatever the case, please don't lose sight of how much they do improve and learn, become 'more able than disabled', as you pursue the 'Holy Grail' of recovery.

The main way we can help our children is through early intervention. In this chapter we will talk about how medicines can be used to control some of the more disabling symptoms of ASD and related conditions, and then delve into the more controversial area of complementary and alternative medicines, the so-called biomedical approach. But first, *evidence-based treatments*, what are they and how you can use them to maximise the effectiveness of your child's intervention program?

What are evidence-based treatments?

Imagine another scenario. You speak to a well-respected paediatrician, an expert in their field. When you ask about a complementary therapy for ASD they say, 'There is no evidence to support its use.' You visit a biomedical practitioner anyway and they say there is 'lots of research' to support this therapy. Who's right this time? Well, it might interest you to know that, technically, they both could be. It's how you interpret the word *evidence*.

There is mind-boggling amount of research out there about ASD but not all of it is of equal value when it comes to evidence of treatment effectiveness. It's all about trying to establish cause and effect. The hierarchy of evidence runs from the weakest (the anecdote) to the strongest (the randomised, double-blind, placebo-controlled clinical trial). (Strictly speaking, systematic reviews of randomised controlled trials are now considered the top of the evidence hierarchy but will be discussed later in this chapter.)

The problem with ASDs is that the most emotionally powerful stories for parents often *are* the anecdotal. Anecdotes are great because they can personalise the stories of the various interventions. But they are not considered good evidence.

For example, say you read a story of a mother whose child starts talking after going on a gluten-free casein-free diet. You'd be tempted to rush off to the health food store there and then in the hope that the same thing happens with your own child. But just because B (child starts talking) follows A (starting of GFCF diet) doesn't definitely mean that A caused B. It might suggest that possibility, but it doesn't *prove* it, because we haven't controlled for all the variables. It could be that the child was just ready to talk (many children with ASD do learn to speak without intervention), or it could be a result of the child's other educational interventions and/or speech therapy finally bearing fruit. We really can't be sure.

So when a specialist says there is 'no evidence' what they are really saying is that there is no evidence of the quality that can really establish cause and effect. So let's look at the different components of a *randomised, double-blind, placebo-controlled, clinical trial* to see why these trials are the most powerful research tools we have.

A *clinical trial* is a research study conducted with patients which tests out a medicine or other intervention to assess its effectiveness and safety.[2]

This is an important distinction. A lot of the research published about ASD is actually not in the form of clinical trials but *descriptive* (or observational) research. Examples might include a parent survey looking at the frequency of gastrointestinal symptoms in children with ASD, or a study which measures the blood levels of the neurotransmitter serotonin in ASD children at a single point in time. This sort of research is absolutely vital but does not provide any evidence of cause and effect; it is a means of generating theories to be tested in future clinical and other research.

Unfortunately this sort of research is often reported uncritically by the media and afforded much more significance than it might actually merit (think about all the 'major cancer breakthroughs' you've heard about but yet we still haven't eliminated cancer). Each of these individual studies is a tiny piece in an enormous puzzle, a very small step towards improving our understanding of ASD, but by no means the 'answer'.

A *controlled clinical trial* is a study testing a specific medicine or other treatment involving two (or more) groups of patients with the same disease or condition. One (the experimental group) receives the active treatment (that which is being tested) and the other (the control group) receives an alternative treatment, *a placebo*, or no treatment.

Control groups are needed to determine whether the intervention actually caused the observed change and to rule out other possible explanations. For example, if a group receiving intervention X improves you might conclude that intervention X is effective. But if the control group (who did not receive intervention X) also improves to the same degree, something other than X was responsible. This was the problem highlighted with the TEACCH research, discussed earlier. There was no control group so we cannot say definitely that the IQ gains reported were as a result of the TEACCH program or just a consequence of natural progression.

Randomisation is a method similar to tossing a coin to assign patients to treatment groups; the 'active treatment' is given if the coin lands heads and the control is given if the coin lands tails (in reality this is usually done by a computer program). In randomised controlled trials each person has an equal chance of receiving the active treatment, which avoids any possibility of selection bias in a trial. *Selection bias* is where the people delivering the treatment might be (subconsciously) tempted to give the real treatment to the people they think most likely to benefit (or perhaps in the case of children with ASD, those whose parents look the most likely to carefully follow the treatment regimen).

Also, if the number of participants in the study is large enough, randomisation should ensure that the active and control groups are well matched for any other factors which could affect the outcome, such as age, IQ etc.

A *placebo* is a dummy or inactive treatment which is given to the control group and must be indistinguishable from the treatment being tested. Giving a placebo to the controls ensures that any changes we observe in the treatment group are not simply the result of their beliefs and expectations or the extra attention involved in taking part in the study, or other unexplained variables.

The best quality trials are *double-blind*, meaning both patients (or, in the case of children with ASD, their families) and researchers are unaware of which treatment group a patient has been assigned to until all the research results have been collected and analysed. (In a *single-blind* trial only one of these groups — usually the patients — is blinded to which intervention they are receiving). Blinding is important even if you have an objective *outcome measure* (such as a reduced cholesterol blood level with a cholesterol-lowering medicine) but in the case of ASD, where you are going to be looking at subjective outcomes, such as changes in behaviour, blinding is even more essential.

Why is blinding so important? Because when people participate in research their beliefs and expectations that the treatment will work can influence the results of the research quite significantly. This is commonly referred to as *the placebo-effect*. Even the researchers conducting the trial can fall victim to the placebo effect, although in their case the correct term for it is *observer bias*. This is not meant to imply that they set out to be deliberately biased when they report their results. It just makes sense that if you have a lot financially and emotionally invested in the research you are more likely to believe that you can see a treatment effect.

So, in a randomised, double-blind, placebo-controlled trial (RCT) the only difference between the two groups is the type of treatment they receive. If the outcome between the two groups turns out be significantly different it is reasonable to conclude that this difference is caused by the treatment — cause and effect.

Non-blinded (or *open label*) studies have actually been found to overestimate the effects of a treatment by about 17%. The effect of randomisation is even greater; analyses have shown that non-randomised studies may overestimate treatment effects by up to 40%![3] So, in theory, an unrandomised, open label study could overestimate the effectiveness of a treatment by over 50%. That's enough to make an ineffective intervention appear effective.

It is still occasionally possible to get a false positive (ie showing that a treatment is effective when it isn't) or false negative result (not showing a treatment is effective when it is) in a RCT; the latter is especially likely if there are only a small number of patients enrolled in the trial. The trouble with most clinical trials in ASD is that they do tend to be quite small. That's why we need the results to be *replicated* (or reproduced) in more than one trial, ideally including patients of different ages and severity (ie high- and low-functioning) so we can see if the treatment is effective in a larger group of people with ASD. If a result is replicated several times over, and these studies are published in reputable *peer-reviewed* journals, you can be confident you are seeing a real treatment effect (or not, as in the case of secretin, discussed below).

To overcome the problem of small patient numbers in clinical trials, sometimes researchers perform *systematic reviews* or *meta-analyses*. These are the absolute top of the evidence hierarchy. In a meta-analysis data from several RCTs are pooled together and the results analysed. The larger patient numbers means you may be able to pick up a treatment effect that was not evident in the individual small trials. Only good quality RCTs should be included in meta-analyses, otherwise the results are pretty meaningless.

> One of the best known producers of systematic reviews is the Cochrane Collaboration. They have performed a number of systematic reviews of ASD treatments, which you can see yourself at *The Cochrane Library*. An easy way to access the library is through the Cochrane Collaboration website: www.cochrane.org
>
> First click on the *Cochrane Library* link. Then it is fairly easy to find these reviews using the search facility; otherwise you can click on the link to *Cochrane Reviews By Topic*. The ASD reviews are located under *Developmental, Psychosocial and Learning Problems*; select Developmental Problems then Autistic Spectrum Disorder. Although these are quite technical documents, each review has a plain English summary of its conclusions. We are fortunate that all residents of Australia can access *The Cochrane Library* for free, thanks to funding provided by the federal government.

Thus, when that specialist says there is 'no evidence' for a particular treatment, it doesn't necessarily mean there is no research behind it. What it does mean is that we don't yet have any proof that it is effective. This may be because the clinical research hasn't been done yet, or sometimes because the research has been done and the treatment hasn't been found to be effective.

The story of secretin — a case study in evidence-based health care

Secretin is a gastrointestinal hormone; one of the hormones that control and regulate the digestion of food. It became the focus of attention in 1998 when researchers at the University of Maryland published a report of three children with ASD whose autism symptoms improved after they received a secretin infusion during an endoscopy. Following the publicity thousands of children with autism received intravenous secretin, resulting in an international secretin shortage.

People started speculating on how secretin could affect the symptoms of autism. It was thought that secretin may act as a *neuropeptide* (a type of chemical signal in the brain). Secretin and its receptors have been found in the central nervous system of animals, although the exact role of secretin in the human brain is unclear.

Therefore there were both anecdotal reports that secretin was effective and animal studies suggesting a theoretical mechanism of action.

However, when researchers began conducting RCTs of secretin in children with ASD they were unable to demonstrate any effect on autism symptoms. In all, over a dozen studies involving over 700 children were conducted and not one found that secretin was more effective than a placebo.[4] Later in the chapter Dr Richard Couper proposes some theories to explain why this occurred.

A *Cochrane* systematic review concluded that secretin 'should not currently be recommended or administered as a treatment for autism'.[5] Despite this, some of the parents involved in these trials elected to continue secretin treatment even after being told their child, according to all objective measures, had not responded, illustrating the power of the placebo effect. Secretin is still promoted as a treatment for autism even today.

Sadly secretin did not turn out to be the 'cure' we all hoped. However, scientists are still continuing to investigate the role of neuropeptides in ASD.

WHY DO WE NEED EVIDENCE-BASED TREATMENTS?

On a societal level, governments like evidence-based medical treatments because they provide them with a more cost-effective way of allocating health spending. Evidence-based medicine is also behind many successful health promotion campaigns.

The federal government makes sure that all procedures and medicines it subsidises through Medicare and the Pharmaceutical Benefits Scheme 'are supported by evidence of their safety, clinical effectiveness and cost-effectiveness'.[6] This is as it should be. I'm sure as tax payers you would prefer that your precious tax dollars were not wasted on unproven treatments for say, diabetes or cancer.

The trouble is that the treatment of ASD is not generally known for its good evidence-base. In fact, it is the very lack of evidence which causes some of the biggest arguments. We have claim and counter-claim that a treatment is effective, or not effective, but without good evidence we cannot always be sure who's right. Also the lack of good evidence makes it easier for governments to justify not funding many ASD treatments. That's why as parents we need to push for better clinical research.

On a personal level, you might like to use evidence-based principles to help you to decide what treatments to use with your child, especially if your own financial resources are limited. This doesn't mean you have to completely disregard treatments without good evidence, but we'd recommend you give priority to those interventions with better quality research behind them.

WHAT ARE THE DOWNSIDES OF AN EVIDENCE-BASED APPROACH?

Well, in the first place, we cannot always conduct clinical trials of the highest quality demanded by evidence-based practice. We can conduct placebo-controlled trials to test the effectiveness of medicines (conventional or complementary) in ASD but for obvious reasons we cannot have a placebo-controlled trial of an educational intervention. We can have a control group, however, (children receiving an alternative intervention; it would be unethical to have a no intervention group these days) and some of the recent trials of early intervention have even recognised the importance of using randomised controls.

Also, it takes lots of time and money to conduct good quality research, especially if we replicate the research several times over. Lots of parents say, 'but we can't afford to wait for the evidence' and that's a reasonable view. So, if you decide to use a non-evidence-based treatment for your child, here are a few questions you might like to consider before you commit.

- What are the potential side effects or risks?
- Does the theory behind the proposed treatment make sense, given what we know about autism?
- Is it individualised, taking into consideration my own child's behaviours and symptoms?
- Is it monitored for effectiveness (based on data) and changes in dose and intensity?
- What training and supervision are needed to administer the treatment?
- How much does it cost?

Prescribed medicines in ASD

We haven't yet found a medicine which can 'cure' autism but sometimes medicines can help alleviate symptoms and manage associated conditions, such as attention deficit hyperactivity disorder (ADHD), anxiety, sleep disorders or obsessive compulsive behaviour. Some medicines which have been prescribed for people with ASD are discussed in Table 1. These medicines appear to work by altering the level or response to important neurotransmitters (serotonin, dopamine and noradrenaline) in the brain.

We need to avoid medicines becoming the 'easy option' for managing some symptoms, especially in the case of antipsychotics used to manage aggression, which is more common in low functioning autism. These medicines should really only be considered if behavioural measures and environmental supports (such as PECS or other visual aids) have failed to bring the problem behaviours under control.

With this in mind, the atypical antipsychotic, risperidone (Risperdal®) was recently listed on the Pharmaceutical Benefits Scheme, but with some significant restrictions on its use:

> *Treatment under the supervision of a paediatrician or psychiatrist, in combination with non-pharmacological measures, of severe behavioural disturbances in a child or adolescent aged less than 18 years with autism. Behaviour disturbances are defined as severe aggression and injuries to self or others where non-pharmacological methods alone have been unsuccessful.*[7]

However, in other cases medicines may help to reduce problems such as hyperactivity, anxiety or obsessive compulsive behaviours, which prevent a child succeeding at school or slow progress of their other interventions. In these situations a carefully supervised trial of a medicine may be justified.

Joe currently takes the stimulant medicine methylphenidate (Ritalin®) and whilst I was initially reluctant to go down this path, the benefits for him (improved attention and therefore better performance at school) do seem to outweigh the downsides (some initial insomnia and appetite suppression).

Of the medicines used in ASD, risperidone has the best evidence of effectiveness, but there are also RCTs to support the use of ADHD medicines and selective serotonin reuptake inhibitors (SSRIs), with lots more in the pipeline.[8-10] We do need some more long term safety studies, however.

Medicines should always be started at the lowest possible dose and increased very gradually, with careful monitoring for response and potential side effects.

Table 1. Some medicines that may be used in ASD*

MEDICINE	INDICATIONS	POTENTIAL SIDE EFFECTS
Risperidone	May reduce aggression, self-injury, tantrums and repetitive (self-stimulatory) behaviours associated with ASD. See the Cochrane Review.	Weight gain is common and can be significant; sedation and Parkinsonism; raised prolactin levels.
Selective serotonin reuptake inhibitors (SSRIs) eg fluoxetine, fluvoxamine, citalopram, escitalopram and sertraline.	Originally developed as antidepressants, SSRIs may also reduce repetitive behaviours, obsessions, restricted interests, and anxiety associated with ASD.	Nausea, sedation, sleep disturbances and behavioural agitation; increased suicidal thoughts in young people when treated for depression.
Stimulants: methylphenidate and dexamphetamine. Other medicines: clonidine and atomoxetine.	Symptoms of attention deficit hyperactivity disorder (ADHD) associated with ASD.	Social withdrawal and irritability; decreased appetite, insomnia. Should be avoided in people with heart problems.

*Epilepsy or seizure disorder is a common co-occurring condition with autism, but medicine treatment of epilepsy is complex and will not be covered here.
.

The role of your doctor in ASD

Many parents feel that, except for prescribing medicines, doctors have little role in the management of children with ASD.

However, children with autism have the same health care needs as children without a disability. A doctor may help with the following medical issues: sleep disorders, toileting problems, constipation, nutrition and weight gain. Other issues that arise for which a doctor may play a role in the life-course of the child include: sexualised behaviour and other sexuality issues (eg menstrual hygiene in girls).

Also, depending on their degree of expertise, a doctor can regularly review the child's progress and may provide a more holistic approach to the child's difficulties than can be given by specialist therapists. A knowledgeable doctor can also keep the family informed of breakthrough reputable research.

A doctor can play a strong role in advocacy for services and help your family access government-funded supports such as the Carer Allowance, Enhanced Primary Care and Mental Health Care plans. With the new Federal government autism policy (page 219) doctors are likely to play an even greater role in providing access to Medicare-funded autism intervention services.

Like all professionals, some doctors are more helpful than others. You may have to shop around to find someone you feel sufficiently understands the needs of your child and family.

Complementary and alternative medicines — the 'biomedical' approach

One of the more controversial areas in ASD treatment surrounds the use of complementary and alternative medicines, which are often referred to as *biomedical* treatments. These treatments are not endorsed by most paediatricians and official autism organisations but are promoted heavily on the Internet and favoured by many parents and a smaller group of professionals.

Biomedical advocates believe that ASDs are not just brain disorders, but that autism is the neurological manifestation of a condition that can affect the whole body; for example, they point to the large numbers of people with ASD who also have gastrointestinal problems, such as, reflux, diarrhoea and constipation. What biomedical treatments seek to do is alter the body processes that result in the symptoms of autism. Most biomedical treatments do tend to be of the 'complementary' type (vitamins and supplements, restricted diets etc) but not all; for example, prescription only anti-fungal medicines are sometimes used to treat 'fungal overgrowth.'

The trouble is that at the present time most of these treatments don't have any good evidence of effectiveness to support them and they are not going to receive widespread endorsement until they do. Also some doctors are worried that, without good clinical trial evidence, we cannot be sure these treatments are completely harmless.

You might encounter an 'us versus them' attitude when it comes to the use of complementary medicines in ASD, but the divide is not as great as it might appear. The mainstream scientific community is prepared to look seriously at some of these therapies and has committed many research dollars towards investigating them (witness the amount of research effort that was directed towards secretin studies, reported earlier, or the National Institutes of Health sponsored research into the GFCF diet, discussed below). It is likely that some of these complementary therapies will turn out to be genuinely helpful — after all, we now have randomised, controlled trials supporting the use of fish oils in ADHD — whereas others will not.

We don't have the time to go into the various complementary treatments here but will discuss the most popular of these interventions: the gluten-free casein-free (GFCF) diet.

Then on the following pages, you will hear the differing perspectives of two paediatricians, Dr Antony Underwood and Dr Richard Couper, on the GFCF diet and other approaches to managing symptoms and conditions associated with ASD.

The gluten-free casein-free diet story

The GFCF diet involves the elimination of all foods containing gluten (wheat, oats, barley and rye) and casein (all dairy products) from the diet.

The rationale for the diet is based on the theory that some children with ASD have a 'leaky gut', and are unable to completely break down selected proteins such as gluten and casein. As a result, peptides are absorbed into the body where they bind with the opioid receptors of the brain, affecting behaviour and attention. Supporters believe that GFCF diets can improve learning, social and communication skills in children with autism.

At present time, the GFCF diet is mainly supported by anecdotal reports and open label studies. A Cochrane Review from 2004 concluded:

> Extensive literature searches identified only one randomised control trial of gluten and/or casein free diet as an intervention to improve behaviour, cognitive and social functioning in individuals with autism. The trial was small scale... Results indicate that a combined gluten and casein free diet may reduce some autistic traits. This is an important area of investigation and large scale, good quality randomised control trials are needed.[11]

Since then, a small double-blind RCT of the GFCF diet has been published. The researchers were unable to detect any significant diet-induced behavioural changes in the group as a whole, although the study was only pursued for 12 weeks and some parents reported improved language and behaviour in individual children.[12]

Currently the US National Institutes Health (NIH) are supporting a double-blind RCT to study the effectiveness and safety of a GFCF diet. Thirty children following a GFCF diet will either be challenged with snacks which contain gluten and casein or receive identical placebo snacks. All children in the study will be receiving intensive behavioural intervention so that the effects of their early intervention program cannot influence the results. Researchers will try to identify the characteristics of children who are responders and the nature of that response. You can read about this trial at: http://clinicaltrials-nccs.nlm.nih.gov

The GFCF diet has its enthusiasts and its detractors. The supporters, such as Dr Underwood, believe it can alleviate the symptoms of autism in many children and is a healthy and safe intervention. The detractors, including paediatricians such as Dr Couper, believe there is insufficient evidence of effectiveness to support its widespread acceptance, that it can further restrict the diet of children who often already have very rigid eating habits and that it may divert parents' energies away from pursuing evidence-based interventions.

Interview with Dr Antony Underwood, a Sydney-based paediatrician with a biomedical practice.

What is your general approach to biomedical treatments for ASD?
Parents come to me because they've heard about my work and what I do is offer them guidance if they choose to go down this path. I make it quite clear that I'm not sure whether their child will respond. A lot of the parents are very well-informed, they've been on the Internet; they've done their own research.

I try to guide them in what I call a 'layered approach'. In other words we don't throw a hundred different things at the child. We try and approach it step by step, and the first step is usually the diet. Then I look at the biochemistry and then we look at any additional supplements like zinc, magnesium and [vitamin] B6. Then we look at how the gut is functioning and whether there are any gastrointestinal problems.

If we just put in one intervention at a time and we look at the response, we can see what's working and what's not working. It's very important that we have this layered or gradual approach to the treatment of the child

It is very understandable that parents want to do everything straight away but one of the problems in racing ahead is that the children can have setbacks, they can react to biomedical interventions. Even though it's only vitamin therapy they can react and they can regress on it. It's very tricky trying to get the biochemistry right and also to prepare them for each step.

I've also learnt that less is more. Often you'll get a greater response by doing less therapy than you will by doing too much. You can actually slow or impede their progress by doing too many biomedical interventions at once.

What are your views on dietary therapy for ASD?
There are a number of different diets. The basic diet is the gluten and casein free diet. That's the first step and then you have to try to work out which subgroups will respond to which different diets like the diet that eliminates salicylates, glutamates and amines. The diet may also need to be refined further to eliminate other foods to

which the child is reacting.

Assessing whether a child will respond to the gluten and casein free diet is difficult. We still at present don't have any reliable tests that can help us in determining which child is going to respond. It's still at the level of trial and error so that we do an elimination diet for at least six weeks to see if there's any response to a very strict elimination of casein and gluten.

My experience and the experience of other colleagues working in this area is that around 60% will report some sort of response to the diet and there'll be also a smaller, but very significant sub group who will have a profound response to the diet.

In fact there is a group of children, and it's only a small group, who have such remarkable improvements on the diet that they really stand out. Food intolerances can induce in certain children marked autistic symptoms, so when you control the diet the child will come much closer to normal.

There are also other food intolerances such as to soy or corn, or to the natural chemicals: salicylates, glutamates and amines. Picking out that sub group is very important because often they'll display behavioural problems if the diet is not corrected.

If children do respond well to dietary changes, can they ever have a normal diet again, in your experience?
I think the answer to this is that you'll never quite put them onto a normal diet again, which is a good thing because a normal Australian diet involves a lot of refined foods, carbohydrates, sugars, additives, colours, flavours, chemicals, non-organic produce, all things which are very unhealthy for the child. So one of the benefits of going through this biomedical approach is that the awareness of the parent is raised in terms of knowledge about nutrition.

After two to three years some of the children have been able to tolerate gluten and casein for example whereas previously they would have reacted to them. It seems to take about two to three years before either the gut heals or their whole metabolic process seems to be corrected and then some of the children can tolerate going off the diet.

What should parents look for to gauge improvements?

There are really three groups. You have the non-responders; then the very good responders — and some of them are in the excellent range — and then the biggest group of the good responders. In this group with each visit they're making good steady progress and that's the majority of patients I work with.

In order to assess the contribution of the biomedical interventions what we are looking for is a jump in the development which is above the expected level of improvement. So usually with other therapies there are steady improvements but often with the biomedical intervention you get this sudden improvement. In some cases the child will have a language explosion within a week or two weeks, so that it really stands out.

Most children are enrolled in early intervention and therefore they'll be improving anyway. The biomedical approach is really an adjunct to the other therapies. If there can be improvement in their cognitive function which opens up 'blocked' pathways in the brain then they'll be more amenable to receive the therapy and will make greater progress.

Can families really be sure that the biomedical is helping, as opposed to the other interventions?

When families stop taking the treatments or if they go off the diet, the child can regress and lose speech and eye contact. Then it becomes apparent to them to what extent the biomedical treatments are helping their child.

This stopping of treatment is something I discuss with the parents to see whether they think it is working. We review that at each appointment and decide what we should keep going.

In some patients the major contributors to the child's development are the other interventions and not the biomedical treatment. In such cases it serves the family and the child to cease the biomedical treatment.

Biomedical treatments are sometimes criticised as being potentially dangerous. What is your experience?

Most of the biomedical treatments are very safe providing they are used in a sensible fashion and monitored by a practitioner. Generally I have encountered greater side effects from the use of prescription medications than I have from dietary interventions or mineral or vitamin supplementation.

What other issues do you think are important in ASD?

Parental mental health is very important and sometimes it's healthy for the parents to stop everything and give themselves a break. You have to have an overall view that we are in for the long haul. We might have a setback or we might stop biomedical treatment for three months just to let everyone recover. If everyone's sick of taking medicines and vitamins and even doing therapy, then for the mental health of the family it can be good to stop everything for a period of time and then reassess the situation. We can always pick it up where we left off and then go forward again.

You need to have that overview. If the mother is under stress, we need to know when to back off and we also need to coach the mothers that they need to look after themselves. They need to understand that they can't help anyone until they help themselves because the mother usually is the key person in the household.

Also, I tell all parents not to put their children in front of the TV. In the autistic group, I explain to the parents that this is even more important because these children are like magnets to technology. They live in a visual world and they'll be very good with computers. A lot of children become addictive or obsessive about certain DVDs; they'll replay the same thing over and over.

So what I try and get across to the parent is that I know that they'll be very good at computers and that method of learning will be very easy for them, but what I'd like them to do is interact with a human being. So if computer and television usage can be reduced this will often benefit the child even if in the short term they are more difficult to manage.

Dr Richard Couper is a paediatric gastroenterologist based in Adelaide. Dr Couper is also the parent of a child with ASD. Here he talks about autism and the gut.

Why do parents believe that the gut may contribute to their children's autism?

Children on the autism spectrum often seem to have altered bowel habits. Some children at the severe end of the spectrum may present with offensive loose bowel motions. Paediatricians and paediatric gastroenterologists are often consulted about these symptoms. Parents not unreasonably wonder whether these problems are either caused by their child's autism or have contributed the child's autism.

What problems do children with autism have with their gut when assessed by paediatricians and paediatric gastroenterologists?

They often do have problems with *continence* (control of bowel movements) as a result of loose bowel motions. This may directly affect toilet training and attainment of continence. Some children are constipated and have retention and overflow which may also directly affect continence and may interfere with schooling.

It is not uncommon for children to be very fussy or obsessive with their diet, although micronutrient (vitamin and trace metal) deficiencies are surprisingly rare. Some children have such a problem with textures that they avoid certain foods. This sensory avoidance may result in failure to thrive and in *extreme* cases starvation. Unusual intake called *pica* may occur with some children consuming paper, soil or other non-edible materials.

Why might the gut contribute to autism?

The gut is often referred to as the second brain. It is endowed with many neural (nerve) circuits and shares many neuropeptides with the brain. These neuropeptides may act as both neurotransmitters and also as inflammatory mediators or *cytokines*. The actions of many of these peptides are poorly understood and it has led some investigators to theorise that disturbance of gut neurotransmission may be responsible for the autistic child's diarrhoea and that similar change may exist in the brain, contributing to the child's autism. If indeed this is the case there would be a possibility of delivering a replacement therapy or designing new autism specific therapies.

Is there any proof that gut peptides may be contributory to autism?

Some years ago Karoly Horvath, a paediatric gastroenterologist in Baltimore, was investigating diarrhoea in a child with autism. He was investigating pancreatic malabsorption and stimulated the pancreas with secretin, a hormone which increases fluid and electrolyte output. The parents noted an improvement in behaviour and symptoms after the pancreatic stimulation test. This led to an explosion of interest in the autism community with unregulated administration of porcine (pig) secretin to children with autism and the development of synthetic secretin for both intravenous and intranasal use. The benefits of this therapy were unable to be confirmed by RCTs of synthetic secretin including an Australian trial. There are a number of reasons why this might be:

1. Secretin has nothing to do with autism.
2. If secretin has something to do with autism determining the effective dose may be very difficult.
3. It is possible that the porcine secretin which is a biological extract has an active contaminant not seen in the synthetic preparations.
4. Nasal administration may be complicated by poor absorption and enzymatic breakdown of the peptide.
5. Delivery across the blood brain barrier may not be easily achievable. These reservations extend to future neuropeptide therapies.

Is there evidence for gut damage in autism?

Many children with ASD appear to have a leaky gut. That is, if we test the absorption of markers which are normally excluded by the gut's surface epithelial cells, we can demonstrate that these cross the gut into the bloodstream. The non-absorbed sugar markers lactulose and rhamnose are detectable in the urine after an oral load.

Why might this be? The population groups are often highly selected — you are more likely to have this test if you have symptoms. It is possible that this could represent in some children a number of things: underlying inflammation, subclinical allergy, trace metal, vitamin and essential fatty acid deficiency.

The fact that the gut is leaky should not be discounted and it might provide a reason for so-called autistic diarrhoea. Whether it translates to therapy is a different story. There is no convincing evidence that dietary or vitamin based therapies help either autism or the autistic gut. Most of these interventions have never been adequately tested. The NIH trials website allows both doctors and the public to scrutinise trials, from what is currently being assessed to the numbers involved, the design and the endpoints

Is there a hope for treating autistic diarrhoea or the increased permeability? Possibly — there is theoretical evidence which shows that probiotic agents such as lactobacillus GG may improve a leaky gut. Whether this would help the individual autistic child with either autistic diarrhoea or their development is debatable.

What can your doctor do for you with your autistic child and their nutrition and gut health?
The adequacy of the diet can be assessed and practical benefit may result. Children with autism are rarely trace metal or vitamin deficient, despite often very limited diets. I recently saw a child whose diet consisted of peanut butter, Nutella, occasional Vegemite and watermelon. Such a diet is surprisingly replete. For example, Vegemite provides most vitamins except vitamin C, which would be present in the watermelon. However, if you are iron or zinc deficient, supplementation can improve both intake and the variety of foods consumed. Similarly, contributors to poor intake ie cows' milk can be reduced (cows' milk is deficient in iron and promotes microscopic blood loss in the gut). Behavioural therapy in a child with severe dietary restriction secondary to sensory problems can be lifesaving.

As mentioned before, probiotic administration may have potential benefit in autistic diarrhoea and would appear safe.

There is also good evidence that fish oil (omega 3 fatty acid) supplementation may in neurodevelopmental disorders (eg ADHD) result in improvements in attention, hyperactivity and conduct disorder. In autism, early trials suggest that both hyperactivity and stereotypy are reduced. Similarly, there are studies which suggest that supplementation may improve cognition in neurotypical children and favourably influence the short-term outlook of schizophrenia and depression.

It is a little unclear as to what the dose should be; various preparations differ in their content of omega 3 fatty acid. There are also problems with administration. There are liquid preparations and also capsules, which can be emptied into fruit juice or milk or placed on toast.

Folate supplementation may also be worthwhile. Autistic children have been shown to be low in folate. Folate is required for the glutame pathways in the brain and it has been shown that there is an increase in a gene variant responsible for reduced folate processing in some autistic children, There is a current NIH trial on folate supplementation.

Toileting behaviours can be addressed. Constipation and overflow may promote undesirable behaviours such as smearing and attention to this may result in improved behaviour at school and at home. Administering stool-softening medicines can be difficult with autistic children, but with persistence and patience, acceptable regimes can be implemented.

Where are we at with our understanding of the autistic gut?

Our understanding is rudimentary. A few abnormalities have been identified but we don't currently know what these mean, either in population terms or for the individual. It remains to be seen if they have any relevance to the neurobehavioral changes seen in autism.

Therapies are best designed on an individual basis for defined symptoms and should not be applied because of some theoretical bias or some unproven suspicion.

THE SENSIBLE APPROACH TO BIOMEDICAL TREATMENTS

It would be a rare parent who is not seduced by the appeal of at least one biomedical treatment. US surveys found the use of complementary and alternative medicines ranged from 50% to over 90% in the ASD population.[13]

The medical profession does recognise the need to offer support to parents if they chose to pursue biomedical treatments. This quote from a recent issue of *Australian Family Physician* sums up the situation well:

Because AD [autistic disorder] is a chronic condition for which there is presently no cure, it has become the focus of unconventional treatments. Often disenchanted by a health care system that appears to be able to do little to help their child, hopeful parents may turn to complementary and dietary therapies. It is important to discuss alternative therapies openly and compassionately. Although one needs to be cognisant of the emotional, time and financial impact of any intervention, if they are not causing harm to the child, there may be possible subtle benefits to the child, especially if the interventions are coupled with an intensive behavioural and/or educational intervention. However, large RCTs have not been conducted to examine efficacy of many of these interventions.[14]

However, if you are contemplating going down this path, please heed these few words of caution.

Complementary is okay; alternative is not.

The strict definition of a *complementary* medicine is one that is used **together with** a conventional treatment. In contrast, an *alternative* medicine is used **in place of** conventional treatment. If you introduce appropriate biomedical treatments to *complement* an early intervention program, your doctor should generally be supportive.

It is not okay to use biomedical treatments as an alternative to an early intervention program. Remember, most of these treatments don't have good evidence to support them, whereas we know early intervention can help your child to learn and communicate. The *only* exception to this rule would be if you're on a waiting list for an early intervention program for a few months. Then it might be okay to try some biomedical interventions while you're waiting, as it is sensible to stagger the introduction of any of your chosen interventions so you can better see if they are effective or not.

Remember the physician's edict — 'first, do no harm'

There is a tendency for some people to associate 'natural' products with safety, as if the two things automatically go together. In fact, some of the most toxic prescription medicines we use today, for example, the heart medicine digoxin from foxglove and morphine from the opium poppy, are derived from natural plant sources. Natural products are *not* automatically safe and even some vitamins and supplements, if given at the wrong dose, for too long, can potentially cause side effects.

Sometimes it's not a case of what you're giving your child but what they might be missing out on. A study of 36 young children with ASD found that they had more essential amino acid deficiencies (indicating poor protein nutrition) than a control group of children with developmental delay but no ASD. However, the researchers also found that there was a trend for the children on the GFCF diet to have worse protein deficiencies than the other ASD children in the study (whose protein deficiencies were probably a consequence of their own rigid eating habits). They concluded: 'Children adhering to these diets may require nutritional monitoring to ensure protein adequacy, otherwise these diets may not be nutritionally sound over time'.[15]

So the message from this is: if you choose to pursue biomedical treatments, please do so under the supervision of someone who is suitably medically trained and keep a close eye out for any harmful as well as beneficial effects.

---

1. Coleman, Mary. Ed (2005). *The Neurology of Autism*, New York, Oxford University Press, x.
2. Bandolier Evidence Based Medicine Glossary www.jr2.ox.ac.uk/bandolier/glossary.html

Bandolier – Evidence-Based Health Care (2001). *Bandolier Bias Guide* www.jr2.ox.ac.uk/bandolier/Extraforbando/Bias.pdf

3. Levy, SE, Hyman, SL. (2005). Novel treatments for autistic spectrum disorders. *Mental Retardation and Developmental Disabilities Research Reviews*, 11, 131–142.
4. disorder. *Cochrane Database of Systematic Reviews*, Issue 3. Art. No.: CD003495. DOI: 10.1002/14651858.CD003495.pub2.
5. Australian Government Department of Health and Ageing. Background to the establishment of the Medical Services Advisory Committee (MSAC) www.msac.gov.au/.
6. *Schedule of Pharmaceutical Benefits* August 2007. www.pbs.gov.au/html/healthpro/search/results?term=risperidone&scope=PBS+STATIC&form-type=simple © Commonwealth of Australia.
7. Jesner OS, Aref-Adib M, Coren E. (2007). Risperidone for autism spectrum disorder. *Cochrane Database of Systematic Reviews*, Issue 1. Art. No.: CD005040. DOI: 10.1002/14651858.CD005040.pub2.
8. Kolevzon A, Mathewson KA, Hollander E. (2006). Selective serotonin reuptake inhibitors in autism: A review of efficacy and tolerability. *Journal Clinical Psychiatry*, 67, 407–414.
9. Research Units on Pediatric Psychopharmacology (RUPP) Autism Network (2005). Randomized, controlled, crossover trial of methylphenidate in pervasive developmental disorders with hyperactivity. *Archives of General Psychiatry*, 62, 1266–1274.
10. Millward C, Ferriter M, Calver S, Connell-Jones G. (2004). Gluten- and casein-free diets for autistic spectrum disorder. *Cochrane Database of Systematic Reviews*, Issue 2. Art. No.: CD003498. DOI: 10.1002/14651858.CD003498.pub2.
11. Elder JH, Shankar M, Shuster J et al. (2006). The gluten-free casein-free diet in autism: results of a preliminary double blind trial. *Journal of Autism and Developmental Disorders*, 36, 413–420.
12. Schechtman MA. (2007). Scientifically unsupported therapies in the treatment of young children with autism spectrum disorders. *Pediatric Annals*, 36, 497–505.
13. Mangley M, Semple M, Hewton C, Paterson F, McKinnon R. (2007). Children and autism. Part 2- Management with complementary medicines and dietary interventions. *Australian Family Physician*, 36, 10, 827–830.
14. Arnold GL, Hyamn SL,Mooney RA, Kirby RS. (2003). Plasma amino acid profiles in children with autism: potential risk of nutritional deficiencies. *Journal of Autism and Developmental Disorders*, 33, 4, 449–454.

Additional references:
15. Perry, A. & Condillac, R. (2003). Evidence-Based Practices for Children and Adolescents with Autism Spectrum Disorders: Review of the Literature and Practice Guide. Children's Mental Health Ontario. Toronto, Ontario, Canada.
16. Pavone L, Ruggieri M. (2005). The problem of alternative therapies in autism. in Coleman, Mary. Ed *The Neurology of Autism*, New York, Oxford University Press.
17. Morgan S, Taylor E. (2007). Antipsychotic drugs in children with autism. (Editorial) *BMJ*, 334, 1069–1070.
18. New Zealand Ministries of Health and Education. (2006). Draft Evidence-based Guideline for Autism Spectrum Disorder. Wellington: Ministry of Health www.moh.govt.nz/moh.nsf/pagesmh/5597/$File/draft-asd-guideline-jan07.pdf
19. Roberts, JMA & Prior, M. (2006). *A Review of the Research to Identify the Most Effective Models of Practice in Early Intervention for Children with Autism Spectrum Disorders*. Australian Government Department of Health and Ageing, Australia.

7

Don't try and be superwoman and think you can do this without getting help from others. Initially you can, but as the months and years go by, there comes a point where it all gets too much. By then people have stopped asking to help because they think you don't need it. So from the word go, swallow your pride and accept any help friends and family offer — cleaning, cooking, babysitting, whatever it may be.

Do NOT compare your child to another, because you will always be disappointed. Instead, focus on and rejoice in the achievements your child makes (however small). These 'small' achievements are the stepping stones to bigger and greater things and must come first. Enjoy the success of his progress before you begin chasing that next goal — your child (and you) have worked extremely hard to have achieved that target, so make sure you take the time to pat yourselves on the back.

Angie Hatcher, mother of Ben

MANAGING THE INTERVENTION MINEFIELD

We've talked about early intervention and occupational and speech therapies, about conventional medicines and biomedical therapies. At this juncture it's probably a good idea to briefly step back, look at the big picture, and talk about how you can manage all these interventions sensibly and efficiently.

DO A FEW THINGS WELL, NOT A LOT OF THINGS BADLY

In those difficult early months after diagnosis, there is a tendency for some parents to get in a panic and try anything and everything, in the belief 'it can't hurt'. The trouble is, it can!

For a start, we cannot be 100% sure that some non evidence-based treatments *are* harmless. But more importantly, a mish mash of too many different treatments has been shown to be ineffective when treating children with ASD. Remember that for many therapies it's not just a case of turning up for the appointment; you will be required to generalise the skills your child has learnt outside therapy hours. You will not be able to do this if every waking hour of your child's life is taken up with some activity or another.

You and your child will much better off if you choose a few interventions — obviously the main one should be an early intervention program — and give these a proper shot at working. For some people four interventions may be manageable; for others, say those with other small children at home, one or two may be all that's possible. If one of these treatments turns out to be ineffective you can scrap it and try another.

If you spend all your days ferrying your child here and there, from speech therapy to music therapy to the chiropractor and so on, and then spend all your evenings baking GFCF foods, you are going to burn yourself out and then you'll be no help to anyone. You will often hear that treating autism is 'a marathon, not a sprint' and it's true. You need to allow you and your child some downtime to rest and regroup.

START ONE INTERVENTION AT A TIME

Remember that no two children with ASD are the same. This means that no two children respond to ASD interventions in the same way. A therapy that works wonders for one child may do nothing at all for yours.

To avoid wasting your precious time and money, you should really try to start one therapy at a time. If you start a whole lot of interventions together you will not be sure which ones are effective and which are ineffective, or even harmful. Try to wait a suitable period after starting one (three months has been suggested) before starting another.

BEWARE THE 'MIRACLE CURE'

As you are researching interventions for your child you may encounter glossy websites promising quick fix 'cures' for ASD. Usually these will be backed up by parent testimonials, but no real evidence.

Please be very wary, especially if the treatment requires that you hand over large sums of cash up front. If it sounds too good to be true, it probably is.

BE ALERT FOR THE PLACEBO EFFECT

Remember when we talked about the *placebo effect* — that's where you start a new treatment and because you *expect* improvement you start to believe you can see it in your child. The placebo effect in itself is not *necessarily* a bad thing. In some countries doctors actually prescribe placebo tablets for non-serious conditions. Also, there is a school of thought that parents of children with developmental disabilities may become more energised and hopeful when they introduce a new treatment and as a result become more attentive to their child. If the child responds favourably to this extra attention it's possible the intervention may produce some genuine positive effects.

The trouble is the placebo effect may occasionally lead you to continue with interventions which are not effective for your child, and therefore prevent you from pursuing other treatments which are potentially more helpful.

Autism is a mysterious condition. While all children with ASD will grow and develop, symptoms can wax and wane from day to day, with no apparent cause. If your child is having a good day or so you might attribute this to a new treatment, whereas in reality the two things may be unrelated.

Complicating this further is the fact that most children with ASD are receiving more than one intervention. Joe's language has come ahead in leaps and bounds recently — is it the result of speech therapy, school, RDI®, his own natural development, or a combination of the above? There's no way we can really know for sure.

So how can you tell if an individual intervention is genuinely making a difference? It's difficult, but taking a more scientific approach should help:

- Start one intervention at a time, as mentioned.
- Have an objective baseline measurement of where your child is at before you start a new intervention. Good intervention providers will do this for you.
- Keep objective measures of progress. Once again a good therapy provider will do this, but you can keep your own

records. However, it's no good making vague assessments like 'improved behaviour' or 'seems more alert'; you need to monitor and record behaviours that are measurable, such as the number of spontaneous verbal requests during a day.

- Record progress via videos. Take a video of your child before they commence a new therapy and then periodically throughout the treatment period — remember, 'the camera doesn't lie'.
- 'Blind' some of your child's teachers or therapists to new interventions. If they don't know that your child is on a new therapy they can't be influenced by any expectations. This method is particularly helpful if you are introducing a prescription or complementary medicine. (Having said that, you might need to tell a few key people, such as the principal of your child's school, just in case a new intervention actually has some unwanted effects.)

If you follow these guidelines, hopefully you'll be able to tell if an individual intervention is effective or not. If it doesn't deliver results after more than a few months, you can stop it and look elsewhere, for something that works better for your child.

To conclude, some words of wisdom from an ASD and biomedical 'veteran'.

Way back when Tom was diagnosed, I was confused and distressed to be told there was 'no evidence' for treatments which seemed to have screeds and screeds of scientific research. People in universities all over the world were clearly beavering away producing mountains of scientific papers. I attended many talks by biochemists and doctors who appeared to know their subjects and offered ideas for autism treatments.

The careful explanations in the previous chapter are the clearest I have read and, we hope, a genuine contribution towards greater understanding between the mainstream and the alternative. There is no room for black and white thinking in ASD, every day we are living its shades of grey.

Why we pursued biomedical treatments

By the time of Tom's diagnosis, I had lost my faith in the medical profession. My GP was not concerned by Tom's lack of speech at two and a half and I had to argue to get a referral to a developmental paediatrician when he was nearly three.

Together with giving some useful advice, this developmental paediatrician advised us to 'wait and see' for six months. At Tom's official diagnosis, we were not informed fully about evidence-based early intervention treatments for ASD. In fact, my impression was that we were wished good luck, waved goodbye and left to fend for ourselves. I know we were not at all unique in feeling distraught that we were given a life-shattering diagnosis and offered no follow-up as we stumbled out into the world of the endless waiting list.

It was such a relief to me to meet some doctors who offered biomedical treatments and who took the time to sit down and talk at length, then offered some ideas for treatment.

When our family's autism crisis struck in 2000, I did what I had always done in life when the **it hit the fan; I plunged into denial and became completely hyperactive. I look back on my headlong dive into biomedical treatments as part of my autism denial; I would totally 'cure' my son, whether he liked it or not!

Of course, I had a huge emotional investment in the idea that my son's ASD was a case of the genes loading the gun but the environment pulling the trigger. Environmental issues seemed much easier to treat and overcome, and also, I had new little baby and wanted desperately to try to 'protect' him from autism.

Like most families, I was also reading about the huge increase in diagnoses, and looking for answers. The arguments that environmental factors are contributing to a real rise in ASD numbers are extremely emotionally appealing to families as they go hand in hand with the idea that these triggers can be eliminated and their effects reduced.

Which biomedical treatments did we try?

In short, almost all of them! I used to say that I didn't want to look back and wish I had done more. Nowadays, being honest, I look back and wish I had done less.

It's not that I regret trying experimental approaches, but I do wish I had taken a much more focused and scientific approach to the many interventions I tried.

Tom's dietary changes

The kind early intervention teacher who first uttered the immortal words 'autism spectrum' to me suggested we could look at diet. We made some changes and they really did help Tom to calm down. Several friends noticed this and 'blinded' preschool teachers did too.

We visited the Allergy Unit at Royal Prince Alfred Hospital in Sydney, where dietary approaches to developmental disabilities are taken pretty seriously. I leapt into a gluten-free, soy-free, milk-free and low-chemical diet. In my madness and clinging to hope of a quick cure, I still thought we could sort out the food issues and — Bob's your uncle — Tom would be FINE.

Tom certainly did seem to improve with dietary changes. We started these well before starting an intensive ABA program. Also Tom was what my biomedically-minded friends and I call a 'gut' kid, lots of very yucky nappies and red, sore bottoms, constipation and diarrhoea. Tom was always a good eater, eating a wide variety of foods, so I did not worry about his nutrition being compromised.

As Tom's life has become more and more typical, we stopped doing so much dietary intervention and he is no longer on any really strict diet. But he does have a generally wholesome and healthy diet — much to his disgust.

Other treatments

In the first years after diagnosis, we consulted with several of the doctors in Sydney who offer biomedical treatments for ASD, and *tried out all sorts of treatments, including several medications. I was a founder of the first GFCF Yahoo group in Australia. When he was five, I took Tom to the US to consult a doctor there.*

In the first few years we also tried a number of other therapies, such as AIT, sacro-cranial massage. chiropractic, homeopathy and... blimey... I can't even remember some of them. Being honest, I have no idea if any of these did any good at all; sometimes I thought they did, sometimes I certainly felt good if I had met a particularly knowledgeable or caring practitioner.

Looking back, I tried too many things too quickly and overlapped different treatments. If only I had been more patient and careful, I could have saved a lot of money and time. It is really important to try something for a good, long time and to only do one thing at a time, with space between treatment attempts. Otherwise you end up not knowing if things work or not and possibly spending money on treatments that are not helping and may be causing harm. Nobody wants their child to be taking lots and lots of pills and powders unless they really are helping; it's unpleasant for the child and too expensive for us parents. I'll say it again but louder:

I could have saved a lot of money and time if I had been more patient and careful.

On the brighter side though, we did have 'blinded' therapists and teachers working with Tom and they were taking copious amounts of notes and data. If they reported he was brighter or could focus better and his data sheets were good, then that was a good indicator of improvement. A couple of things really did seem to have a bit of a 'wow factor.' But, in my son's case, intensive early intervention has made the biggest difference.

Although people might think that parents are always hoping for a 'miracle cure,' I do believe that this is an idea that fades over time. After we had calmed down a bit, myself and my many friends who have followed the path of biomedical treatments came to realise that improvements are small and incremental but that they can add up to make big changes over time.

What worries me now about the biomedical approach

There is no limit to the amount of money that can be spent on biomedical interventions. This is fine if you have a bottomless bucket of cash, but most people do not. I look back now and feel we spent far too much money.

Over the years, I have talked to lots of families who have found trying the biomedical approach to be very stressful indeed. They had fussy eaters who would rather starve than eat new foods on a GFCF diet, or they spent lots of money on supplements and then found there was no way to get them into their child. Often the parents have then felt dreadful, as if they were letting their kids down. Families attempting biomedical interventions need lots of support and certainly do not need to feel worse for not managing to succeed with them.

There is also the tricky issue of families hearing about treatments and then trying them with no medical supervision at all. This is not wise. It really is vital to have a good medical practitioner to work with you as you try biomedical interventions and to make sure that they know everything you are doing. Some seemingly innocent treatments eg zinc are anecdotally known for making some children demented.

Finally, be careful of ANYONE who claims that they and they alone have the answer to autism. My advice is that if anyone is saying that they are right and all others are wrong, or if they are charging vast sums of money for small bottles of liquid yet have no scientific data at all… throw your arms in the air and run away screaming.

Where are we now?

These days, what I think is most important to the health of my son are: a lot of physical exercise, plenty of sleep, a healthy and varied diet, a good school environment, and some extra vitamins, minerals and fish oil. And, I think this is vital for my son, there are strict limits on the hours spent watching TV and playing video games; too much of either can send him troppo.

Absolutely critical to my son's wellbeing and to that of my other three children is my own mental health. When I start to fall apart, so do they all. If I get depressed, Tom seems to me to be more autistic — it is painful to accept but it's true.

*Over the past eight years I have met and become friends with all sorts of families, who have taken all sorts of approaches to their child or children's diagnosis with ASD. **Lots of my friends do not use any biomedical treatments at all; many have had terrific improvements in their children, and some haven't. Lots of friends have done all the biomedical treatments possible: many have had terrific improvements in their children, and some haven't.***

Most of the people who were enthusiastic biomedical mums alongside me in 2000 have calmed down just as I have. Very few keep to a strict diet now, only those who feel they absolutely have to in order to keep their children healthy.

I look back on myself in that year or two after diagnosis with enormous compassion, and when I meet the parents of newly diagnosed I am also full of compassion for them. There is a real autism crisis, and there have been recent steps put in place to ease this, but families are still bearing the brunt.

I am a passionate believer in unity, in all parents and professionals working together with compassion and understanding in the best interests of our kids with ASD. There is no room for complacency in the world of autism and no room for bickering and in-fighting.

I believe it is absolutely crucial that biomedical and other treatments are properly tested and trialled and that the studies generated are communicated to families in an accessible manner. Some Medicare support would be very welcome, but will only come when treatments are conclusively proved to be beneficial.

There is a long way to go, but if you want to feel more hopeful, click onto the website http://clinicaltrials-nccs.nlm.nih.gov/ct. If you look for current autism trials you will find many. Currently, there is no easy method to find out about Australian clinical trials and other forms of research, but I am sure that will change. At the very least attempts are being made, and things are moving along. The trick now is to be able to access reliable information.

On that note, it is a terrific idea to make some effort, once life has settled down a bit, to read up on medical matters in general, to learn about research versus treatment efficacy and also about the placebo effect.

One final thought, we do believe that if evidence-based, family-centred intensive early intervention programs were universally available then families would not be thrown into the vacuum that tends to follow diagnosis and which leads to that infamous desperate search for a cure.

1. Siff Exkorn, K. (2005). *The Autism Sourcebook*, Regan Books (Harper Collins), New York.
2. Sandler A. (2005). Placebo effects in developmental disabilities: Implications for research and practice. *Mental Retardation and Developmental Disabilities Research Reviews*, 11, 164–170

8

Don't isolate yourself from friends and family thinking they don't understand. Your ASD child will benefit from the experience of being with them, and there is no better education for them than going through it with you.

Solange, mother of Matthew (aged 15)

FINDING THE RIGHT SCHOOL

Children, parents, teachers and bureaucrats
— ASD is an education for us all

Education is absolutely crucial for our children as it is in itself a treatment for their autism. Experts agree that just as early intervention is the best treatment approach for children as soon as their diagnosis is made, their school-age education has a vital role in improving their symptoms and quality of life overall.

The education of children with ASD is a vast topic which raises a lot of emotional as well as practical issues for families. In this chapter, we aim to give an overview of what is generally agreed to work best and what options are currently available in Australia. This is followed by some thoughtful advice from families on what to look for in a school and how best to prepare your child and yourself for the school years.

If you have a young child who has recently been diagnosed with an ASD then the school years may seem very far away indeed. But children with ASD grow up as terrifyingly quickly as their peers and a look ahead with a view to planning early is a good idea. If your child is a bit older and diagnosed with Asperger's then you may already have had some dealings with school. There are some specific thoughts from parents in this chapter about this. A booklist at the end gives ideas for further reading.

My advice to any parent is not to believe your child's education is someone else's problem. You need to research, to learn, to get involved, to invest time and money. No one else will do what a parent can do. The parent is the child's best advocate... and the one in the best position to navigate the ship through all sorts of stormy waters.

I was very active in my daughter's schooling environment. It took great relationship building skills, the desire to want to learn (even if I didn't always agree with the method), the desire to look for other help and to put the effort in at home.

Do not expect the school to know about ASD in general, or how it manifests in your child. Every kid is different in their symptoms. A big issue could be the school that thinks they know ASD, and then is amazed that your child does not fit the mould.

Educate yourself on ALL the options — there are so many mainstream, alternative and special needs/ASD schools it can be overwhelming. A general rule could also be that you may need to seriously consider private schooling with small classes. Be prepared for the endless effort of advocating for your child.

We visited many schools, talked to parents who had trod the path before us, and attended a talk on schooling special needs children run by the local assessment centre. The parents there sent out some powerful messages, my take-home one was: your child's needs may change, for the better or worse. The school they start at isn't necessarily where they will end up. It isn't setting their future in stone, it can be changed. Just make the right decision for now, for your child and your family. That lifted a lot of the pressure from us, and in the end, after all that, we enrolled him in the local public school.

MY FAMILY'S SCHOOL JOURNEY

Funnily enough, as I write, I am also looking in earnest for a good high school placement for Tom. I have two and a half years left, and can already hear the clock ticking. The process is bringing back lots of memories of the year I spent looking for a primary school. Only this time, I don't feel half so vulnerable nor half so apprehensive.

There were many moments of excruciating pain during that primary school-searching year, several schools were at best thoughtless and at worst ignorant and ill-informed. But there was great joy too, when schools and teachers were willing, welcoming and warm.

Tom was born in March, and so it was easy to decide to hold him back and send him to school when he was nearly six. That extra year of early intervention made a big difference. Later is often better with regard to starting school for ASD kids.

Tom had been doing an ABA early intervention program and we needed a school which would let the professionals and ourselves be very involved in his transition to school. This ruled out the local state primary school. I had a meeting with the principal and deputy there and within minutes it was absolutely clear that they were not willing to work collaboratively in the way we hoped. Much gnashing of teeth and pulling of hair!!

In my experience, when you talk to school personnel they will have one of two attitudes: arms folded closed or arms open wide. Being a person who prefers to avoid conflict at all costs I had already decided that I was not going to battle with any schools but would hunt until I found the right one.

I visited many public schools and found great variety in their approaches. It really does seem that each school has its own way of doing things. There were tremendously welcoming schools who could guarantee us an out-of-area place, others that looked marvellous but couldn't guarantee a place and several that said 'thanks but no thanks' to the very notion of accepting an out-of-area special needs child.

So I started on the private schools and basically had the same three reactions as from the public schools: sorry, we can't help; yes but we do things our way; yes and we'd welcome your help and the help of the professionals working already with your child.

In the end, we chose Tom's school primarily for the small class size and for the warmth of its welcome. The school had a genuine desire to work in a real partnership with our family and our early intervention team, and it was not bogged down in a large bureaucracy, which certainly suited me well.

Tom had a massive amount of support in his early school years. Aides helped him to attend in class, and most importantly, helped him to socialise in the playground. This worked very well and by his second year at school, there was never a playtime or lunchtime where Tom was playing on his own.

Classroom aide-time was also faded out over time. This is not to say that Tom is learning just like the other children in the class. But the class size is small enough for the teacher to adapt the curriculum and to help him when needed, and Tom does a bit of 1:1 and small group work with the lovely special needs staff. In a few of his subjects Tom needs no extra support or adjustments. He is especially keen on sports and loves art, science and music: anything taught visually.

Tom doesn't do any outside tutoring at the moment. I really don't want to work him to the bone just to improve his grades by a few percentage points. I would like him to enjoy his life, to play with friends, to play lots of sport, to battle with his brother and do typical kid stuff. That seems to me to be the best path to follow in the pursuit of a happy life.

Children with ASD and schools

There is not a great deal of research available. However, in the debate over whether mainstream or specialist education is best for children with ASD, there is some broad agreement about what is important in the classroom. Families who are interested in this subject can read more in the 2006 review by Dr Jacqueline Roberts and Professor Margot Prior which deals mainly with early intervention but does have a very readable section on schools.[1]

Below are some of the things which are generally accepted to be important. Many will be familiar to you from the Early Intervention chapter:

- **Individualised support** for the student. Each student with ASD will have their own unique skills and needs and therefore require individualised support. Depending upon the child, support could be in the form of a list of school social rules, augmentative communication (see page 77) or a 'safe spot' they can escape to if stressed. Experts also recommend that teachers incorporate a child's special obsessions (whether it is birds, trains or whatever) into learning activities to encourage motivation and interest.

- **Environmental and curricular modifications**. Environmental modifications might include allowing a child to wear a hat inside to reduce distress caused by fluorescent lights, or letting them spend time in the library rather than join in a boisterous social game. Curricular modifications could include *pre-teaching* (that is previewing information before it is taught to the whole class), providing hands-on learning activities to teach abstract concepts or allowing a child complete shorter, less difficult assignments than others in the class.

- **A structured learning environment.** For example, having an uncluttered classroom with clearly defined work areas. Structure can also be provided through consistent programming (maths lessons always in the morning etc) with picture scheduling and other supports to help with transitions.

- **Systematic instruction.** Identifying educational goals, outlining the teaching methods required to achieve those goals, evaluating the effectiveness of these methods and making adjustments based on the data. Effective teaching methods include incorporating choices, modelling the correct way to do things (and also the incorrect way for kids with a need for perfection) and pre-task *sequencing* (giving a child a series of short, easy tasks to reinforce motivation, followed by a more difficult task).

- **A functional approach to problem behaviours,** as discussed in our Early Intervention chapter. *Self-management*, whereby students are taught to recognise and monitor their own problem behaviours (such as leaving their seat when they're not meant to) can also help reduce challenging behaviours.

Other helpful factors include:
- good team co-ordination amongst the educators
- a high degree of home–school co-operation
- trained teacher's aides available when needed
- in-service training for teachers and aides in ASD
- peer-tutoring for both academic and social skills
- smaller class sizes
- social skills training and support
- regular evaluation of progress
- a positive attitude towards inclusion (for inclusive settings).

Although all of the above sounds pretty marvellous, do not hold your breath. Few schools will be able to offer all of these to all of their students. Special education settings probably fulfil a lot more of these criteria but it's likely most children with ASD will end up in mainstream education. This is because the biggest number of children with ASD are in the higher functioning/Asperger's syndrome end of the spectrum and by definition do not have an intellectual disability. We have a long way to go before all children with ASD in mainstream settings are getting an optimum education:

> *Inclusive education requires significant resources to implement; complaints of lack of resources are ubiquitous. Studies in NSW indicate that teachers feel they lack the necessary time, skills, training and resources to implement inclusive practices.*[1]

Be realistic about what your child can and can't do then visit schools you think will suit them and that you have heard about from other parents. It is always good to listen to the recommendations of other parents. Go with your gut feeling, if you like the school and they are willing to help then give it a try. The most important thing for us is that our son is happy. When he is unhappy he will not do his best. Always judge whether it is working by the happiness of your child, especially if they are non verbal.

I haven't found that teachers are really skilled up to help our kids learn to be more social. And why should they be? Teaching social skills to children with ASD is a huge topic and not part of any general teaching degree. Having a plan on how to use aide time to help with social skills in the playground is essential and you may need a specialist to draw up that plan.

I had spent a lot of time getting the teacher prepared to teach my son. I had made a book for my son about what would happen at school, so I also made one for the teacher about how my son might behave. This meant we got off to a really good start.

Our school was fantastic. The teacher had a chat to the other children in the class about my son and in the first year he arranged a buddy system so that someone was always there to encourage him to play. We used video modelling and would show my son lots of video of him playing with the other kids (the bits where he ignored them were left on the cutting room floor!)

I try to help out in the classroom as much as possible so that I build up a relationship with the teacher, the teacher feels supported and I can subtly observe how my son is going. Most schools provide lots of opportunities these days for parent involvement. The best form of communication is always 'face-to-face'. Emails are a good back-up.

What sort of an education does my child need?

As parents, we need to look at our own child's strengths and weaknesses, then to look at all the available school options and find the place that suits our child and our family best. It is good to become familiar with the entire range of options and to know when and how to make a change if it is needed. Of course in many parts of Australia, especially in rural and remote areas, there are very few if any of these options available: see the state-by-state listings for contact details in your state.

GOVERNMENT, CATHOLIC AND INDEPENDENT GENERIC SPECIAL SCHOOLS.
In special schools children with disabilities of all kinds are taught together in small groups with teachers who are generally trained in special education and supported by teaching assistants. In some states, children can divide their week between a special school and a mainstream school. Students at special schools generally have more than one disability and require a very intensive level of support.

A very few special schools have boarding options for their students, generally Monday–Friday boarding.

GOVERNMENT, CATHOLIC AND INDEPENDENT AUTISM-SPECIFIC SPECIAL SCHOOLS
The only state with government autism-specific special schools is Victoria. Two state autism associations also run specialist autism schools, these are Autism Spectrum Australia (Aspect) which runs six schools in NSW, and Autism Queensland which has two in Brisbane. There are Giant Steps schools in Sydney and Tasmania and Woodbury, the very new ABA school in Sydney.

GOVERNMENT GENERIC SPECIAL NEEDS SUPPORT CLASSES
Based on the campus of a mainstream school, these classes are smaller and generally have teachers trained in special education, supported by classroom assistants. Children with ASD will generally be found in classes for children with an intellectual disability. Children in

support classes usually (but not always) share a playground with the other children in the school and are integrated into mainstream classes for some of the day.

GOVERNMENT, CATHOLIC AND INDEPENDENT AUTISM SUPPORT CLASSES

NSW and ACT state education departments operate their own autism-specific support classes. These generally have teachers trained in special education and a classroom assistant working with a small number of students. In NSW, Aspect schools manage many of their own satellite classes which are located within both state and Catholic schools. The aim of these support and satellite classes is generally to slowly integrate the student into mainstream classes.

GOVERNMENT, CATHOLIC AND INDEPENDENT MAINSTREAM SCHOOLS

Many students with ASD, perhaps the majority, are fully included in a regular classroom. In most schools, the student and their teacher are supported with the provision of a classroom aide for some of the school day. Assistance can also be sought from specialist autism or special needs teachers who can visit the school as needed. There is generally less support funding available in Catholic and Independent schools.

It would be a very brave person indeed who dared to say that the assistance given to children with ASD in regular classes is adequate at this time in Australia. Whilst many parents and children are happy with their school situation, most are aware that the children's educational and social outcomes would benefit enormously from a large increase in resources. Many teachers would welcome more training and extra help and resources in the classroom. Parents would very much like to see their children being assisted by aides who are specifically and extensively trained in ASD.

INDEPENDENT AUTISM OUTREACH SUPPORT FOR ALL SCHOOLS

Most state autism associations have a schools outreach service. Private practitioners are also operating in some states.

HOME EDUCATION

Last but very definitely not least, home education is a solution found by many families of children with ASD. State education departments can give information about what is required of home educators in their state.

More information about home education can be found on these websites:

Home Education Association: www.hea.asn
Home Education Network: www.home-ed.vic.edu.au

Homeschooling has been working for us, I find that it gives us plenty of time to work on all the things we need to be addressing in order to remediate autism. Rather than my son spending six hours at school each day to meet the academic requirements (and coming home too tired to do much), we find we can meet the academic requirements in about an hour a day (it is much easier to teach concepts to two children than to a class). The rest of our time is then free for us to remediate autism and socialise with other homeschooling families.

This time involves lots of free play in parks, at pools, beaches etc and it also involves lots of small group learning activities which we set up. This way, my children get to learn what is required academically but also have lots of opportunities for socialising. The best thing about it is that I am there, and I can step in and help my son if a social situation gets beyond what he can currently manage. I can monitor what is best for both my children. Rather than me working on autism at the end of the day when he is tired from school, I get to have the best hours with him.

Children's rights

Children in the United States seem to have very different rights in terms of education to children in Australia. Under the US *Individuals with Disabilities Education Improvement Act 2004*, children have the right to a free and appropriate public education which meets their unique needs. Because of this Act there is much public debate about what sort of education is appropriate for children with ASD and much litigation occurs. There is no similar education act here in Australia.

However, Australia does have clearly defined Disability Standards for Education. These were written in 2005 as a way to make clear both the rights of students with a disability and the obligations of their educators. It is worthwhile becoming familiar with these. The Federal Attorney General's Department website has a very clear description of them (see website link below).

In summary, the Standards explain the sections of the *Disability Discrimination Act* 1992 (DDA) which pertain to education. The intention is that students with a disability have the same right to education and training opportunities as all other students. They have the right to the same services and facilities, and education providers have an obligation to make 'reasonable adjustments' when necessary and to ensure that harassment and victimisation of students with disabilities does not occur: 'An adjustment is a measure or action taken to assist a student with disability to participate in education and training on the same basis as other students.' The US term is 'accommodations' rather than 'adjustments'. However both the DDA and the Education Standards say that changes need not be made if they would cause 'unjustifiable hardship' to the organisation.

These days, most teachers and educational organisations will be aware of the Standards and that they are required to make adjustments. But how much expertise there is in making the optimum adjustments for the student and, vitally, how much extra funding is available to help make adjustments are much thornier issues.

For a full description of the Standards, go to:

www.ag.gov.au/www/agd/agd.nsf/Page/Humanrightsandanti-discrimination_DisabilityStandardsforEducation

So How Do I Choose?

Often of course, many of us don't really have much choice. First of all, family finances may mean that all the fee-paying options are simply out of reach. In addition, autism-specific schools and classes are very much in demand and it can be very difficult to secure a place. Sometimes it may not be clear whether a place will be available until quite late in the year so parents need to have a few options up their sleeves.

The conventional wisdom is that you should mainstream children with high-functioning autism and my husband and I were fully aware of that. However, Joe's ABA supervisor expressed concern that, because of his attention problems, he would struggle in a regular school setting without a full-time aide. She pointed us towards a fairly unique school, linked to a Special Education department at a leading university. I'll admit I was a wee bit disappointed at first, but I knew by this time that she was usually right about most things so I set aside my prejudices and went along to see this school. Once I observed the school, the teachers and the happy, productive children in the classroom I was converted. Nothing I've seen since that time has convinced me that we've made the wrong decision. Joe is learning at a rate of knots and greets the teachers each day with a broad grin. So my message is when it comes to schools, decide what is best for your child and your family. Nothing is set in stone and you can always change things down the track.

The most important thing is finding a class suitable for your child. There is no use putting a child in a class that they are not at the right level for. It may make you feel better they are in a higher level class, but ultimately they will be behind everyone else, and may not achieve as much. Any child can try mainstream, but in the long run, only the children with moderate behaviours, no more than mild intellectual delay and a good understanding of rules and boundaries will survive.

I had worked and hoped for a mainstream education for my child. She had done the early intervention hard yards and I thought she would make it. Eventually the time came for a meeting with the school and various representatives from the Department. It was at this meeting that the bombshell was dropped... she was advised not to start off at a mainstream school. If she improved, then she could be integrated in the 'normal fashion'. It was a bitter pill to swallow. I could have continued to fight the mainstream system but I had to conserve energy and fight battles wisely.

Individual Education Plans (IEPs)

The use of IEPs seems to be varied. In general, special education schools and classes do use them, but many children in mainstream environments do not have them, although there is usually an annual review of funding. IEPs are a huge subject, for further reading, we recommend the relevant section in *The Autism Sourcebook* and contacting your state education departments.

The IEP is a document which should state your child's strengths and weaknesses and explain what measures are being taken to remediate the weaknesses. It is most desirable that **measurable** outcomes are described and that reviews are conducted regularly to ensure that changes can be made if outcomes are not being reached.

> *Experience to date in NSW suggests that regular class teachers who make the time and effort to develop strategies for the students with autism in their class frequently find that strategies such as the provision of structure, routine, visual supports and the teaching of social skills, often benefit other students with learning problems in the class/school and potentially all students in the school. Teachers have also reported that successfully rising to the challenge of having a child with autism in their class has made them better teachers.*[1]

I suggest that the parent needs an advocate in meetings, this person needs to be a strong person, who is non-confrontational but knows their way around negotiation. Parents need to be armed with all the information regarding Individual Education Plans and their right to input into this process. Be clear on how the Education Act covers disability and make sure schools comply with this. The most important thing is to document every meeting and conversation because there may come a time you need this.

It's important to find a way to educate the other parents so that they feel more comfortable about my child's behaviour and know how to best support him and his parents and teacher. My own bewilderment, shame and fear of my child's extreme behaviours and its effect on other children and their shocked parents got in the way of being calm and clear to other parents. Make a fact sheet about how ASD manifests in your child and how they can help. Explain your child's social needs and quirks if s/he wants to socialise but has no idea how.

One of the early things we did was insist that my son was never to play alone. But you couldn't force that on every child, it could be counter-productive. Each child does need their own socialisation program at school and sadly I can't imagine many schools in Australia are able to manage this without outside help. As ever, it is up to us parents who understand the child best and where he or she is up to and what they can deal with next.

We chose to send our son to a NSW Department of Education Autism Support Class. His older brother was already attending our local Catholic school, but the classes had 30 kids, and there wasn't going to be much extra support if we sent our son with ASD there. He was well supported in learning the school routine, as well as in the playground, and he was learning with visuals with other kids that also had autism. He loved school and it was exactly the right place for him to learn. He had a class of six kids, one teacher and an aide, and worked along side the IO class in

K–2. They integrated with normal kids in sport, dancing, playtimes, assemblies and excursions. Again, not all ASD kids are up to this level, and unfortunately there are not many good options at levels below this one.

School can be a fun place to learn, with lots of rewarding activities for when the kids do their work. My son's class got to play learning CD-ROMs on the computer when they completed their work. They also had a 'blue chair' where the child had to sit when not behaving. A good behaviour management program along with good working environment with incentives is the best for our kids. It also helps to have a good teacher/student ratio, as when working in smaller groups the children get more attention.

Give your ASD child some 'mental health' days at home. School can be very exhausting for kids on the spectrum, especially days that are different from the usual routine (like excursions, athletics carnivals etc). One or two days off a term can make all the difference.

At home it is much easier to tailor the work to his special interests and I find that all outcomes can be addressed this way. My son is high functioning and extremely bright, I am not concerned with his academic knowledge, it's his social skills that remain the problem. We address this through cognitive behavioural therapy, occupational therapy and a small social skills group we are lucky enough to have found.

If your child is a candidate for mainstream education, then you should at least consider your local public school. Convenience is a major advantage, not to mention the opportunity for both child and parents to make supportive friendships in the local area. One of the really nice things about public schools is that they typically have an incredible mix of kids from a range of ethnic backgrounds. Some children will start school with no English at all. There are so many 'different' kids that the ASD child doesn't really stand out from the crowd too much. Public schools typically *place a high value on diversity. While my son with ASD is 'different', I feel that the vast majority of kids and teachers are very accepting of him.*

Some ASD kids need a very small school and a quiet classroom environment due to sensory issues. If sensory problems are not a binding constraint, bear in mind that large schools do offer some advantages. A child with eccentricities is more likely to find kindred spirits if they can choose friends from a larger pool. A big school will have more resources to devote to special needs. A large school also typically has a split campus so that big kids are not playing in the same area as the little ones.

In a public school there are systems in place to support ASD kids. Some funding is available for integration aides, to train teachers and for special learning resources. I am yet to meet, however, a parent that is completely satisfied with the level/quality of support. This means that you will have to be your child's advocate to get the best out of the education system.

You will need to take the initiative to get your child the support they need. That's why it is imperative to find a school that is willing to work with you; that is, willing to discuss problems as they arise, to discuss possible strategies for resolving them, that respects your views and ideas and will allow you lots of opportunities to visit and observe.

We negotiated with the school for our son to have extra aide time beyond that funded by the Dept of Education. We made a donation to the school each term to cover the extra cost. In the early years we negotiated with the school for partial attendance. My son would come home after lunch three days a week so that he could do other essential therapy at home. It meant that he didn't get too tired.

Try to take your partner (or another suitable person) along to meetings at the school, especially if you are discussing difficult issues. Two heads are better than one. When both parents are involved the school really takes notice.

SCHOOLS AND INCLUSION — INCLUDE YOURSELF IN!
Caroline McCallum is a primary school teacher and the mother of a daughter with Asperger's syndrome.

The thing that stands out a mile is that everyone wants what is best for children. Any conflict that does arise often comes from the fact that a parent only has a few kids to think about and a teacher has a class to cater to.

We must remember as parents that our child is only one of many in the class. In other words — give the teacher a break. They have their job to do and the vast majority are doing the best they can for our children. You only have to listen to the way teachers talk about students to know that they care. Also, remember they are only human, just like you. Try to remember how you felt when you found out your son or daughter had a problem and all the learning you had to do. When faced with a new child in their class, teachers may feel the same apprehension and have similar concerns as you did at that time; it's only natural.

As parents we have expectations and hopes of what our children will achieve. Sometimes our expectations are different to the teacher's and it is up to the parent to help the teacher in any way they can to show the true potential of their child. Along the way some compromises may have to be made, but it is important to keep the end goal in sight. I have found one way to overcome this potential conflict and to build a shared vision, is to establish good communication links with the school and class teacher.

Why build good communication?
Good communication with the school makes life much easier for everyone. Parents and teachers can support each other. The more the teacher knows about the child, the more the teacher can tailor the curriculum for that child. The more the parent knows about what happens in school, the more they can support the child with homework, projects and in aspects of behaviour and social development. No matter what we do, problems will arise and they are easier to deal with if you already have a good relationship with

the teacher and school. For the child also it is important to have consistency and continuity.

How do we communicate with school?

The first thing I try to do is actually ask the teacher how they would prefer to communicate. Some options are notes in the reading folder, or an actual home/school communication book or school diary, or even by email. I like to use what my daughter and I call our 'rememberall book'. We use it as a reminder for afterschool activities, going home by bus, and handing in notes. It is also a space where the teacher can jot down anything I might need to know or if she needs to see me about something.

Remember that if you do have a communication book, it may not always have something written in it. Don't be disappointed, it may be that there is literally nothing to write home about!

Obviously there will be times when you need to talk to the teacher, in which case the best thing to do is make an appointment. It may be useful to give the teacher some idea about what you want to talk about so that they can be reasonably well prepared. For example, if you were particularly concerned about maths the teacher will have a chance to collect both thoughts and resources that may help. Or if it is some social aspect the teacher may be able to observe a little more closely before you meet and so on.

It is always better if both parents can come to any meetings — this takes the pressure off one parent remembering what was said! If you are not able to take a partner it may be that the teacher will agree to your having a friend accompany you. Always ask before you go as the teacher may feel you have come mob-handed.

If you have questions you want to ask, jot them down so you can refer to them. There is nothing worse than remembering after the meeting!

What do we need to communicate about?

As a teacher I can say that in general we like to know if there is anything inside or outside school which may affect your child's behaviour or ability to learn, anything from a late night, through to illness or a death in the family.

As a parent when I am sending a communication book back and forth for a particular reason, such as encouraging good behaviour or developing a positive attitude towards maths or writing etc then I make sure that I make as many positive comments as I can. You will probably find that the teacher will do the same. It is important that you also communicate this to your child. Read the comments with them and praise and encourage them as appropriate.

I also tell the teacher the strategies I use at home when a particular problem arises. It may not be practical to use those exact strategies at school, but the teacher may be able to adapt them. Teachers are great hoarders of ideas and anything they can add to their collection is always welcome.

CLASS ROUTINE

I try to know the class routine so that I can be consistent in remembering library day, sports day etc. It also gives me an idea of what to talk about at dinnertime.

HOMEWORK

If I don't understand what is expected, I don't guess, I ask. I try to make sure that I support my children with their homework and let the teacher know if it was a struggle. If homework is not done, I send a note or tell the teacher why, otherwise the school might assume that we can't be bothered.

If your child is having problems remembering to bring home homework assignments, ask if they can be faxed or emailed home as a back-up. It may be that your child is asked to do some extra homework to help them practice something they are struggling with. Try to make sure that these extra assignments are done, remembering all the time that the teacher is only trying to help your child reach their potential. Make sure your child knows that it is not some sort of punishment. Remind them that, for example, when you want to learn a new sport you have to practice the skills at training so you can use those skills to play a game, it's the same with homework.

Having a routine at home really helps, so your child knows when it is homework time. Take all the advice the school gives you about the right environment to give your child the best chance.

MEDICAL

It is important to inform the teacher about any medical issues that may affect your child, however small: for example, hayfever medication which may make your child a bit dopey or livelier than usual. Sometimes it may be a bit embarrassing, but it is always better that the teacher knows.

Other tips

At the start of the year, before school starts, go into the school grounds a few times with your child to get orientated. Then, if you are new to the school or have a new teacher or if your child has more specialised needs, write a little book with your child to introduce them. Not only does it give information, but it also gives the teacher some idea of where the child is at through the drawings and the handwriting.

Through the year have regular meetings with the teacher and regular IEP meetings. If you have a child who faces many challenges please try to be realistic about your goals. Use these meetings to identify and prioritise the goals and don't try to work on too many at a time. The last thing you or your child needs is to feel frustrated by a lack of success. That is not to say that you should not set goals at all. You must have expectations for your child and be positive about what they can achieve. At these meetings, ask what you can do to support the achievement of the goals that are set.

Another way you can help your child at school is to help out where you can, for example, going on school excursions, class reading, canteen etc. Even if it is only occasionally, everyone from your child to the principal will appreciate it. Many parents assume that their kids, especially when they get older, would prefer their parents to stay away, but a local school actually surveyed the older primary students and a huge majority were for greater parent involvement. Another reason to help out in the classroom is to see how the teacher works and pick up on the way they handle different situations, or explain a concept. This can really help you help your children at home.

So, to sum up, we should endeavour to *include ourselves in*; in our children's learning and development, in our community and in our own lives.

References
1. Roberts, JMA and Prior, M. (2006). A review of the research to identify the most effective models of practice in early intervention of children with autism spectrum disorders. Australian Government Department of Health and Ageing, Australia
Available at:
www.health.gov.au/internet/wcms/Publishing.nsf/Content/mental-child-autrev-toc
2. Roberts, J. (2004). Autism Spectrum Australian (Aspect) Satellite Class Project: A Proactive Transition Model for the Inclusions of Students with Autism in Regular Education Settings.
3. Harrower, JK and Dunlap, G. (2001). Including Children with Autism in General Education Classrooms. *Behavior Modification*, 25, 5, [page refs].
4. New Zealand Ministries of Health and Education. (2006). Draft Evidence-based Guideline for Autism Spectrum Disorder. Wellington: Ministry of Health www.moh.govt.nz/moh.nsf/pagesmh/5597/$File/draft-asd-guideline-jan07.pdf.
5. Iovannone, R, Dunlap, G, Huber, H, Kincaid, D. (2003). Effective educational practices for students with autism spectrum disorders. *Focus on Autism and Other Developmental Disabilities*, 18, 150–165.

Further Reading:
Each State and Territory has its own Department of Education, and each has a lot of useful information to read on its website. That is a terrific starting point, as are the publications offered by some Education Departments and available for download.

'Making It A Success' by Sue Larkey is aimed at teachers working with students with ASD in an integrated class, www.suelarkey.com

'Practical Sensory Programmes' by Sue Larkey has strategies and activities that can be used at home and at school, www.suelarkey.com

Sue Larkey's website also has DVDs and other resources for teaching professionals.

'Transition to School Manual' by Susan Dodd, Libby Brennan and Melanie Fryer is designed for use by families, preschools, therapists and school personnel. There is also a shorter Aspect handbook: 'Effective Support Strategies for Students with Autism Spectrum Disorders Transitioning to New Educational Settings.' www.aspect.org,au

'Which School' is written by five mothers from Aspergers Services Australia and can be purchased from their website. www.asperger.asn.au/

Understanding Autism by Susan Dodds, Elsevier 2004, has useful information and strategies both for parents and teachers.

9

I do regret very much my obsession and denial in the early years after diagnosis. Life got so much better when we let go of that and embraced the lovely boy we have. He was always cheery and delightful; I wasn't.

Seana

THROUGH GRIEF TO SELF CARE...

How to look after yourself and your family...

JUSTINE WATSON
*Justine was born in the UK and emigrated to Australia in 1992.
Qualifying as a counsellor in 1998, Justine has maintained a
private practice and worked with individuals and families on a
wide range of issues, specialising in autism and families/parents
with ASD children. She has a son with an ASD.
Justine is part of the Carers NSW NCCP (National Carers
Counselling Programme) which provides low-fee counselling for
carers. Justine runs regular support groups for parents of children
with disabilities in various locations in Sydney. Read more at:
www.counsellingforall.com*

If you are reading this book, it is highly likely you have a child, close
family member, pupil or friend with autism. You may be the parent
and feel that this complex disorder consumes your entire life, nearly
all of your energy, thinking time, resources, finances and emotional

wellbeing. You may be a relative or friend, who is aware of the challenging nature of the disorder. You see the management of the child taking its toll on the family and have a desire to understand more about it and ways you may be able to help.

Although a diagnosis of ASD may feel like the end of life as you knew it, it need not be. There are ways to navigate the emotional as well as the practical maze of autism. The shock and grief will lessen and this will enable you to regain some measure of control in your life. Picking up this book is evidence that you are on your way; congratulations on taking the step. There are new skills you will be able to learn as you read on. You may surprise yourself at the talents you already have and the ones you will acquire.

There will be good days and bad days, good weeks and bad weeks. Caring for a child with ASD may overwhelm you from time to time. Finding a balance in your life is the key. If everything is 'spent' in the first year, what will be left for the years to come?

Why do parents feel such a mess?

I saw autism as a 'black hole'. In the early days, it took everything I had and gave me nothing in return. I taught my son as much as possible and got little in return, very few smiles and cuddles just blank looks and appalling behaviour.

I remember feeling just one big mess after receiving the diagnosis. As the developmental paediatrician delivered the 'verdict' I felt as though my life suddenly changed to slow motion. I felt removed, distant and numb, to the extent that the rest of the paediatrician's words left me feeling like I was the dog in the popular comic strip listening to a human and hearing only 'blah, blah, blah...'

This stranger had, in seconds, delivered me a life sentence — AUTISM. 'A life long condition with no cure,' was the description I read. I felt that my heart was being ripped out and stamped on. I was in shock.

My days and nights became a whirl of trawling the Internet, talking to other parents, reading books and spending the little sleep time I could get dreaming about autism. This time served a purpose, education, which did help to temporarily soothe my anxiety.

The intensive early intervention path I chose took up every waking hour. I became a mini speech therapist, a Makaton trainer, a mini occupational therapist, an ASD researcher, a behavioural therapist and often a mini medic 24 hours a day. This didn't leave much time for me, time to consider how I felt. The anxiety that had been triggered inside me just kept building.

Questions would regularly race through my mind:

What about the future?
Will he ever talk?
Will we ever have cuddles?
Will he tell me he loves me?
Will he live independently — have a job — get married — have children?
Will he ever play soccer like his brother?
Will we ever get to know each other?
Will he ever care what I think or feel?

All these potential losses came crashing into my consciousness, exacerbated by the loss of the 'normal life' that was slipping away from me, rapidly, as I burned both rubber and cash consulting a variety of health professionals seeking much-needed support.

The anxiety I already carried was being triggered to levels well beyond my ability to cope. If I hadn't been in the counselling industry, I really don't know if I would have coped at all. I had the support of a therapist, some colleagues, and good friends at that time but the missing link for me was other parents in a similar situation, the other unseen heroes, all in the same boat as me.

Eventually, I found a couple of other mothers and they listened to me, soothed me and guided me through the maze of different therapies, treatments and professionals. In time, I would do the same for others and we all learned from each other. This has been an essential ingredient in my journey.

The intervention plan I put in place soothed my anxiety as well, as it enabled me to begin to feel some form of competence again. Everything I had been doing as a 'normal parent' wasn't working — it was just giving me a feeling of being useless and de-skilled! This pain lasted for 12 months or more, until my son started to make a little progress and I was able to see the fruits of my efforts, in the form of words and simple self-care skills.

My maternal instinct was to keep my son at home to 'protect' him from the world. It took my trusted speech therapist to convince me that this may not be the best course of action. I chose some care outside the home and some assistance in the home to give myself, other members of my family and importantly, my son, some balance. This was when I was able to start taking some time for me, and giving myself some thinking space for our future.

Once I started to take some time out, I began to think of myself as a counselling client. I thought about what I would be encouraging a client to do for themselves. What would someone need when they were walking into the unknown world of autism?

Firstly, I had to address the crippling anxiety and sadness I was trying to suppress. I began to be very firm with myself and banned myself from thinking about the future. I was not to think more than six months ahead in the beginning. This timeframe was allowed to grow, gradually, to thinking up to 12 months ahead. At the present time, with my son aged nearly eight, my next nervous breakdown is booked in for commencement of high school! I allowed myself my tears and frustration, and gave myself permission to grieve, permission to be angry.

The process of grief can be likened to the care of a physical wound. After the accident/trauma we need to assess the damage, often whilst in shock. We know we will need to attend to our injury. We may have to pick out gravel or dirt from the wound. This hurts and takes time and care. We then apply an antiseptic, which causes pain again. We may then dress the wound and make attempts to protect it, this takes time and a lot of care. This may be a daily routine until a scab forms to protect the wound. The head may be knocked off the scab or it may crack and hurt again. We may have to go back to the antiseptic and daily care routine once again. With time and tender, loving care the skin grows back over the wound and it becomes a scar. The scar is a reminder of the wound and a reminder of how that area will never be the same again. Like a scar, grief takes time to heal and does so best with care and attention.

I was lost for ways to nurture myself. I had become isolated, having lost friendships whilst we were living under 'house arrest'. I had stopped all the fun things I used to do through lack of time, energy and cash. I had become obsessed with autism and a shadow of my former self. I simply had to regain some 'self'.

I had neglected my self-care. I was constantly anxious, exhausted, irritable, unable to 'switch off' and certainly not able to sit still and 'just be'. Here I was getting my son all the help in the world — what about me? I thought back to the things I used to love to do: walking, meeting friends in coffee shops, shopping, dancing, watching movies, going to the gym, reading, enjoying sunshine, eating well and sleeping etc. I was just doing autism, 100%!

Once my son had a comprehensive program in place I forced myself to start to take better care of myself. I wrote a list of 'things that nurture me' on my kitchen wall and my mission was to complete at least one thing every day. This was, of course, excruciatingly painful in the beginning. I constantly felt I should have been doing more for my son and any time I took for myself was time taken away from him improving.

The guilt I experienced was something I had to overcome if I was to survive. My inner voice was also telling me that if I carried on in this way I was heading for some kind of a break down, as my new ASD-obsessed lifestyle was not sustainable for the long term.

My self-care actions were invaluable to my wellbeing. In my experience of facilitating support groups and working daily with parents of kids with ASD, I have found that once mum is willing to put herself first, family life changes. Happy mum = happy family.

I have seen tremendous transformation once grief, guilt and shame have been addressed professionally, within the safety of a trained professional's office. A weight gets lifted and parents feel as if they can breathe again.

Parents, especially mothers, usually arrive at counselling exhausted and desperate. Once they can grasp the concept and importance of self-care they often start to see a difference in family life, relatively quickly. And, importantly, they start to minimise some of the guilt they feel for taking time away from their child. It is not unusual to feel guilty when we first leave our child with anyone else, even if it is our child's immediate family. In order to survive autism, this is a skill we MUST learn and practise.

For some mothers, going back to work is one of the ways to bring normality back into their lives. I know it helped me to get my life in perspective and have something for myself outside of the home and family. It has crossed my mind that if I hadn't been a parent of an ASD child I may not have had the opportunity to learn how to take care of myself emotionally and physically quite so well. I had to learn to give myself permission to relax and enjoy other activities. I now see the blessing in this, and have discovered the importance of allowing myself 'thinking' time, relaxation and fun! I needed to learn how to make myself happy, despite life's attempts to pull the carpet from under me. I learned how to appreciate the little things in life and not to take anything for granted.

I feel that the parents of kids with ASD are highly susceptible to depression. We all suffer from lack of sleep, the exhaustion of the 24-hour care these children demand of us, and strain on our physical and mental health, and nervous system.

In addition, relationships with these children are often severely impaired: parents don't receive much in return for their efforts. Although we want to give unconditionally, we have a desire for reciprocity. We get emotional feedback in day-to-day relationships with others and with our typical children. But with children with ASD in the early days 'unrequited' love can be demoralising.

We all know children are hard work and usually, it's those 'special moments' that make the effort worthwhile:

- smiles and hugs — the 'I love you Mummy/Daddy'
- team sports
- reading to us
- music they play for us

- the thought of our future grandkids
- listening to their dreams for the future
- academic achievements

When we lack some or all of these moments, the task of parenting can feel thankless.

For example, when we have babies they consume all of our time, feeding them, settling them, nappy changing and staring at them. Within weeks all that hard work is rewarded with smiles and gurgles. With an ASD child in the formative years, the rewards, if we get any, are normal child behaviour (eg toilet training, feeding themselves) often accompanied with crying and resistance rather than with smiles. I always explain to parents of typical kids: all the skills your child learned by osmosis, I had to teach to mine.

Another reason we, as parents of ASD children, are under so much strain and susceptible to isolation that can lead to depression, is that our kids often look normal on the outside. If you spend any time with an ASD kid you will quickly observe that everything is not quite normal on the inside. When we attempt to shop in the supermarket and our child has a sensory meltdown people might glare at us and feel compelled to pass comment on what they consider our bad parenting skills. We are judged in public by people's ignorance, time after time. The lack of support in the community can be very isolating and diminish our own self-worth, and can lead to social isolation.

DOES MEDICATION HAVE A PLACE?

Dealing with loss, grief and depression is debilitating and often means we don't function as well as we would like to. Some people have a resistance to medication for depression. Some are happy to embrace it. Others might overuse medication and other substances to keep their feelings at bay and not deal with life in general.

Any one of us may be vulnerable to the overwhelming impact of the grief of having a child with ASD, the loss of the 'normal' child and the loss of normal life.

Although we may want to 'tough it out' or feel we shouldn't

'need' medication, anti-depressants may have a place in this journey if we find ourselves too overwhelmed and unable to cope.

Not everyone is born with the same of amount of serotonin. Many are born with high levels (serotonin is the happy hormone in our brains) others are not. It is worth checking with a medical professional or your doctor as medication, even in the short term, may improve YOUR situation.

HOW TO TAKE CARE OF YOUR RELATIONSHIPS

The current notion of 'family' embraces a variety of relationships and genders: two-parent families, one-parent families, same gender parents, grandparents, adoptive parents.

If you are a sole parent it is important to take on board the principles of taking care of important relationships in your life; the most important being the relationship with yourself. When you're giving to children with such high needs all the time, and there is no partner to give to you, you must give to yourself to even out the balance.

Many relationships suffer on this journey and some break down. I have seen a variety of coping mechanisms partners take on during the crisis of diagnosis. In order to understand this I explain to parents the things I learned in studying family therapy. It is believed that when we are in an ongoing love relationship we bring to the table, the bedroom, and our day-to-day lives, the thoughts and feelings of our forebears. Our family of origin, our childhood family, has imprinted many thoughts, feelings and beliefs on life and how it 'should' be.

So when a crisis, trauma, loss or tragedy occurs we revert back to how our family of origin would have dealt with it. Think back to a time when one of your primary carers experienced a trauma. Maybe they lost a parent, lost their job unexpectedly, got sick with a terminal illness, had to move cities or maybe countries. How did the family respond?

Was there much communication?
Were your fears, worries or tears addressed?

Did you feel supported while the grown ups in your life fell apart?

How do we deal with the crisis of a child whose needs are so great, coupled with the loss of the anticipated 'normal' child we all expected? How do we handle the impact that has on the family and our relationship?

Most of us hang on for grim life, like 'white knuckling it' on the roller coaster, hoping and praying that when this gets better all will be well. But how do we minimise the collateral damage?

I teach parents to be detectives. Look at how your partner and their family of origin deal with trauma and have dealt with it in the past. This will give you insight into coping mechanisms.

Has your partner just shut down and withdrawn?

Are they constantly weepy and unable to focus on a task?

Have they started to drink every day to cope?

Are they putting in longer hours at the office to avoid coming home?

We all cope with trauma in different ways. Problems arise when the ways we choose to cope are driving a wedge into our relationship.

It is during any 'tough times' we discover the fabric of who we are and how we cope and the same about our partners, family members and friends. If your body was sick then you would go to a doctor. If your relationship is suffering wouldn't you go to a relationship doctor too?

For some of us this is a tough call. Admitting we are having relationship issues is hard to do. However, it is liberating when we do. If you were to break a bone you may have to do rehabilitation or physiotherapy plus a series of often painful exercises in order to facilitate the healing process. Relationship therapy is similar.

Exercises may include:

- how to listen and be heard effectively
- how to communicate your needs and have them met

- understanding each other's coping mechanisms in grief and trauma and the impact they may have
- reminders of what made you fall in love in the first place.

This is a tough process, but a good way to stay engaged with your partner and, importantly, to model good relationship values to your children.

Having a 'date night' is essential. A night out together every week (or fortnight) that is solely for your relationship is a way to reconnect and is vitally important for both parties. The time is not for discussions about autism or difficulties, it is to relate to your partner and remind yourselves that you are human beings as well as parents who take time out for each other because you matter. It's also really important to have some fun, engage in activities you love and take turns to choose the agenda.

The golden rule is to keep in mind you both have a broken heart due to your child's autism. Everyone deals with a broken heart differently but how you react has nothing to do with how much you love your partner.

For me, our lives began to resemble our 'new normal' in the first year my son went to school. I am fully aware that this isn't everyone's story but at some stage, life has to regain a sense of 'normality'. I returned to work, and my other son was able to take on more enjoyable activities as well as receive more of my time. My ASD son improved and the school system shared some of 'the burden'. Things became more 'normal' and bearable.

By normal I mean:

- base level needs are being met — everyone in the family is sleeping, eating well, resuming normal activities etc
- the financial resources are more evenly spread through family members — holidays and other activities are possible again
- Mum/Dad have resumed work (if they gave it up initially to cope with their child)

- respite is in place
- parents both have time out as individuals
- parents have time out together and time with other children
- siblings are receiving an equal share of time from the family
- the family becomes more accepting of the child's autism.

It may be easy to feel resentful hearing my story if you have a severely autistic child. You may feel the whole idea of getting to a stage where you felt you could implement some strategies for a 'better life' is very remote. You may be so comfortably numb in the 'hard life' that there is no longer light at the end of the tunnel. My heart goes out to you.

In my practice I have had parents of severely autistic kids who have, against all odds, completely changed their lives and the future of their family. They have had to make hard choices: some have moved home, involved a respite service in or out of the home, surrendered some control/care of their child. Ultimately their bravery has resulted in them changing their lives and they have started 'living' again. It is possible with support.

Another thing I learned on this journey is that you need to be comfortable with all the professionals you allow into your child's life and sometimes into your home. It is imperative to trust them professionally and feel that they will be able to provide the best care for your child. If you don't, you could waste a lot of time and money on a path that isn't right for you or your child. Developing that parental intuition or the 'all knowing voice inside' is crucial on this journey.

Summary
My life will never be the same as it was before autism.

Without autism, I would never have learned to be in awe at a spoken word. I may never have been able to see the wings on the backs of the children who passed the parcel for my son at parties. I too may have judged those 'terrible' mothers in supermarkets whose 'horrible' children throw tantrums instead of speaking!

Without autism, I may not have had the honour to meet some of the most determined, courageous, tenacious superheroes (disguised as parents).

Today I have a more normal family. My son is weird. He does strange stuff, he's funny and quirky and has special gifts that other kids don't have. He is our gift. I still feel sad at certain times. I take care of my grief by knowing that sometimes I may feel sad at the loss of the 'normal child' I didn't have. At the school Christmas concert I cry more than the other mums. That's normal. I take better care of myself at those times.

Two things I hold sacred now:

Look after me first, because if I don't, then who will look after my children when I cannot?
Autism is a marathon not a sprint.

Journey towards healing

Wendy Rafferty and her husband have three sons, the eldest now are young men in their twenties, the youngest son is 13 and has an ASD.

In the early months after diagnosis there are various methods that parents use to cope. Denial and anger, feelings of guilt that you somehow brought this on your child and all the other stages of grief are part of an unstoppable road train that has to run its course. Self-care is the last thing on your mind as you are overwhelmed with panic and despair in the quest to fix your precious little one. However, nature has a way of making us relax at times, and you may find yourself lying around a lot despite your panic, albeit not without guilt. As long as this doesn't spiral into full-scale depression, please let yourself have some time off from trying to be perfect.

You will find yourself bombarded with information from many different sources and will probably feel overwhelmed and unable to take it all in, let alone know all there is to know. Do and learn things at a pace that will keep you sane. I remember feeling like the most uninformed, unmotivated and hopeless mother on the egroup, compared to the up-beat dynamos who made regular new and exciting discoveries and couldn't wait to share them. All I ever thought about that was, 'great' another bloody thing to do! Nevertheless I dutifully printed it off and filed it in that enormous and growing pile called 'I'm a hopeless mother'.

Amazingly I did slowly absorb it all, and started to make better decisions about what to learn more about and do, and what was just not worth the effort. I tried to do just one thing at a time and do it well. When it was chugging along, I chose what to try next and so on. I prioritised the things that I thought would help my son the most, which is different to the list of things that are easy to do, but infinitely more productive. Now my son is nearly 13 and I have tried everything on the list that isn't completely weird (and a few that are). You too will eventually get there, and don't be disheartened by those who seem to do it all effortlessly. From experience I can tell you that as far as those people are concerned, everything is not always as it seems.

Coping depends on a lot of things, sleep for one! Yes, glorious sleep is a biggy, as are money, relationships, family support, access to services, career (or lack of it), friends and levels of sainthood. If you have all that sorted, you'll be fine. If not, you may be like most parents of children with autism and occasionally fall apart. That is normal, healthy and perfectly understandable. If anyone tries to tell you to buck up at these times, just clearly tell them to… well, you know. You deserve and need the occasional emotional release. Please remember that if you are always down, depressed and obsessed, you are in danger of becoming a total bore.

Occasionally ask yourself these questions:

Am I always bringing others down with the difficulty and injustice of my situation?
Do I always bring the topic back to autism?
Do I want people to think of me as 'poor (boring) Jane' or would I like them to see me as fun company?

It might be time to actively avoid the topic of autism, and even the topic of your child other than to say 'he's fine thanks, how is yours?' Focus on being fun company and a good friend to your friends. Even loyal relatives deserve to enjoy the best 'you', whatever you are going through. If you are tough and mostly bright and cheery, you will definitely have more fun, make and keep friends, attract support from those who like and love you. If you are always gloomy, you may find yourself getting increasingly lonely.

Many children with autism do incredibly well with a good intensive behavioural program. My child is one of those who is severely affected with autism, and for him, doing well means not self-injuring or attacking others, and learning to speak in halting sentences. These are miracles for him and therefore for us. So we are one of those families who will always stand out in a crowd for all the wrong reasons.

The up-side of this is that my husband, myself and our other two sons are all totally unembarrassable. This is very liberating! Do you know how many people spend a large part of their day worrying about what others think of them? Until you have been pinned down on the floor of the supermarket by your enraged ten year old, had him start fondling the breasts of the fat man on the next towel at the beach or had to scoop the floating poo from the water under the disgusted upturned noses of the kiddy pool parents, you can't reach the nirvana of not caring what people think. I think my son is wonderful and I love him dearly. Our lives will never be normal again, but they'll also never be dull!

A sense of humour is your greatest tool in coping. Friends are too, especially the ones who also have children with autism. You can laugh together and really look beyond the disability to see the beauty in each other's children. Treat yourself as often as you need to with whatever 'fills your cup', as someone wise once said to me. Get a facial, take a walk, get legless, watch daytime TV, whatever!

It took me years to reach a point I call acceptance. It's not that I have given up, far from it! My son still has many more mountains to climb. But instead of resenting and resisting every step, I have accepted that I will be there to forge ahead for him with sword ablaze! It's going to be tough, no-one can alter that. I can either embrace it wholeheartedly, enjoy it whenever possible, laugh at every opportunity and revel in the rewards, or be a beaten sad sack. It's a no-brainer really!

10

Never give up on your ASD child. Even if your child is considered 'high functioning', which is a serious disability that can limit your child's potential for relationships, independent living and work, you, as parent or carer, can make a difference. Be prepared to learn and change your life so that your child has the best possible chance for a fulfilled life. It's a big commitment for any parent but the rewards are enormous.

Anne Little, mother of David

WHAT NOT TO SAY ... AND HOW TO HELP

A few words of advice for relatives and friends of families with a newly diagnosed child

To friends and family

Your friend or relative has a child with autism and they are going to need you to be there for the long haul. When their child has just been diagnosed, the parents may go through many different stages of denial, grief, anger and despair. Following this, there will be panic about time slipping away, interspersed with depression and inertia, and many long-winded dissertations about this or that treatment.

All you have to do is follow their lead. DO NOT give advice! This parent has a long and difficult journey ahead, and even though it will seem like they are possessed or completely insane at times, they will get to an even keel eventually and be the person you loved again. In fact, after going through all that is ahead of them, chances are they will be a wonderfully tolerant, accepting human being, who you'll treasure even more!

Chances are, your friend will at times appear boringly obsessed with autism, please forgive them. Remember when you had a brand new baby and you were so exhausted that you couldn't think or talk about anything else? Well it's the same, except with the worry that life will only get harder and your precious bundle may have a desperate and lonely life. You cannot really understand what it's like for them so don't compare your child's 'despair' at not making school captain with their child's autistic meltdown at the sound of a motorbike passing. OK, this is an extreme example but you know what I mean!

Don't tell them how 'marvellous' they are. Of course they're bloody marvellous! They have no choice! Tell them instead when their child does something which shows some improvement, how clever, amazing, cute and gorgeous their child is and how well their child is doing. But make sure it's true! Parents of children with autism can spot a patronising attitude a mile away.

Under no circumstances say 'I could never do what you're doing'. This is the single most offensive statement in the history of the world! As if we had a choice!

Many fathers take a step back after a diagnosis of autism. Men are notorious for needing to fix things, and as this is not easily fixable, they busy themselves with their careers, sometimes martyring themselves to make the necessary money. This may result in some venting to be done by mothers. Be careful not to put the knife in as the loyal friend. It's going to take a mammoth effort from both parties to keep the relationship together and this person needs a partner.

Many parents of children with autism are extremely reluctant to accept help, or even accept that they need help. They do, however, need bucketloads of it, and will eventually tearily accept that they need a break, however small. If your friend or relative has declined your kind offers many times over and suddenly calls to see if you are free for two hours next Sunday night please make yourself available even if it's inconvenient. They are desperate and they need you. The gratitude you will receive will far outweigh and outlast the inconvenience it causes you.

Seeing the child, not the diagnosis

I think the most useful thing that any family or friends can do at first, is not ask too many questions and not offer any advice. This sounds harsh, but in reality it is the parents that need to get their heads around the diagnosis and what it means. Family and friends just need to listen and reassure for the first few months.

I say this because there is so much conflicting advice out there, and it can be overwhelming and confusing without everybody trying to be 'helpful' as well. Parents need space to decide what they are going to do. If family and friends can look after the children whilst the parents have a few days just to talk that is a great help.

Of course, diagnosis is a shock and causes sadness for the both family and friends. Try to hang on the fact that the child is still the same child they were before the diagnosis: the only thing that has changed is how we look at the child. It's important to remember that ASD is a 'syndrome' which means every autistic child is different — just like the rest of the human race.

My family were very accepting about my daughter's diagnosis and I helped them to understand by giving them the reading material that I had read. What is not helpful however is when family friends and teachers etc say 'well, all kids do that' when I am trying to explain what it is my daughter is struggling with at that particular time. I mean, yes, I try to normalise her behaviour as much as possible BUT it seems like people are sometimes trying to tell me I am making more fuss over something than I need to.

The best things family and friends can do is to treat a child with autism the same way as they would treat any other child, with only a few modifications. In our case the modifications are more to do with sensitivity to those aspects of my daughter that she did not choose and may never be able to change. For example, loud music and crowded places freak her out so avoiding these or being close by when it cannot be avoided are all she needs. It is just a matter of being considerate.

One thing we need family and friends to really understand and actively support is that we do not want to modify our behaviour expectations for our daughter. It is wrong to let her get away with poor behaviour that her brother, for instance, would never get away with. We have adapted our response to how we deal with poor behaviour but her diagnosis does not give her the right to be rude and unkind. We think of it like this: Would that behaviour be acceptable when she is older, say 18? If not then we have to start to teach her NOW because it may take a bit longer to get the appropriate behaviour than it took her brother.

Family and friends can best help by remembering that as parents we know our child better than anyone and that our struggle to give our daughter the best future possible is something we need to share, but on our terms. We have been open about our child's diagnosis in the hope that we can spread some knowledge to the community, so that she, and children like her, are understood, accepted and supported, not by so called services, but by that community.

In the end autism is just a label, look beyond that to the needs of the child as you would with any other.

To grandparents

I am a grandmother of twin boys that were diagnosed in 2000 with mild to moderate autism. They had lost all speech. If I was to give advice to any grandparents that might be starting out on the autism road, I would suggest that you ask the parent what they would like you to do.

My daughter and I decided our roles from the very outset, we split the responsibility as we thought this would be easier. I mainly did the biomedical research as I had a knack for that. She did the education because she had been a teacher and this role was best suited for her. My husband and the boys' godfather shared in babysitting and odd jobs.

On the biomedical pathway, the first thing we did was start on the gluten/dairy free diet and I did a lot of the cooking for the boys. I also researched, mixed and paid for their supplements and managed their biomed protocols.

We babysit as well, from just a couple of hours to ten days so that their parents can get a break away from the children. We are on tap to praise and encourage the boys. We are a full time support system for them and their mother.

My husband is a handyman and fixes things around their house or helps with deliveries. The boys' dad has to work overseas, so my husband puts the boys to bed and tells them stories.

We have had the pleasure of watching one grandson doing really well, and the other improving greatly. It has made all the effort worthwhile. We often take holidays together and really love being with our grandchildren.

Family get-togethers — for ALL the family

It is hard for a parent of a severe ASD child to trust anyone — you can't take your eyes off your child for even a second. Once you do find family or carers you can trust it is wonderful to have some time off, besides just school hours.

I have always asked for help when I really need it, but really only rely on my mother, or another close friend who also has an ASD child. I have a lot of support from family with my two boys on the spectrum, but as one of my sons is such a handful, I don't really like asking very often. Also, my mother and mother-in-law would have trouble catching him if he ran off, so I only ask them to babysit at home. I don't really trust anyone to help in a public place.

Our families help us by having a lot of family functions at someone's house rather than out in the community. This means there is easy toilet access, and gardens are fenced. Public parks can be hard when you have a 'runner'. Some parents of ASD kids don't go out unless they have to, as it is often more trouble than it is worth. I have found it great when our family has offered to take the boys' big brother (who is typical) out to movies, parks etc, so he can get some extra outings that we are often unable to do with the other boys.

My advice for extended families when organising a family outing is to take into account the crowds, fencing, toilet facilities etc. Making it too hard for the family with the ASD child will either mean they struggle on the day or do not bother to come at all. And always make sure front doors are locked if there is a function at your place!

Learn to really know the child

If I was a stronger person than I am, I would have said straight out to everyone who knew me before my son's diagnosis, to respect the fact that he is an individual, before they tell me what to 'do' about him. Not that I don't want their advice. I do. But it's all in the word choice and the timing. ASD isn't just a disorder, it's a context.

We know our son does odd things sometimes. We know he's on a different timeline to the other kids. We know him better than anyone else on this planet. All we really want is for everyone else to get a chance to meet the excellent boy we know. It's just that a lot of the time, this just isn't possible. Sometimes, the world is too loud, too hot, too scratchy, too... much.

Having said all of that, our son has taught us some valuable lessons. We have learned to live a life with a lot less stress than before. We are very Zen now. And if people want to join us, they might learn a few things from him too.

We're in this together

If you have a relative or friend whose child has just been diagnosed with as ASD, you can expect them to be feeling really fragile and probably not acting normally. It's a bit like being in a car crash; their world will be forever different, whatever the child's long term outcome.

Ask what books they have been reading and then ask to borrow them. Read the books with the understanding that every child truly is unique. Ask them to write down a long description of the child, or write it for them as they tell you. Learn all about the child's quirks and preferences, and what the family is working on with the child at the time. A written list is helpful for everyone.

Offer respite… families really need this but it can be very hard to ask friends and family to look after a child who is behaving very oddly or who can have massive meltdowns. So, realise that if you do help, you need to get a real handle on the child's behaviour, likes and dislikes. It may take lots of little steps to get an ASD child to be happy to stay with others, so start small — slow and steady will always win the race.

We families fear above all else that our child may live a life with no friendships… so befriend that child and get to know them well. Your friendship will be a great gift to the family as well as to the child. Expect odd behaviour and some over-enthusiasm perhaps. My son has to be restrained from visiting our lovely neighbour at 7am most mornings and once climbed through an open window in his keenness to say hello.

As families with ASD we need to realise that our friends and family are feeling as confused as we are and that we need to pass along all the information we have. It's not easy to look after kids with ASD, so it's no wonder that people might be reluctant to offer. But it's no good waiting to have help offered — most people don't mind being asked at all.

Bridging the knowledge gap

Sadly, most of my family weren't able to be helpful in the very early days after diagnosis. It's hard to believe it now but back in 2001 no one I knew, knew anything about ASD. Most were unable to support or comfort me in any way except to say they thought it must be a mistake. Friends and family not accepting the news did not help.

But, my father was fantastic! When I told him, he said he knew nothing of autism and that he would get back to me. He hung up and within 24 hours phoned back with names of people he had sought out and within 36 hours I stumbled upon ABA.

The greatest help from family and friends is given by just listening, not judging or giving advice. Try to understand the confusion and anxiety. The feeling of uncertainty about the future is very unnerving. The realisation that it is not a phase and they won't 'grow out of it' is not easy to bear. Once parents discover the road they need to take, they will feel a little better although financial constraints and pressure can and will take its toll.

You can communicate with an ASD child

I find that many friends and relatives have problems knowing exactly how to speak to my little boy, who can talk but has a fairly significant language delay. It's probably because they feel ill at ease, but people tend to prattle on, saying far too much and speaking far too quickly.

A helpful rule to follow is to speak the way the child speaks. So if a child speaks in short sentences or phrases, try to limit your speech to the same. You'd be surprised how much many ASD kids can understand if you just slow down and shut up a bit! Please try not to ask too many questions of an ASD child either. Answering questions can be really hard work for a child with language delay. If you can limit yourself to making comments about things and try to be 'fun', you may find that communicating with an ASD child is easier than you thought.

Advice for dads from another dad

Having a child with ASD left me feeling emotionally battered and bruised, but a stronger person for it. I know it can strain relationships, especially marriages. Fathers often have to work more to cover the cost of therapy, especially as their wives may not be able to work or at least have to work less. On the positive side, I have found that, by my taking an active role in his intervention program, my relationship with my son with ASD has developed into a very intense one, different to that with my neurotypical sons. I find great pride and succour in the hands-on role I have had, and improving 'his lot' has become important to me. It has made me re-evaluate other things I used to consider important.

Comments that are REALLY NOT HELPFUL

'Well, he looks all right to me.'

'Oh don't worry about that, all children... chew their clothes/tantrum/spin objects in front of their eyes.'

'You've got to look after yourself you know, dear.'

Also, lengthy descriptions of children who are doing so well at ballet/school/music lessons etc can be a bit hard to hear, especially in the early days.

(You know that you are getting back some sense of perspective when you listen to your friends' descriptions of their kids many activities, friendships and fantastic Lego creations, and don't want to rush off and vomit in a toilet whilst weeping copiously.)

Comments that are REALLY HELPFUL

'Why don't you sit down and let me make you a cup of tea.' (Popular with any parent)

'You need a night out, show me what to do and I'll babysit.'

'I'm just dropping off this casserole for you, for now or pop it in the freezer.'

'I knew you'd appreciate a nice bottle of wine/bar of chocolate.'

11

It is crucial that you get to know your 'individual' child with autism: for example, where they are breaking down in development, their learning strengths and the therapy strategies that they respond to, particular stressors in their life, which teachers/therapists they respond to and why. If you focus on getting to know as much as you can about your 'particular' child then you will not waste time and resources on therapies that your child does not need or will not respond to.

It really pleases me when I come across families with a child with autism who have a fun and balanced life. Sure they have their challenges but they keep 'the autism' in perspective. Not only are they focusing on 'autism intervention' but they are also focusing on how their family can have the 'happiest and most fulfilling' life possible. I find this very inspiring and often these children do incredibly well because the parents are happy and balanced.

Monique Simpson, Connect Therapy

WHERE ARE THEY NOW?

If you are the parent of a newly diagnosed child, you may well be wondering what on earth the future holds for your family. Below you will find personal stories from 10 Australian parents who have a child with an ASD.

In the early days I felt so lost and fearful, I couldn't see at all what sort of a future my little family might have. In the bleakest times, I didn't even really want a future. I longed to meet families who were a few years ahead. When I did, I stuck like a leech and tried to absorb their knowledge, their wisdom and their cheeriness. These friends gave me a sneak peek, a preview of what might be coming next for our family. This was especially useful when school approached, and I am so glad now to have friends whose children will start high school a year or two ahead of mine.

In the early days, I was also desperate to know how Tom would 'turn out'. Although some of the best clinicians might be able to offer some thoughts, at the point of diagnosis there is no real way of knowing how a child will progress exactly..

Hopefully the stories below will offer some comfort as you

read how each family has come to terms with their child's ASD. Whilst still striving to do their best for their child, each has found contentment and happiness in their family's 'new normal'.

We have tried to put together a range of stories, from a young man who is at this time leading a completely typical life to more severely affected children. We have a piece from a lovely mum who has two children with ASD.

Ineka at age 6
– by Therese Potma. Therese and her husband have two young daughters. Therese is a graphic designer and used her skills to create 'Inekards', see p. 236

The impact of ASD on my life has led to an appreciation of small things and to a sense of never taking anything for granted. As a parent of an autistic child, the joy that comes from watching both of our children take even small steps forward is wonderful and amazing. In this way, this year has truly been a good one for the whole family.

We have two children Ineka 6 and Hannah 4. Up until now our lives have been anything but normal. For some time autism has been our focus — not by choice but out of a necessity to understand and help our little girl. After lots of tears, continual stress and endless hours of hard work on intensive early intervention, our lives have turned around and we can now function as a relatively normal family. I have found myself once again dreaming about the possibilities of Ineka's future.

Ineka's first year at school has far outweighed our expectations. She attends a special education school where the teacher-student ratio is one to five. This environment has been a good transition for her, providing the attention she requires to continue learning. We are so deeply pleased to watch her academic skills progress like a normal developing child; she is reading, writing and — to our disbelief — even doing well at maths!

Ineka still finds it hard socially with her peers in the playground, but is always excited to be in their company. She does not talk about classmates at school unless I ask her a specific question and even then her answers are mostly very factual: 'Jenny has earrings;' 'John played basketball; or ' Charlie is a naughty boy'. Emotional attachments and the desire to be with other children are definitely missing. I often wonder what her capacity for friendship and relationships with her peers will be in the future. The strange thing for Ineka is that she has no problem forming emotional connections with adults. Maybe we are a little more predictable?

Ineka's communication has come a long way. She will tell us: 'My shoes hurt'; 'it is sunny today'; 'Hannah is my friend'; 'I want dinner now'. The list goes on. Her expressive language is improving all the time and she can answer most questions we ask her. We are constantly surprised by her newfound knowledge, not to mention her ingenuity!

Only last week we were having an unusual battle to get her to go to bed. It was already way past her bedtime and she wanted an apple. This resulted in a major meltdown. Soon after, my husband Paul went into to her room to comfort and settle her. When she regained her composure she said: 'Daddy, in your brain you're angry and that makes you sad. In my brain I am angry and that makes me sad. In your brain and my brain we need to be happy'. Paul was blown away. He lent down to kiss her. It was then she whispered in his ear, 'Now give me the apple'. Kids!

When a child turns three, then four and doesn't speak many words, you begin to think they don't understand what is going on. I was often guilty of speaking in front of her as if she was not there, now I see that Ineka was soaking up the world around her up like a sponge; she just couldn't express herself. No wonder she was so frustrated through her early years.

Living in the everyday world is going to be one of Ineka's biggest hurdles. In most circumstances she never ventures away from me and often covers her eyes and ears when we're among unfamiliar people or in a playground full of children. As a mother who wants to see her child embrace the world I still find it hard to come to terms with these fears and uncertainties. I know my child likes to have fun, but her autism stops her. I always find myself asking: 'Why can't she just have fun?' I know she wants to experience her surroundings, but there's an inner barrier that sometimes seems so immovable. I remain hopeful that as her language improves we'll be able to talk through some of her anxieties and try and work out ways to improve her confidence.

When it comes to family outings, this year has also been full of constant and pleasant surprises. After so many disasters at the shops, the zoo, the swimming centre and the park you start to believe that it's easier to stay at home. I am glad that we did not give in during those trying times. Ineka now really enjoys going out, asking us to go to the beach, take a bus ride or go to the museum. The other day we took a long walk through the Botanical Gardens and then along to the Opera House. Just over a year ago I could not even walk around the block with her! That night I cried tears of happiness. I now actually believe that we will be able to do a lot of things I thought we never would.

Sure we still have meltdowns and anxieties, but it is so much easier having learned Ineka's triggers, how to prepare, how much to expect from her and how to get through it without too much fuss.

So far my journey as a mother living through autism has been painful and unpredictable, but also strangely rewarding. I know there are many challenges ahead. The fact is that Ineka's autism will always make our lives much harder than it might have been.

When your child is diagnosed with autism your dreams are shattered and you feel that your life and your child's life are never going to be what you imagined. Three years on, having moved through many stages of grief, I am actually starting to see more positives than negatives. I am starting to accept Ineka's autism. Although I will work very hard to help her improve, I have come to accept she will always be a little bit different. Although saddened by her disability, I now rarely cry about wanting it to be different. Instead, I find myself focusing on helping Ineka fit into our life as a family, so we can find a sense of fulfilment in our lives, together.

Joe aged 6 – a weekend away with the family
- by Benison O'Reilly.

As I write, we have just returned from a weekend away. We stayed with my parents for a night and then in a nice hotel down the coast. If you don't know already, you'll soon discover that ASD kids tend to behave worse on holidays than they do at home; the change to their routine seems to upset their equilibrium. Of course all kids play up on holidays but the difference is that playing up in the context of autism might mean a full on meltdown in an airport or hotel lobby. Not fun... Consequently, many parents find it easier to stay home.

Fortunately we're pretty much over that phase with Joe and go away often as a family. We had a particularly great holiday in Fiji last year and now have another one planned. Interestingly, Joe also loves the dreadful theme parks that other kids seem to adore. It's remarkable how a boy with 'sensory issues' can brave the crowds at the Sydney Royal Easter Show and line up eagerly for the noisy rides with flashing lights, whilst his mother is the one who wants to run screaming from the place, protesting sensory overload!

But back to our weekend away...

> First we stay with my Mum and Dad. When Joe was first diagnosed he was very aloof with his grandparents but now he loves Gran and Grandad (and Nanna and Pop). His first action upon arriving is to yell out 'Hi Gran' and wave eagerly from the car. He adores my Mum because she is a former teacher and instinctively knows how to play with him. I know he loves her because he told me so: 'Joe loves Gran'. We are still working on perfecting that 'I' pronoun but we never needed to teach Joe about love. He worked that one out all by himself.
>
> We head down to the beach with Joe's brothers. Whereas a year or so ago he would have 'stimmed' with the sand, this time he joins in a game to cover his biggest brother with it. TICK

I go shopping with all three boys, against my better judgment. My 13 year old is looking for clothes so we visit the trendy surf shop. He gets embarrassed about Joe's loud voice (nothing unusual here — he gets embarrassed by everything the family does these days) so I make mental note to work on Joe's voice modulation. I entice Joe off with a promise to visit the toy shop. We are looking for Buzz Lightyear, as we need a companion for Woody, who Joe plays with all the time (simple but real pretend play, unthought of a year ago.)

But the toy shop is closed. Oh no!!! A year ago Joe would have been inconsolable. I brace myself for the histrionics. But today, remarkably, he is okay about it. BIG TICK

Then things go awry. Joe has a thing about numbers and in particular those restaurants that have numbered tables. Table number 5 is his favoured spot. He spies one of these and he's off. Next thing I find myself ordering an ice-cream for him, to justify our occupancy of Table 5. He sees a girl buying an apple juice and demands one of those too. The café workers are probably thinking 'what a brat' but I'm too tired to argue and pay for the juice.

Joe picks up on my tense voice and set jaw and realises he's gone too far. 'I love Mummy', he pleads and gives me a kiss. This is kind of cute so I soften, but his funny little obsessions remain a big issue. Mark that down as a cross.

That afternoon we head for the hotel and Joe reads out the road signs as we drive the 45-minute trip to the hotel — not bad for a kid who was assessed as having a 'moderate to severe developmental delay' at age three.

We check in and then it's off to the hotel pool. Joe loves the water and will happily paddle around in it for hours. 'Mum! Mum!' he yells, but the water is cold today and I resist his entreaties to join him. He's always been scared of jumping in the pool, but today he hops out, sits on the side and pushes himself in. 'I'm splashing in', he calls. He does this several times over, to my applause.

A father arrives and lowers a small toddler with an unruly mop of black curls into the pool. Joe loves babies and makes a beeline for them. 'That's a baby girl' he says, pointing and smiling back at me. 'No, it's a baby boy', his dad explains. It's an understandable mistake and I marvel at the way pointing to share things with me has become second nature.

Then I warn Joe: 'five more minutes'. Five minutes pass and I tell him time's up. He sneaks me a sly look and starts his negotiations, 'one more minute?'

Just before we leave he gathers up all his courage and jumps in the pool from a full standing start, not once, but twice. I clap and whoop and yell 'Hooray Joe!' The other parents probably think I'm mad, but I don't care. His shy smile of pride is worth bottling. It's a good day.

The weekend sums up my little boy, now aged six and a half. Not 'cured' — far from it — but a very different child from the one who lined up trains and parroted video talk only three years ago. These are the fruits of early intervention, although ironically Joe seems to have made the biggest strides since his fifth birthday; after the so-called 'window of opportunity' (3–5 years) where the experts suggest the greatest improvements are to be had.

With Joe's transformation have come flow-on effects for our family life. Trips to the shops and restaurants are no longer ordeals. His big brothers, Matthew and Nicholas, include him in their play and tolerate his eccentricities with mostly good humour. His dad has a little buddy who helps in the garden and can play 'pretend doctors' with him at the surgery. And I have been able to write this book, which will hopefully help others.

So life with Joe is not so bad. It's certainly better than I thought it would be. Things will probably get rocky in a few years, when hormones and high school loom on the horizon. But our little boy has come so far. Who knows where he'll end up?

Alex at 10 and Jack at 7 years old
– by Elena Barnes. Elena and her husband have three beautiful boys and live in western Sydney. Charlie the eldest has developed typically, Alex and Jack have ASD.

When I was growing up, all I wanted was a little girl. I had three brothers, so with the birth of each of my three boys, I secretly hoped for that little girl. I got used to the fact I had three beautiful boys, then I found out my middle son Alex has ASD. I didn't even know what it was, and had been very casual about the fact he was late to talk and a bit hyperactive.

We began an ABA program a few months later, when we realised that sitting on waiting lists wasn't going to help. Then, when Alex was just four, we found out my baby Jack, who was not even two was also showing symptoms of ASD. How could this happen twice? I really had wished too hard for that little girl...

Alex had made wonderful progress with ABA, so we started a program with Jack too. We also tried diet, supplements and all. I couldn't ignore what helped some kids make wonderful improvements, so I dabbled in what ever I could, with the guidance of our paediatrician.

Now Alex is ten and still has mild ASD. He was lucky to start kindy in a NSW Department of Education Autism class, and now is in Year 4. He learns well at school and is quite smart in some areas. He can speak well, but he is just not into conversation and lacks many social skills. He is fantastic at Nintendo games though, and could beat anyone! He is also a fantastic drawer.

He plays well with older brother Charlie who is 11, and loves it when our cousins come over. He loves being around other kids, and will play video games, swim and play with them, just not have normal conversations. He is so easy to look after though, as he has so many interests, plays well on his own, understands rules, time and can dress himself etc. He is a beautiful boy, with a lovely gentle nature. He is a bit fussy with food though, and loves junk food!

Jack is now seven and although he has had the best early intervention, is still quite severe; he has no language, and is still very hard work. It is like having a toddler, as he ALWAYS has to be watched. He is messy, raids the fridge and cupboards, and has to be helped with all of his living skills. He still has some toilet accidents and he likes to take his clothes off. He has been to a special school where the teachers even struggled with him, as he doesn't really like doing academic work. He is now at Woodbury, an ABA school and we are hoping for a rise in his abilities; every improvement counts.

We have tried biomedical treatments with both boys, and it is true to say that they do help some kids, but not others. I think both boys are better off for having help with their digestion, having fish oils and multivitamins, but nothing even got close to making them normal again.

I love my boys dearly. My husband and I didn't ask for this, no one does, but this is what we got, and we have no choice but to make the best of our situation. The boys love swimming, so we have a great, solar heated pool!

We know now to steer clear of family outings that might be too hard work. We used to go to the zoo a lot, as Charlie loved animals, the other two were not interested in them – but they liked the hot chips! We love to get up early on hot days in summer and go to the beach. Then by the time the beach gets too busy, and it gets too hot, we are on our way home to our pool.

We were very lucky to get some regular respite a year ago, and now Jack goes out with his lovely carer for four hours each Saturday, which gives us that extra break, and time to do other things that Jack is too difficult to include in.

Both our families are very supportive, and we feel we can count on them for support and companionship. Most of our friends now are other parents of autistic kids. We don't feel bad going to their places, as they understand us.

We don't have family dinners at the club and we will never know if we would have. Our lives are not normal, but we never got to taste what normal was before autism came into our family.

I don't like to think too much into the future, but we do know for sure Jack will always be with us, and I think Alex could be semi-dependent too. We are blessed to have one normal child I suppose, to hope he finds love and happiness.

I am lucky my husband works hard for us, so I don't have to find time to work as well. Autism costs a lot!! The three boys are at three different schools, and looking after the house takes a lot of time. I also organise support group meetings for other parents of kids with autism, and help Jack's school with fundraising and other jobs.

If you were still trying to have a normal life with these circumstances, you would be disappointed every day. Life is not easy, but we enjoy our boys and they do give us a lot of love and we adore all of them. All I hope for is more awareness and funding so there is more in place for our kids when they finish school. In the meantime, life will be a challenge, but one we keep finding the strength to face!

A Christian perspective
– by Kate Hurley. Kate and her husband have three young children.

We have three beautiful children, each one a much-loved precious gift. William is our second child and has autism. We started down the path of autism when William was practically a baby. He was nine months old when we began to be concerned about his development and by 15 months we were convinced he was deaf. After a perfect hearing test result we first heard the words 'autistic characteristics'. By the time he was 18 months old the reality of autism hit and we felt shattered. We had barely come down from the elation of his birth when all of a sudden joy was snatched from us.

My husband and I cried and grieved. We prayed for help and comfort and asked God why? We waited for these feelings of grief to pass and for acceptance to come. We wanted to 'get over it' and to 'move on'. We felt this was what was expected of us.

We poured all our energies into early intervention programs hoping we could reclaim our son as 'normal'. We often felt racked with guilt that we were never doing enough. Sometimes we celebrated impressive gains. However, as I write, our son is nearly six and he still has significant difficulties.

William brings our family much happiness. He is fun loving and affectionate and at times his antics make us double over with laughter. But in a sense our deep love for him heightens our grief which has not disappeared with time. It is now our companion, a part of who we are. There are times when grief is buried deep beneath the joys of life, and other times when we feel it acutely. His birthday, his first day of school and seeing other kids playing team sports all trigger these feelings. Sometimes, in day-to-day life, we feel pushed to the limit, on the brink of not coping and desperate for help.

So where do we find comfort and help? In difficult times I read Psalm 121 from my bible. Its words encourage us in our journey of life knowing that times can be tough. It starts like this:

'I lift up my eyes to the hills —
where does my help come from?
My help comes from the LORD,
the Maker of heaven and earth.
He will not let your foot slip —
he who watches over you will not slumber;'

In ancient times the hills often represented a place of trouble and fear due to the unknown nature of what could be hidden. Living with autism, we too can have many challenging hills and uncertainties: arduous therapy programs, communication and behavioural challenges, sleep deprivation, toileting disasters and worries about the future. Sometimes these hills can be emotionally overwhelming — like the time William scaled the back fence and escaped.

Despite all the difficulties my help comes from God. As our maker and sustainer He cares for all he has made. He hears our cries for help. He never slumbers. He will never let my foot slip from his care. He cares so much that he entered our world in the person of Jesus Christ.

My hope and comfort is grounded in knowing Jesus. He sought out people who, like us, were grieving, and he wept with them. He also healed people and transformed their lives. Some of these people had disabilities, just like William. But whether 'cured' or not, Jesus promises true healing to all who trust in him, the kind that endures into eternity, where all of us, including William, will one day be made whole. It's in this promise that I find strength.

Maybe it's not so important that William doesn't measure up to society's definitions of 'normal'. If we're honest, we all bear the marks of brokenness in some way. Yet God continues to love us. And it's because he loves us that he has promised one day to heal and renew this broken world. Perhaps if we loved, as God loves us, having a disability might not be such a worrying hill after all.

Carina in Year 4
– by Caroline McCallum. Caroline and her husband Ian emigrated from Scotland to a farm near Esperance, WA. They have a son and a daughter who has Asperger's syndrome.

This year Carina reached Year 4. I knew this would be an important year for a few reasons. Firstly, I knew that although Carina was a fantastic reader, the comprehension of texts was going to become more challenging. This is the stage where children are asked to deduce, infer, understand simple motivation, empathise with characters etc, all quite difficult for a child who takes most things literally.

Another area of potential difficulty was going to be problem solving in mathematics, homing in on the essential information for solving the problem and ignoring unnecessary detail. This is the reverse of what autistic people typically do!

Our other area of concern was Carina's social interaction. Kids were noticing more and more that her behaviour was not quite like theirs. Cliques were beginning to form and exclude her for her 'difference'. And she was beginning to notice it. My husband and I decided it was a good time to have Carina evaluated.

Darrell Wills and Paul Cain are education consultants who work for a parent group based in Bunbury called PLEDG (Parents Learning Education Development Group). I was already an active member of the group in Esperance and we had provided workshops in our area for parents and teachers to talk about issues surrounding Inclusive Education.

We are STRONG believers in Inclusion and the group not only acts as advocates for that but also as mutual support for parents wishing to be the senior partners in their children's education and development. We are not an autism support group; we are a parent support group for parents who feel that, for one reason or another, their children's potential is not being met.

So Paul and Darrell tested Carina and the results were pretty much as I predicted, except for maths, which came as more of a shock. She was a lot less skilled in basic arithmetical skills than I expected. I had assumed it would be her thing, but I was wrong and regret not starting a maths program sooner. Still, every mistake is a learning opportunity!

We worked through a comprehension program and later added an addition program. This is work we do after school for about 30 mins each session, four sessions a week. I do the instruction, and send a video of the occasional lesson to Paul and Darrel so they can give advice on pace and praise etc.

We recently re-tested Carina and she has really improved in all areas especially comprehension — she moved up two years in just four months! We are now working on subtraction, and in an exciting new development, on money. This is because Carina has enjoyed working in the soccer canteen, but was a bit wobbly on the change etc. This extra work at home will make her more secure and will provide an excellent social situation for her to practise her skills.

As to other social aspects of Carina's education, well, that came from her. Carina told me that she wanted Darrell to go and talk to her peer group about Asperger's syndrome and her. Darrell did this with his usual flair and lightness of touch, talking not just about Carina, but about how to be socially inclusive to all kids.

The benefits of this have been two-fold: Carina feels she has been listened to and that her point of view is valued, and her peers have a better understanding of who she is and how (and crucially) when and if to help her. I hope this leads to a little more tolerance. It is early days yet but there are some children who are already showing a bit more understanding. Recently Carina was in a bit of a paddy about losing her cardigan and we were looking in the lost property bin. She was upset. Some of her class were passing and asked what was wrong and if they could help. This calmed her immediately. Before, they would have been wary of approaching, particularly with me there.

I have also had some positive comments from some parents, so the talk must have had enough impact to be part of dinnertime discussion. The longer-term aim of this is that Carina learns to live with her Asperger's with the help and support of her friends and the community in which she lives, not despite it. This is **vital** for her future mental health.

If we had lived in the city where we could access social skills groups, psychologists and other therapies then I think Carina's life would be poorer. Instead of physio and occupational therapy we do dancing and gymnastics, instead of social skills group and speech therapy we do drama. It just needs a short talk with the teachers to put them in the picture and a willingness to be involved.

Another aspect of Carina's challenges is her ability to control her emotions and to behave appropriately. We have tried all sorts of reward charts and systems. She was wise to them all. We also mulled over the fact that my son needs to feel that he has parity with his sister; absolute fairness is required for a boy of 12, no matter how understanding he is.

So what we came up with was a simple earning system where we would not spend extra money, but the children would have to actually earn a term's drama or really specco footie boots etc. They do chores and there is also a good behaviour component. This is working pretty well, but we are by no means beyond the weekly dose of meltdowns. But at least they are weekly not daily or hourly.

When we first realised that Carina was 'different' we were devastated. I am fortunate to have met people who shared my vision of Inclusion. I see the world as a huge ocean in which you either sink or swim, and school is like a swimming pool. It is my job as a parent to provide the skills and knowledge to help Carina and my son so they not only survive, but thrive in both the pool and eventually the ocean.

Right back at the start of my journey, I heard a parent of two boys with acquired brain damage give a speech. The first thing she said was 'Take your ear off the ground, the cavalry ain't coming!' She was right. We are all so used to doctors, psychologists and all the rest of the 'services' coming to our rescue we forget to look at what we can do for ourselves.

These days I really advise all parents of children with special needs to give themselves a break. Don't waste time and energy blaming anyone, especially yourself. Also, don't get too tired for your kids. Sometimes I think we run around so much after our kids taking them from one activity to another (all with the best educational, social and developmental intentions) spend hours looking up special diets and reading labels in the supermarket to get them the best nutrition — but then **we** end up sick, tired, malnourished and irritable.

One of the most important things you can do for your kids is to keep yourself fit, happy and healthy and that is why our support group has fun activities balanced with the informative ones. Keep a sense of perspective! It is very easy to become obsessive about our children.

My husband sometimes feels he is at the bottom of the list. I tell him that that spot is mine! It is difficult to practice what we preach, but we do try to get away as a couple when we can and our friends and families are good at helping us do that. Without these short breaks we would not survive as a family... and that would be no help to our children at all.

As I look back I see how much we have learned as a family because of Carina. I am a better teacher and parent than I would have been. My husband is a more involved father and my son more tolerant and thoughtful than his peers. We have gained skills that will not only help Carina, but others in our community.

Life with Harry — a marathon, not a sprint
– by Jennifer Couper. Jenny is a paediatrician in Adelaide. She and her husband have four children, the youngest of whom has ASD.

Our youngest started to concern us somewhere between two and three years when he became dangerously hyperactive, lost language, and stopped playing, so that by three years I didn't know what to get him for his birthday. But even at four years there was still doubt from professionals who held to the diagnosis of a language disorder. By the time he was diagnosed with autism at five years I suspect everyone in the clinic waiting room knew what was wrong.

After years of discussion over all his problems it was a relief when we were able to get specific help from a behavioural psychologist. At last there was a plan and I had some hope again. Looking back it was amazing what she did. She came into our exhausted family who didn't know what to do, and calmly set up a program for Harry who by then could do very little.

In fact, some things I was doing intuitively weren't so bad. Harry sang rather than talked and sometimes in context (eg 'open wide come inside it's play school' when he wanted to get into the bathroom occupied by his sister) and I found if I sang back he seemed to understand and connect a bit. But it wasn't going to turn him around. Behavioural therapy (ABA) got us back on track and made therapies in general possible. It still remains the intervention with the most data.

There were some drawbacks with behavioural therapy for Harry though. It was great for getting rid of interfering behaviours but it placed so much emphasis on responding correctly that it put a lot of pressure on him. He had lots of difficulties retrieving words and he became very dependent on prompts. It wasn't until he could read and type that we learnt how much he actually knew. Now at 11 years we realise he is very good at some things that were not revealed by ABA. It did improve his IQ (so called static intelligence by some psychologists) but not his emotional intelligence.

We did meet some amazing people through the program we set up, students in their early twenties with maturity and commitment way beyond their years. When Harry was nine years old he had a bad reaction to a medication making him so obsessive he could not go to school or really do much for months. They could have quietly walked away and found an easier job but they stayed with us through really difficult behaviours.

There are so many things that interfere with these children showing their abilities and reaching their potential, but it is well worth persevering. Lots of people have understandably given up on Harry but there have always been those who were happy to hang in there. We've also learnt how easily these children can become dependent on someone prompting them to do something so that they don't experience competency which is so essential to develop motivation. There's really no long-term advantage to being good at maths for instance if you don't find it rewarding and aren't motivated to do it.

For a while I convinced myself that the talented students and teachers were helping Harry more than us as a family, but a few videos ended that idea. I saw that he often learnt more with his brothers and sister in the pool than in the bedroom doing an ABA task. So we began Relationship Development Intervention (RDI®) two years ago. It's a developmental approach that, rather than teaching discrete skills and behaviours (behavioural therapy), aims to rebuild the developmental stages for interacting in relationships that neurotypical children learn in the first few years life. This supposedly builds dynamic or emotional intelligence essential for quality of life, regardless of one's static intelligence. We send regular videos to a RDI® consultant in the US for review. The videos we make teach us a lot too. But the jury is still out on whether it will substantially improve life for children with all degrees of autism.

Like too many autism interventions the research on RDI® is sparse: there is a lot of anecdotal evidence and one encouraging study of 16 fairly high-functioning children, but if you are waiting for top-level evidence for most autism interventions you will probably be waiting a long time. The money just hasn't been invested in carrying out definitive trials, so you have to glean what you can from the literature, other families and professionals. There remains a lot of disagreement amongst professionals which is frustrating for families. Do be beware of anecdotes or magic bullet treatments. If it sounds too good to be true it probably is! As parents you are the most important guide for your child. Ultimately your child will learn more from you and spend more time with you than with anyone else, so beware of any program that suggests otherwise.

It is said that siblings of children with problems usually cope well and while our three older children have had their issues they and their friends do cope well with Harry. Likewise the neurotypical children in his school class have a remarkably good understanding of him, thanks to integration. They have been his best advocates at school (and at the local supermarket!) and more tolerant and able to see the good in him than children who have never known a child with autism.

There have been many times when I thought Harry had stopped making progress but after any rough spell he has improved again. He still struggles emotionally and socially, which is hard to watch, but most months we see definite changes. He ignored our first dog but he is very interested in our second dog and very involved in his care. It is very rare for us not to understand how he is feeling and what he means now, even if that is high anxiety when he wakes up to find his 19 year old sister has not returned yet from a party the night before.

We have made mistakes along the way: sending him to preschool too early before he could imitate and benefit from children's company, persevering with some behavioural drills for too long, and prompting him too much (too easy in a busy family). However, the information about what to do is clearer now and community (and hopefully government) awareness has improved. 'He has autism and is doing well' silences most uncalled-for comments from strangers and most people are pleased to help once they know what is wrong.

Music is another new find for him; he is quite rhythmic on the drums when not being silly. Music can open up all sorts of possibilities. He always sang beautifully in tune, but only recently did he start to sing at the same time as the other children in the choir (rather than a few minutes after everyone!)

I have found trying to fit into systems such as education one of the hardest things. Despite autism being relatively common there are remarkably few options for autism-specific approaches at school (or at least in our state) so we are always trying to work around the system and ' keep up appearances' rather than just concentrating on making progress step by step.

A friend once said to me it will be two steps forward, one step back, and this has been very true for us. We have learnt to savour enthusiasm from the good weeks and to keep going during the hard ones. Harry at 11 years is still learning a lot of new language and reading our expressions more easily. His eye contact is spontaneous and for a purpose rather than in response to that unhelpful command people love to use 'look at me'. He is also showing a lot more cunning and can be quite devious and lie to find a way to trick us, great developments for an autistic child.

Don't listen to those who tell you if they don't talk before five years they won't. Harry lost almost all of his language between two and five years despite a lot of speech therapy, and now he speaks in sentences spontaneously. Don't listen to those who tell you that you must start therapy and achieve results by seven years or whenever... the brain is neuroplastic thoughout life. Most of what Harry has learnt has been after seven years. It's obviously much much easier to begin as early as possible, before there is too much development to catch up and before there are lots of difficult behaviours. It's also much easier to fit into the school system if you begin as early as possible. However it is wrong that older children can't connect and make real progress. And we're keeping going.

Teenager alert — planning for the next phase
– *by Seana Smith*.

Our lovely boy Tom is 11 years old now, eight years have passed since we realised that he has ASD. Our family life no longer revolves exclusively around Tom, what a relief! His ASD used to fill up all the spaces, but these days ASD is just one part of Tom and one part of our family life.

There are four children in the family now and each needs a turn on centre stage, whether that means a toddler who is starving or needs a nappy changed, or our second son needing some special snuggle time with Dad.

Our 'new normal' as a family of six, is often pretty damn normal. We certainly look normal from afar and sometimes I get a real shock when things happen that make me see how clearly ASD still does impact our lives.

Sometimes we 'forget' that Tom has ASD and we expect him to behave just like a typical child. We get annoyed with him if he is clumsy and drops things, or doesn't understand what we are saying to him or if kids come round and he gets overloaded and withdraws from them.

We had a huge fright recently when he became horribly obsessive and then threw a series of massive, explosive tantrums, and we had to rapidly make some changes to bedtimes and sensory stimulation levels. We also dusted off our trusty copy of Boardmaker and made some visual schedules again. It was weird to have a child who could be so very autistic one week and then go off and have a terrific and problem-free time at school camp the next week. No wonder we're still confused.

But that's high functioning ASD, Tom looks so normal and is so normal some of the time, why can't he just be OK all the time? Does he really have to converse around the topic of milkshakes quite so much… and what's the thing about having a pork pad thai EVERY Sunday night? I still do sometimes wonder whether he couldn't just pull himself together and snap out of it. Oh dear.

Having the twins in 2006 threw a real spanner in the works in terms of having time to be with Tom. Over the past two years, we have done very little that is therapeutic and are lucky that he has still progressed, probably thanks to his very positive school environment.

But the time is coming to focus on Tom a lot more. There are two more years before high school. Finding the best school will require much effort and mental fortitude. Preparing him and making the transition process will need a lot of time and effort. Planning for puberty and adolescence must also be done and we are sure to need a lot of help with that.

Tom also has lots of learning difficulties, and he does have some 1:1 and small group lessons at school. It was a relief when we let go of the idea that he could keep up with the rest of the class in all subjects. He can't, and we knew that even if we worked him to death academically, he would always have issues, the ones typical of his type of ASD, plus learning difficulties with maths. Nowadays we always chose family time, time to play sport and time to relax over working him to the bone.

The spectre of the teenage and young adult years can bring us out in a cold sweat. Probably the best thing we can do as parents is to be in the best mental state as possible ourselves and to make sure that we work as a team. That's a pretty big ask! The good thing is that with our eldest child being the one on the spectrum, we will, as ever, learn the hard way with him and be able to put those experiences into practise with the other three. Well, here's hoping…

In the longer term, we don't know what the future holds for Tom, nor for the rest of the family. This of course, is true for everyone. It does concern us that Tom functions well enough to live in mainstream society but he lacks so many skills that one needs to survive in it: 'street smarts', negotiation skills, knowing when someone is ripping you off.

However, we chose, most days, not to have fears for the future nor regrets over the past. We have learned that all we really have is the present, and it's best to make that positive and fun for us all. Let the future take care of itself.

The children who do very well in IBA programs are sometimes referred to as the 'best outcome' kids. At the end of his program Tom still tested as having a massive speech delay and an IQ test showed a score of about 70 (borderline for intellectual disability.) So that is definitely not 'best outcome.' But I think that our family had a terrific outcome from early intervention and from intensive support at school in the first few years. It cost us a fortune, but it has been well worth it for us and in ways that cannot be gauged by language and IQ scores.

So here are a few of my personal assessment scores on where we are today:

The Kids Club Score: When we send Tom to holiday programs or to kids' clubs, he needs no support. I sometimes tell the carers that he has a language delay and suggest they speak slowly and clearly if he seems not to understand something. But all those hours, weeks and years of teaching imitation skills have certainly paid off. If Tom is unsure of what to do, he just copies the other kids.

The Cricket Club Test: In his third year of cricket, Tom is doing really well. If we told the other parents he has ASD, I'm sure they'd think that he was fine, but that we had Munchausen's Syndrome by Proxy. However, any canny ASD parent would see that, when not on the field, Tom doesn't chatter away and socialise like the other boys do, and a knowledgeable observer might spot the odd stim.

The Go Anywhere, Do Anything Criteria: There's really nowhere we would avoid going and nothing we would avoid doing because of Tom.

I can't say the same for the twins!

There are still a few assessment criteria we need to work on though:

The Playing with Toddler Siblings Test: It is so easy to see the core deficits of ASD in Tom's interaction with his twin toddler siblings. Tom just doesn't have the intuitive ability to adjust to their level and to their rapidly changing moods. He can be far too rough with them, even though he really loves them.

The 'What's He Up To Now' Test? Tom is not great at keeping himself gainfully employed and we like to know exactly where he is and what he's up to. Otherwise we can get surprises like 'Do you know your son is on top of the roof' or 'Mum, I was just seeing what happened if I poured the honey into my hand.' Our radars are always switched on as they have to be with much younger children.

Putting People Before Electronics Assessment: If he had his way, Tom would spend all his time playing PS2 or computer games and would lose all his social skills. We are very strict about how much 'screentime' he is allowed and have to deal with this very behaviourally.

The Table Manners Test: We need to work hard on this one as Tom is a messy eater, uses his hands, jumps up from the table etc. We do know EXACTLY what to do: comedy video models of good and bad table manners, clear descriptions of how to eat well, video self-models of Tom eating properly, then tick charts for good table manners with the reinforcer being a meal out with Mum. We know that will work; we just need to get a grip and do it.

The Taking Mum a Cup of Tea in Bed Test: This is the big one, and we have a long way to go!

Personally, I have a few plans in place for keeping healthy and happy. Sleep comes first, it's not unusual for me to go straight to bed after putting the four kids to bed. Even if I don't go straight to sleep, just lying in bed reading or watching TV feels like luxury.

Over the years I have realised that I need to self-soothe, so I have a little list of things to do when I start to get harassed, starting with a cup of tea and going all the way up to getting away for the night with a friend. I also attend a weekly self-development group meeting which I find invaluable. It isn't religious, but it is spiritual. And I do pray, not sure who I am praying to, but it is always a great comfort to me in times of distress. I think it's important to have lots of little things in life that you find enjoyable, things that are meaningful just to you. I really do try to stop and smell the roses, not to rush around and to keep calm. I love the book *Buddhism For Mothers* by Sarah Napthali and keep it in my bedside drawer to regularly dip into. Having been seriously depressed in the past and seriously hysterical too, I know I need to look after my mental health, for my own sake and for the sake of the kids.

We know that our family has been let off very lightly by ASD and we are tremendously grateful. ASD is a very serious thing to have, but at least we have the milder version to deal with. I believe that Tom can always keep improving, and that Paul and I can keep on growing as people and parents too. It's been a relief to let go of the idea of total recovery. We don't expect perfection in our lives, not in ourselves not in the kids…and come to think of it, not in this book either.

Jack in Year 6
– by Nicole Rogerson. Nicole and her husband have two sons, one of whom has autism. Nicole ran a home-based ABA program and 'loved it so much she bought the company' setting up the Lizard Children's Centre in Sydney. Nicole is also the founder of Autism Awareness.

These days I do not spend a minute thinking about Jack at school; whereas when he was in kindergarten, first and second grade, that's all I could think about. I'd check and re-check the time. At 2:30, I would drive to the school, just to sit outside wondering what he was doing in there. Was he hitting another child, screaming or perhaps running about and out of control? All of those worries now are such a distant memory. In fact, I am starting to forget what it felt like, to be perpetually on edge like that.

Challenging behaviours seem like a long time ago. I think behaviour is the biggest one for me and probably because it was the biggest hurdle for us to overcome. Jack was so incredibly hyperactive. He could not stand still, even for a moment. Think of a wind-up doll on Speed having a bad day, and that may have been one of our good days. Always alert, hyper-sensitive to sounds, he would just snap. It was horrible. Jack was so impossibly difficult to live with life was pretty awful.

There would have been few parents more relaxed about parenting, before autism, than Ian and I. We never wanted to be those parents who set rules and live and die by schedules — we hated that idea. But with autism our life became so increasingly miserable that I said to our ABA provider, 'just tell me what to do, and whatever it is, I'll do it'. I took notes and went home. We followed everything to the letter. We never wavered, and I believe that is why we have turned around the most hyperactive, God-awful autistic child with a major language disorder into the most gorgeous and well-behaved pre-teen. I might want this all rewritten when he's a teenager, but Jack is the most delightful child now and he has such empathy — I am just proud to be his Mum!

Jack's only really obvious autistic symptoms now centre on his language difficulties; he has a chronic language disorder. His desire to speak is phenomenal, he doesn't shut up anymore. He understands communicative intent, he WANTS to tell us things, he loves to tell us about his day but he just has such trouble doing it. I always say Jack has English as a fourth language!

Jack's very sociable at school. He's got his core set of mates, and has really befriended another autistic boy, who has done really well. He and Jack are firm friends. When I arrived at school last Friday, I saw Jack playing with this boy and it made me really teary because I remember when they were both two years old and so frighteningly autistic. It is astonishing to watch these two play, a testament to the countless hours of therapy. Jack has no idea his mate is a Lizard 'old-boy'. Those children have been lucky enough to have had the Rolls Royce of intervention, and autism has very little effect on their family lives anymore.

Jack has been on school camp three years in a row now. The kids get on big buses and go out of Sydney for two or three nights. Jack has to take all his own belongings in a bag and his teacher says he tries pretty much everything camp has to offer. He tends to find the first night a bit harder but given no aides accompany him on camp I think he's doing pretty well. Jack gets put in with his mates and they really help him out. Granted, we are blessed that he goes to a school with possibly the nicest bunch of kids in Australia. If he doesn't hear an instruction or doesn't understand it, he knows to follow their lead.

We spent years teaching Jack how to imitate others and this is how it pays off. I know a lot of new families look at the ABA imitation drills and think *what the hell are you people doing? This is ridiculous, what do you mean 'do this!'*. But all the hours we have spent doing the 'do this' has paid off and means Jack can go to camp and 'do this' without us or his therapists, with his peers, just like any other kid.

Our family loves to go out for meals, however when Jack was little we could never eat out, we were virtually housebound. If we left the confines of home everything focused on managing his behaviour, but now we can go out anywhere. A couple of weeks ago my father-in-law turned 97 and we held his birthday lunch in a posh restaurant at the Art Gallery of New South Wales. First, we did a tour of the art gallery and then we sat in the restaurant for three hours and proceeded to have a fabulous time. My boys came along, they joined in conversation, they drew on their notepads, they went outside and played on the grass, they surveyed the art and then came back to tell us what they'd seen. It was the most civilised day I think I've ever spent in my life. It makes me cry just thinking about it. Every effort, every therapist hour, every ABA drill = my boy Jack at 12.

I appreciate that everyone carries their own personal expectations and what they consider to be a level of success. I am sure some days people look at Jack with me and think 'oh that poor woman, she's got that disabled child'. Whereas, I think I've got the best autistic kid in the world. He gets on beautifully with his brother. They are so caring and thoughtful, they are an absolute joy.

Wherever your child is at, you've got to look at the positives, because the alternative will get you nowhere. Make a list of whatever your child is able to do right now, and don't let it become a list of what they can't do. Look at the things they can do, the one's they couldn't do before. These are all skills that you have taught them and how exciting is that! Don't stress out about it; just make sure that that list gets bigger. It is only then that you can make a list of what is left to teach them and that is the most powerful feeling in the fight against autism.

It took me a while to understand that Jack is not going to keep up with his peers and I'm okay with that. We finally accepted Jack was going to be different only after fighting as hard as we could to give him the possibilities that all the other kids get for free. We're fortunate to be in a financial situation which allows us to give him the most appropriate therapy available; while also having an aide to accompany him part of the time at school.

Recently, we found out about a special education unit at a private school on Sydney's North Shore. This unit will enable Jack to continue learning within a mainstream environment. At this school other activities will replace the subjects in which he cannot keep up. So, we've gone from an extremely expensive therapy to an extremely expensive private school. Unsurprisingly, running a comprehensive intervention program and having some support costs are more than we would like. It's meant sacrifices in other areas; we live in a tiny house, we don't have flashy expensive cars and we both work — a lot.

I think you get to a stage, and it's no doubt different for everyone, where the panicking just ceases. I can't explain how it happens, it's very subtle, but the panic stops. For me, it was when I accepted that I'd got Jack as far as I could within our circumstances. I accepted that I had done everything I could do, that ASD was not going to stop, but that the perpetual panic had to. The franticness has to stop; no one can keep going at that pace. I spent seven years, every night of the week, sitting in my home office making flash cards and work sheets, all designed to teach him language. Now I do it every school holidays and with a glass of wine. Don't let autism have the last say in your family — we kicked it out of ours.

Finishing high school on a high note
– by Kim. Kim and Dana live in Melbourne, Dana is the youngest of five children.

Although I had noticed my son did a few 'weird things' sometime between 12 and 18 months, I was not really concerned. After all, he had done all the 'normal' things like crawling and walking at all the average ages. But he hardly spoke. He had three older brothers and a sister who would predict everything he wanted before he even had the chance to ask.

He would sit for hours, swaying his head whilst listening to music, but I think I enjoyed the break from his general over-activity. Cuddling was always done on his terms — he would tuck in his legs and arms and I had to have both arms around him. He was difficult to get to bed at night. Sometimes he would bang his head on the wall next to his bed. He had regular night terrors, and often would wake at night.

He seemed to have hallucinations and would scream for no apparent reason, his lack of speech making it difficult to figure out the problem. He had little sensitivity to pain. Often he would wander off and just keep going in whatever direction he was facing. He would seem to ignore most people, except for his immediate family or close friends. My mother would occasionally ask: 'Are you sure he's not a little bit autistic?'

By the age of four, we started to become concerned. He never played with the other children. His teacher commented on how he would seem to be 'in a world of his own' when listening to music. He would dance and the other children would join in and make a group activity of it. My son would be totally oblivious to the other children dancing around him.

By this age he had some speech, but did not form his words correctly and was receiving speech therapy (but did not co-operate with the therapist). The head swaying continued while watching TV, listening to music, in the shower, when he was bored or tired and in bed. He would often have tantrums if he didn't get his own way or was frustrated.

His first year at school was difficult. He could be seen at play and lunch times sitting by himself, although he would play with other children if they asked him. He wouldn't speak in class or ask for help. If he broke a pencil, he would just sit and not do anything. Reading was a significant cause for concern.

If we were late for school or things were not routine in the morning, he would scream and have to be dragged into class. In winter, he would insist on wearing summer clothes and would throw a tantrum if he didn't get his way. I started to think my mother could be right and started to read every book I could on the subject of autism. Finally he was given a diagnosis of PDD-NOS.

At first I was relieved, I had suspected an ASD and it explained my son's behaviour. But I was soon to find out that no-one had heard of PDD-NOS, let alone understood what it meant. I blamed myself for not seeking help earlier when my son probably would have been given a diagnosis of autism, and would have received the help he so desperately needed.

Looking back, everything my son had done fitted into the mysterious syndrome called autism, but at the time things didn't seem so bad. I did have five children, and all of them had done some strange things and had difficult behaviour at times. I resolved to help my child reach his full potential.

Writing this now, Dana is 17. Things have changed dramatically; he is a completely different child, well, young man. Five years ago we just took one day at a time and were never really sure what the future would be. Now it looks very bright.

Just over five years ago, after 12 years of hard work and some strict dietary intervention, things began to turn around. His violent meltdowns disappeared, he told us his thinking was clearer, the need for routine slowly abated, and his health improved. He started secondary school and, due to some dedicated teachers, received the understanding he needed.

Although he didn't qualify for assistance, he was placed in remedial classes for both Maths and English and received assistance whenever possible. By Year 9 he had improved so much in Maths he was placed in an advanced class. He is now in year 11 and is excelling in the creative subjects such as Media, Photography, and Computing. The only symptom that remains academically is difficulty with reading comprehension.

Teachers, although commenting that he is a little too quiet, often tell us that they wish they had a whole class of 'Danas'. Last year he received one of the major awards for his level, being for 'Hard Work and Determination'. This year he became a Peer Leader, assisting Year 7 students with the transition from primary to secondary school and helping to deal with any other difficulties.

Just over a year ago he started a part-time job as a cashier at our local supermarket. I was a little apprehensive at first, but he was so confident and has had no problems at all dealing with customers. He really enjoys having his own spending money, which, typical of teenagers, has gone on items such as CDs, a mobile phone and an iPod.

After-school activities include drama and dance classes. He is a member of a theatre group and performs several times a year. Until recently he was a member of a swimming squad, but had to give that up due to all his other activities and homework commitments.

All-in-all, despite being a teenager, Dana is a delight. He is an amazingly accepting, sensible, caring young man. The future has proven to be a lot different to the one we envisaged.

Living, loving and surviving with an autistic child
– by Dorothy McRae-McMahon. Dorothy McRae-McMahon is a retired minister of the Uniting Church in Australia. She was the first woman to be a moderator of the World Council of Churches Worship Committee. Dorothy is also the author of Rituals for Life, Love & Loss and Memoirs of Moving On.

When our son was brain-damaged at the age of two and half years, he went into a total autistic withdrawal. The fact that his autism was due to brain damage meant we were not in a position to hope for many changes in his behaviour. The medical profession and other health workers knew very little about autism in those days anyway. Christopher will turn 50 this year and has been in 24-hour care since he was 16.

When he was at home, I cared for a child who had no speech, was often significantly distressed with head banging, screaming and little sleep. He had 'pica', that is, he ate everything in sight, like paper, soap, nuts and bolts, rubber gloves, cigarette butts, his siblings' homework sheets and of course anything in the way of normal food at a phenomenal rate. He did things like emptying rubbish bins over the neighbour's fence, was not toilet trained at 16 years and would run away if anyone left the door unpadlocked.

We had three younger children who learned the hard way to care for themselves and to live with dysfunction around them. In some ways it troubled me that on their report cards there was inevitably something about their unusual maturity.

When Christopher was about eight, we found a Steiner Day Care Centre, which meant that I had a few hours in the middle of the day to rush around, wash sheets (we had three bed-wetters), tidy the house, get to the shopping and generally do what mothers do.

In the midst of all this, I decided that, if I was to survive, there were two areas in my life which needed to be cherished. I needed to find a way of 'living', of giving meaning, purpose and expression to my life outside the pre-determined caring for Christopher and his brother and sisters. I needed to affirm that I 'existed', that I was more than the carer of my son.

In the early years, when Christopher was at home all the time, I decided to do two matriculation subjects. Even though this meant later nights and grabbing bits of time when Christopher was relatively calm, it stimulated my mind and carried me beyond the endless practical caring I was doing. I passed both subjects with high marks because that activity meant so much to me.

For several years, I volunteered to go on the Lifeline phones, and later visited people who were suicidal. I and two friends from our church ran a monthly group luncheon in our homes for older people confined to their homes. I joined the local Labor Party and became politically active. There were other church and community activities as well.

Paradoxically I found that, to add to my life in ways of my choosing, renewed and refreshed it in the middle of my tiredness. It lifted my heart to be doing different things with other people, to be doing things I really liked to do, rather than what I needed to do.

In the early days, I was less good at finding ways to relax — this came later. I learned how to reflect on what it was that really renewed my spirit. Sometimes it was just escaping into a book, sometimes it was heading to where I could see a mountain or the skyline of the city. I gave myself permission to play and have treats — a bit foreign to my Scottish Methodist upbringing!

Then I learned to meditate and to dare to stay in the silence of my heart and feel my pain and grief. That took courage, but it was worth it. The reality is that, when life is so full of stress and sadness, you just keep going. It feels as though you can't afford to stop in case you can never start again: if you cry for your life and your child, the tears may fall forever. In fact, it is not so, especially if your have some wise company as you do it.

I also found that sometimes to laugh at things Christopher did was ok. I will always remember our youngest daughter, Melissa, running to me and saying, 'Come quickly Mummy! Chrissie has eaten Mary and Joseph and the angels and he's just going to eat the baby Jesus!' She had made a cardboard nativity scene for our mantelpiece and Christopher was just finishing off consuming it!

It was only when we placed Christopher into care that I knew what my life had been like — not just for me but for my husband and three younger children. Christopher began to have severe epileptic seizures, which these days require him to receive oxygen. We were also at the stage when the friends of his younger siblings were resisting coming to our place to play because they were a bit anxious about Christopher. Not that he was ever anything but gentle and relatively defenceless, but he did unexpected things and made strange noises.

To place him into a government facility was one of the hardest things I have ever done and I deeply respect that many other parents will choose differently. We chose a state-run facility because we felt that there were likely to be trained staff and a continuity of care. As it happens, not long ago, there was a government move to 'devolve' the people in Christopher's facility into community homes with smaller numbers in each household. This sounds reasonable, but when we looked into it, none of these households were to have trained staff and we knew that Christopher was really unable to relate to the community anyway.

In fact, institutional life suits him rather well. He likes things to be in a regular routine and was troubled when that could not be sustained at home. Food is regulated for him as well as exercise and the medication provided has calmed him down considerably. The staff members were able to toilet train him and he is given outings and holidays which he seems to enjoy. I don't know who he thinks his family are — he just looks at us vaguely and gratefully accepts any food provided. On the other hand, he does have some sense of 'belonging' to his companions in the care facility and keeps near to them when out walking and watches their activities.

I am eternally grateful to those who now care for Christopher and that he seems as happy as he ever could be. Melissa takes an active interest in his welfare. She goes shopping to buy him clothes, adds nice things to the furnishing of his room and CDs as he has always responded in a positive way to music.

To those who share something of the life which we have had with our son, I would say two things. From hard experience, I know that we do need to care for ourselves when we walk this journey. Stop and smell the roses or find some way to cherish yourself. This is no easy task. The other thing I would share is that I have often wondered, especially as a religious person, what the purpose of Christopher's life could be. I guess I always hope that he will have another chance to live more fully in some mystery beyond our seeing. However, I also believe that he, and people like him, bring out the best in the faithfulness of care and compassion in others, even if their own lives seem so limited.

12

RESOURCES AND SERVICES GUIDE

Listed here are all of the services and resources we are aware of. The first sections cover the whole of Australia: federally funded help, Australia-wide information and resources and a short guide to finding professionals. Next are state-by-state listings. Most of the services are autism-specific, since young children benefit most from autism-specific interventions.

It is inevitable that details will change. Luckily, we live in a multimedia world and this book is supported by a website. New information and updates will be available on:

www.autismhandbook.com.au

Website addresses have a habit of changing, so in this Resource Guide we have given the home page of most of the organisations listed. These home pages have search facilities so that you can, for example, go to www.centrelink.gov.au and then search for 'Carer Payment'. Updated full website addresses can be found on the address above.

If you are starting a service, or have some service or resource which you feel is suitable for inclusion in the *Australian Autism Handbook*, please do get in touch via the website and submit your details.

FINANCIAL HELP FOR CARERS

Helping Children with Autism

www.fahcsia.gov.au/autism

1800 289 177 *Helping Children with Autism* Inquiry Line

The Helping Children with Autism (HCWA) package is an initiative of the federal government which has committed $190 million over four years to June 2012. The package seeks to provide earlier and more accurate diagnosis of children with ASD; increased access to early intervention programmes for children and school students with ASD; as well as further support services for these children and students.

HCWA is described here in brief, listing components in the logical order in which families might use them and giving web links and contact details from which the latest information and applications can be obtained.

ASD Website

www.raisingchildren.net.au/autism

Information about all aspects of the HCWA package can be found on the website which is a part of HCWA. This is a large website and the first national one for ASD. It has factsheets, reliable information and interactive functions to support and inform parents, families, carers and professionals.

Medicare Rebates for Assessment and Diagnosis
www.health.gov.au/autism
There are two types of rebates. The first is for a paediatrician or psychiatrist to make a diagnosis and develop an autism treatment plan. This can only be used for children under the age of 13 years. You need a referral from a GP to the paediatrician or psychiatrist. The paediatrician or psychiatrist may also refer you to psychologists, speech pathologists or occupational therapists for up to four visits for the purpose of diagnosis and treatment planning.

Autism Advisor Program
www.fahcsia.gov.au/autism
Once a child aged 0 to 6 years has a formal diagnosis, the next step is to make an appointment to speak to the Autism Advisor service in your state. Your Autism Advisor can assist with information and support about: early intervention funding and options, parent support groups, playgroups, resources and all aspects of HCWA. Each of the state and territory autism associations has a team of Autism Advisors- see your state autism association for contact details.

Early Intervention Funding
www.fahcsia.gov.au/autism
All children with a diagnosis of an ASD aged 0 to 6 years has access to early intervention funding of up to $12,000 (up to $6,000 per financial year) regardless of whether or not they have commenced school. Families can use this funding to access services provided by members of the Early Intervention Service Provider Panel. Families who reside in an outer regional or remote area may also be eligible to access a one off payment of $2,000 per eligible child to cover the additional expenses associated with accessing early intervention services.

Early Days Workshops
www.earlydays.net.au
1800 334 155
Early Days workshops assist families and carers of children aged six years and under who have an ASD. The workshops explain ASD, give practical strategies for helping your child's development and parenting your child. They give information about therapies and services and can also be useful for forging support networks in your local area.

PlayConnect Playgroups

www.playconnect.com.au

Playgroups Australia is funded to run 150 PlayConnect Playgroups around Australia. PlayConnect Playgroups provide play-based learning opportunities for children with ASD or ASD like symptoms, and create and extend social support networks for their families and carers. Children will not require a formal diagnosis of an ASD to attend.

Positive Partnerships

www.autismtraining.com.au

Positive Partnerships: supporting school aged students on the autism spectrum delivers the two components of the HCWA package being implemented by the Department of Education, Employment and Workplace Relations (DEEWR). Its aim is to improve the educational outcomes for school aged children with ASD. The two components are: two-days workshops for families and carers of school aged children and five-day professional development programs for teachers.

Medicare Rebates for Therapies

Once an autism treatment plan has been made, each child can access 20 Medicare rebates (in total, not annually) for treatment from a psychologist, speech pathologist or occupational therapist. The treatments can be a combination of all of these professionals. These can be accessed by children up to the age of 15 years so long as their diagnosis occurred before they were 13 years old.

Carer Financial Support

Carer Allowance

Disability, Sickness and Carers: 13 27 17

www.centrelink.gov.au

Carer Allowance (child) is a supplementary payment for parents or carers who provide daily care and attention for children with a disability or severe medical condition at home. It is paid fortnightly by Centrelink and is not means tested. Carers and a medical professional need to fill in the form. This is usually done when a child receives a formal diagnosis. Carer Allowance commences from the date the form is lodged, not the date of diagnosis, so it is a good idea to get it in ASAP.

From 2007 for the next five years there will be an additional annual $1,000 payment to the carer for each child with a disability for whom they are receiving payment of Carer Allowance (child). This payment is made by

Centrelink automatically each 1st July.

Carer Payment
Disability, Sickness and Carers: 13 27 17
www.centrelink.gov.au
Carer Payment (child) is an income support payment for people who cannot support themselves through participation in the workforce while caring for a child with a profound disability who has extremely high care needs. This payment is means tested.

Health Care Card
Disability, Sickness and Carers: 13 27 17
www.centrelink.gov.au
When Carer Allowance (child) is paid then the child is also eligible for a Health Care Card. The card is usually sent out to the child automatically once the Carer Allowance has been set up. The card entitles you to reduced cost medicines under the Pharmaceutical Benefits Scheme (PBS). Many GPs and some specialists will bulk bill Health Care Card holders. Some cinemas, theatres, fun parks and major events will allow Health Care Card holders reduced entry fees, or allow free entry to the child's carer.

Medicare Entitlements
Medicare Safety Net
13 20 11
www.medicareaustralia.gov.au
Medical costs can be very high, especially in the first years after diagnosis, or when a diagnosis is being sought. Families can register for the Medicare Safety Net. After the safety net threshold is reached, Medicare pays higher benefits. These are definitely worth applying for so be sure to register for the safety net ASAP. If your child has a Health Care Card then your safety net amount is lowered and you get higher benefits sooner.

Enhanced Primary Care (EPC) Medicare Services
Medicare Enquiry Line: 13 20 11
www.health.gov.au
Your GP can refer you to an allied health professional (eg physio, OT, speech therapist) and you can get 5 EPC Medicare rebates per calendar year to help cover the cost of those visits. Although this is not a great deal each little bit adds up: help with the cost of five speech pathology visits is certainly better than no help at all.

The referrals can only be done if you have what used to be called a 'care plan' prepared by your GP. These are now called GP Management Plans (GPMP) if less than three health professionals are involved, or Team Care Arrangements (TCA) if three or more health professionals are involved. You will also need a EPC referral form prepared by your GP. This needs to have the name and contact details of the allied health professionals on the form. This form is signed when you see the allied health person and you take this to Medicare to get your rebate.

If your GP is not familiar with writing these 'care plans' they can ask Medicare for more information on them.

GP Mental Health Care Plan

Medicare Enquiry Line: 13 20 11

www.health.gov.au

Your GP can also refer you, your child or indeed the whole family to a psychologist and Medicare will pay a rebate which will partly cover the cost of the visit. Your GP needs to prepare a GP Mental Health Care plan, which is also referred to as item no. 2710. ASD itself is not a condition eligible for this plan, however anxiety, depression and other conditions sometimes found in children and adults with ASD (and their families) are eligible.

You do not need to take any forms to the psychologist, just pay them as usual. You can then go to Medicare with the receipt and they will give you a rebate. You can claim a Medicare benefit for up to 12 visits a year per person. There will usually be a gap payment of some sort payable by you. A review by the GP is necessary after the first six visits to keep getting the rebate. This plan can also cover visits to some OTs or social workers.

Tax — Rebates and Trusts

Medical Expenses Tax Rebate

Australian Tax Office

Personal tax enquiries: 13 28 61

www.ato.gov.au

Taxpayers can claim a tax rebate for a percentage of their family's net medical expenses. Net medical expenses are the medical expenses you have paid less any refunds you got, or could get, from Medicare or a private health fund.

You can claim a tax offset of 20% — 20 cents in the dollar — of your net medical expenses over $1,500. There is no upper limit on the amount.

Included in the list of eligible medical expenses is: 'for therapeutic treatment under the direction of a doctor'. This covers speech therapy, OT and ABA therapy (but not educational materials.) You need to have an annual referral letter indicating that the services are necessary. Of course, it is best to make sure you have an accountant help you with claiming this tax rebate.

Special Disability Trust

Centrelink: 13 10 21

www.fahcsia.gov.au

Special Disability Trusts can be set up by self-employed persons only for the benefit of young children with a disability. You will definitely need a good accountant to help you with this.

Child Care

Inclusion Support Program

www.fahcsia.gov.au

FaHCSIA operates the inclusion support program in all federally funded child care centres, these include:

- Long Day Care
- Outside School Hours (including Vacation Care)
- Occasional Care
- Family Day Care
- In Home Care.

Funding from this program can provide training, the employment of support staff and equipment. The website has links to the 67 regionally based Inclusion Support Agencies (ISAs) which employ Inclusion Support Facilitators (ISFs) to work directly with child care services to build and develop skills. Use the link above to find your local ISA.

Preschool Support

Whilst long day care centres are funded by the federal government, preschools are funded by state governments and each state has a different scheme for supporting the inclusion of children with additional needs. You will need to talk to your local preschool about how to access support funding.

In Home Care

National In Home Child Care Association: 02 4353 5322

www.inhomechildcare.com.au

In Home Care enables parents to access child care when other child care services are unable to meet their needs. This means having a carer look after children in their home. Under this system families can access Child Care

Benefit and also the Inclusion Support Program funding mentioned above.

If a child has a disability then families are eligible for In Home Care. Although this is a national program there is no website at present giving details on the services which support In Home Care in each state. However, the NSW website above gives all the basic information and details of agencies in other states.

Carer Support and Respite for Carers

Respite means having a break, and we are sure that anyone reading this book deserves one. Unfortunately there is no simple method of finding out which services might be available to you. Some useful places to start your search are listed below. Word of mouth is also a terrific way to find out way through the respite maze, so if you can locate a family which is further down the track, pump them for all the information you can.

Your state autism association may also be able to provide help and advice with respite, as may your state Carers Association — see state listings for contact details. Your state Carers Association will also have brochures and pamphlets.

But let us not forget that friends and family can, if we are lucky, provide us with much-needed respite as well. See the Advice for Family and Friends chapter.

Commonwealth Carer Resource and Respite Centres
1800 059 059
www.healthconnect.gov.au
DoHA has a National Respite for Carers Program (NRCP) which aims to support and assist relatives and friends caring at home for people who are unable to care for themselves because of chronic illness, disability or frailty.

The program provides both information and support for carers and respite itself. There are approximately 90 Commonwealth Carer Respite Centres and outlets established across Australia and a Commonwealth Carer Resource Centre has been established in each state and territory capital city. There is one national Commonwealth Carer Resource Centre. The Resource Centre for each state is listed under each state: in NSW see Carers NSW, in WA see Carers WA. This state Resource Centre can send out information to you.

The central number given above will connect you to your nearest Respite Centre. This should be able to provide emergency respite and possibly some short-term planned respite, and should also be able to give you details of local respite services.

The National Carer Counselling Program is also funded. This is administered by the Resource Centre in your state. It allows carers to access a counsellor for short periods at no cost. This is a really useful service and one that has been tremendously helpful for many families.

Carelink
www.commcarelink.health.gov.au
Carelink is another information source. Go to the website and click on Search for Services and search for 'respite' using your postcode. This should provide a number of listings for you to explore.

Home and Community Care (HACC) Program
www.health.gov.au
HACC is a joint Australian, state and territory program which provides community care services to frail aged and younger people with disabilities, and their carers. The services funded through the HACC Program include, but are not limited to:

- nursing care
- allied health care
- meals and other food services
- domestic assistance
- personal care
- home modification and maintenance
- transport
- respite care
- counselling, support, information and advocacy
- assessment.

Some services charge a small fee that varies from state to state. Most families with young children who access this service receive assistance with home care, and some in-home respite care. There are over 3,000 organisations which administer HACC, to find out your local provider call your state disability department and/or your local council who ought to be able to point you in the right direction.

MyTime Groups
1800 889 997
www.mytime.net.au
MyTime groups provide local support for families caring for a young child under school age with a disability or chronic medical condition. MyTime gives

families the chance to socialise and share ideas with others who understand the rewards and intensity of the caring role.

Parents can meet with people in similar circumstances to have fun, swap information and find out about available community support. Research-based parenting information is also available at group meetings. Each group has a play helper who can lead children in activities such as singing, drawing, playing with toys, blocks or sand so parents can spend time catching up with others.

INFORMATION AND RESOURCES

ASD General Information

Australian Advisory Board on ASDs (AABASD)
www.autismaus.com.au
The Australian Advisory Board is the national peak body representing people who have an ASD, their families, carers and helpers. The board's member organisations are the state autism associations. The focus of the board is working with governments to develop appropriate policies for people who have an autism spectrum condition, their families and carers, disseminating information about ASDs and working with the Australian ASD community to build skills. The important 2007 report commissioned by the AABASD 'Prevalence of Autism in Australia: Can it be established from existing data?' is available on this site.

Autism, Asperger's and Pervasive Developmental Disorders
www.autism-help.org
This comprehensive and reliable Australian website has a wealth of information about autism, Asperger's syndrome and PDD-NOS. There are over 350 fact sheets of information, with much practical help and advice offered. Many personal stories from parents and from children, teenagers and adults who

have an ASD are given. Highly recommended site especially for its emphasis on assisting families who cannot access expensive therapies.

Autism Help
www.autismhelp.info
This initiative of Gateways, a Victorian disability support service, is a very thorough website. The aim of the site is to increase awareness of ASD and to provide practical strategies and resources to benefit preschool, primary and secondary teachers, child care workers, integration aides and health professionals.

ASD Advocacy
A4 — Autism Asperger's Advocacy Australia
www.a4.org.au
Autism Asperger's Advocacy Australia (A4) is a national grassroots organisation comprising and representing people with an ASD, their families and associates.

A4's Vision.
1. People with ASD in Australia, their families and carers will:
    a. live as independently as they can and
    b. choose and achieve their personal goals and aspirations.
2. People in Australia in collaboration with stakeholders will:
    a. remove barriers to the participation and achievement of people with an ASD, their families and carers
    b. value and respect the contributions and diversity that people with an ASD, their families and carers bring to their community and
    c. ensure people with ASD, their families and carers can receive, in a timely manner, the treatment, services, support, protections and opportunities that they need.

A4's Mission.
Autism Asperger's Advocacy Australia will:
1. advocate nationally for progress towards our vision
2. educate and inform people in Australia about ASD and
3. monitor and report on issues and outcomes relating to people with an ASD and their associates.

Membership of A4 is free and regular newsletters are distributed by email. There is much of interest to be read in the archived Newsletters on the website.

Autism Awareness

www.autismawareness.com.au
Autism Awareness is a Sydney-based parent group which raises awareness and lobbies at a national, state and grassroots level.

Early Intervention

Early Childhood Intervention Australia

www.ecia.org.au
This national organisation has links to all the state early intervention peak bodies. You should be able to find your nearest generic early intervention service through these websites.

Child Care

Child Care Access Hotline

1800 670 305
This is a national service which provides information and contact details for Commonwealth-funded child care services in all local areas. Information about help with the cost of care and with programs to assist children with a disability in child care is also available.

Disabled Parking Permits

These may not be the first thing you think of when your child is diagnosed with ASD, but they can help make life a bit easier for families and carers. Walking a long way to the car when carrying a tantrumming child is to be avoided whenever possible! Each state has different rules for eligibility entitlements. VicRoads, the Roads Corporation of the Victorian Government has a very useful brochure: Disabled Persons Parking Schemes in Australia (see www.vicroads.vic.gov.au).

Sibling Support

Some state autism associations run sibling support programs. Check details in state listings.

Siblings Australia

www.siblingsaustralia.org.au
Siblings Australia is a unique national organisation committed to enhancing the wellbeing of the siblings of children with disabilities and chronic illness.

Siblings Australia has developed a number of resources for parents and providers. These include:
- a brochure for parents on supporting siblings
- a manual for facilitators wishing to run sibling groups
- a participant booklet for children attending the group
- Directions for Sibling Support: A Guide for Disability Organisations
- a library of books for loan

Australian Autism Resources

If you are receiving the Carer Allowance and wondering what on earth you will spend the annual $1,000 allowance on — just joking — then look no further, there are many useful Australian resources. If you know of others, please let us know via our website at:
www.autismhandbook.com.au

FREE RESOURCES

There are a number of free resources to be found. Many of the state autism associations have electronic information sheets. Find details in the state listings. The ACT-NOW website (see p 338) has a large number of very useful information sheets including: toilet training, visual supports, preschool teachers and families working as a team, choosing and evaluating treatments and fussy eaters. There are helpful for families and good for giving to preschools, schools, relatives and friends.

Helping You and Your Family — Self-Help Strategies for Parents of Children with a Disability

www.acd.org.au/information/content/HYYF_2001.pdf

This is a free PDF download written by the Association for Children With A Disability and designed as a companion volume to 'Through the Maze: A Guide to Benefits and Services for Families of Children with a Disability' written for Tasmania, NSW and Victoria (more info in state listings).

Helping You and Your Family has practical ideas and advice and is useful for families all over Australia.

Bookshops and Book Sellers

Book In Hand

PO Box 899
Redcliffe Qld 4020
07 3283 8214

1800 505 221 Landline only (Leave message if unattended; all calls will be returned).

www.bookinhand.com.au

Book in Hand stocks and sells the majority of books relating to ASD that are published in the English language. Mail order is available, and if the item is on the shelf, delivery to most cities is within 1–2 working days. Prices, book lists and postal charges are on the website.

Experienced staff will help individual customers choose the most useful book if this is required and will assist with selections for libraries and schools on request. As well as emailing, customers are encouraged to make phone contact as this is more flexible and interactive.

Book in Hand attends conferences and seminars in all states, and can make appointments to visit organisations when in your area. On approval service is available. There is a part-time shop front available in Redcliffe, Queensland for locals and visitors to SE Queensland.

Co-ordinates Therapy Services

PO Box 59,
West Brunswick Vic 3055
03 9380 1127
www.autismbookshop.com
www.therapybookshop.com
www.therapytoyshop.com
www.sensoryshop.com
www.speechtherapyshop.com

Coordinates Therapy Services is a Melbourne-based supplier of specialist books and equipment, with a particular emphasis on toys, sensory equipment and occupational and speech therapy aids. The proprietor, Jenny Reed, is an OT and is able to talk to potential customers about their child and what items might be useful.

If in Melbourne, you can call ahead to make an appointment to look at books and other items at the warehouse which is open to public by appointment only, Monday – Friday 9am – 5pm.

Innovative Communication Programming

9 Oaklands Avenue
Beecroft NSW 2119
www.innovativeprogramming.net.au

Innovative Communications produces many useful resources for the topic of augmentative communication (using visual aids and sign language). Many of the resources have a specific autism focus. Training courses and workshops are also run and private services can be accessed. The company produces a software program called Softpics which is a lovely library of clipart type images for creating Augmentative Communication Displays. It contains over 2,500 images and a large range of design tools, which allows you to create displays that can be tailored to individual needs.

OT Resources

See **Co-ordinates Therapy Services** above

Easy Kids

10 Millaroo Drive
Helensvale Qld 4212
07 5519 4566
www.weightedblanketsandvests.com
Easy Kids manufactures a range of weighted products which were designed and trialled with the help of OTs. The range includes weighted vests, blankets, shoulder wraps and wrist bands.

Kids Therapy Network

623 Glenhuntly Rd
South Caulfield Vic 3162
03 9532 7509
www.kidstherapynetwork.com.au
Kids Therapy Network is an OT practice which also sells a range of therapeutic toys and activities from its well-presented website.

Life Skills 4 Kids

www.lifeskills4kids.com.au
Debbie Hopper is an OT based in Forster in NSW. From her website, she sells weighted wheat packs for use around the neck and shoulders and for laps. She also sells a Canadian product, Stickids, an interactive software program which can be used to help support children with sensory integration, processing and motor challenges.

DVDs

See **Professor Tony Atwood's** website www.tonyattwood.com.au for a list of his DVDs.

Autism Spectrum Australia (Aspect) Building Foundations

www.aspect.org.au

Aspect has produced an information pack with a manual and DVD specifically for families of children newly diagnosed with ASD. This features four young children and their families and explains simple initial steps that all families can take to assist their child. 'Building Foundations' is available in seven languages.

Autism Essentials DVD Program

www.autism-essentials.com

Created by Monique Simpson, who runs Connect Therapy in Sydney, The Autism Essentials DVD Program is relevant for children functioning across the autism spectrum. The program includes eight educational DVDs and a training manual designed to increase parents' knowledge of their own child's sensory, emotional, thinking, learning, communication and behavioural patterns. Throughout the program parents are asked to pause their DVD and complete exercises that help them identify exactly where their child is breaking down in development. It then shows parents how they can work on these deficit areas in the home environment using fun, effective and practical therapy techniques.

Being Responsive — You and Your Child with Autism

www.uq.edu.au/sbs/responsivity

Click on About The DVD

This 45-minute-interactive DVD was produced by University of Queensland education and health researchers. It provides information and instructions on how to use techniques that increase opportunities for social interaction in everyday situations.

During the video component of the DVD, four families who participated in the program talk about the techniques they used with their child and demonstrate how these helped to improve everyday interactions. Members of the research team provide additional information and tips about how to enhance communication and social interaction. There are Activity Sheets on the DVD and also at the website. The DVD can be purchased via the website.

Bridges ABA DVDs

www.bridgesabatapes.com

There are several ABA training programs available in the USA. This one has an Australian distributor.

Imagine Having Asperger's Syndrome

www.glenirispsychology.com.au

'Imagine Having Asperger's Syndrome: A First Consultation' is based on presentations made by clinical psychologist Richard Eisenmajer at professional development sessions in schools throughout Victoria and at information sessions for carers and families. Using anecdotes and case studies from his clinical practice Richard explains the main features and common presentations of people with ASD. The DVD aims to provide parents, teachers, and other professionals insight into how people with ASD experience the world, and practical and effective strategies for interacting with and managing people with this condition. The DVD (also available in video format) is available through his practice, Autism Victoria or at selected bookshops.

Kid Can Do

www.kickstartkids.com.au

Kid Can Do is a video modelling DVD for Australian kids. Developed by a OT, a speech therapist and a TV producer, it is an entertaining developmental tool for kids. Focussing on key pre-school social skills, Kid Can Do encourages the development of sensory motor development and language skills. It has an original score, with a few remixed traditional songs thrown in for familiarity. The DVD is full of kids and games, and comes with a comprehensive guide for parents/carers to help kids maximise their kid skills. While it has been created as a tool for kids on the autism spectrum, Kid Can Do is perfect for helping any preschooler develop life skills.

Systematic Behaviour Management

Flinders University Early Intervention Research Program (EIRP)

www.socsci.flinders.edu.au/psyc/research/autism/trainingmaterials.php

The Behaviour Intervention Implementation Guide (BiiG) is useful as a home-based therapy companion. The BiiG shows the progression of a beginner program through to intermediate, then advanced levels. Users are guided step-by-step through each individual program, with full descriptions and video examples.

Tom's Toilet Triumph

www.familiesandcommunities.sa.gov.au (Search for Tom's Toilet Triumph!)

Tom's Toilet Triumph is a humourous cartoon for children about toilet training. It is part of the 'Are You Ready?' toilet training package produced by Disability South Australia for parents, carers and educators.

Video Modelling
www.video-modeling.com
Offering educational DVDs from Australia and the USA eg the Watch Me Learn series and Fitting In and Having Fun, this site offers general information about video modelling.

Language Teaching Cards

Inekards

www.inekards.com.au
A comprehensive flashcard library system developed specifically for children with autism and language difficulties. This progressive learning series enables you to teach a child effectively through clear photographic visuals and help promote communication and language skills.

Inekards can be used as stimulus in many educational and therapy settings including: speech therapy, special education, preschools, ABA therapy, OT and schools.

All flashcards are:
- laminated for durability with rounded corners for safety
- designed using clear consistent photographs without confusing backgrounds.

Each volume is boxed for easy access and compact storage.

Winning Connection

www.winningconnection.com.au
Winning Connection has developed a flashcard system to ensure sound results when teaching children with ASD. The flashcards are also used successfully with children who have pervasive developmental delay and language delays.

The flashcards are carefully designed by specialists for targeted, developmental learning for your child. The range includes 828 superb clear images, available in a variety of convenient sets: emotions, verbs, sequencing and categories.

The pictorial representations in the flashcards are clear and without irrelevant or confusing background information. Each card is laminated for extra protection ensuring a long-lasting durable resource ideal for schools and resource libraries as well as in the home.

Visuals — Software

Flash Pro
www.helpingtogrow.com

Flash Pro is an Australian-produced CD-ROM with thousands of photographs and templates.

Free Visuals

You can also collect visual images from the Internet. Here are a few ideas of where to look:
Supermarket and shopping websites
http://pics.tech4learning.com
http://images.google.com.au/
www.do2learn.com

Visual Supports and Communication Systems

Spectronics Australia
PO Box 88
Rochedale Qld 4123
07 3808 6833
www.spectronicsinoz.com
Spectronics Australia sells Boardmaker and many other inclusive learning technologies. For information on Boardmaker see p. 77. A 30-day trial period is available from the US parent company.

See **Innovative Communication Programming** above for information on their Softpix visuals.

PECS — Pyramid Educational Consultants
www.pecsaustralia.com
For information on PECs – see p 78.

See-n-Speak
PO Box 473
Winston Hills NSW 2153
02 9620 7345
www.seeandspeak.com.au
See-n-Speak produces visual supports for children with ASD, speech and/or language disorders, English as a second language. The visuals can assist with acceptable behaviour, communication, interaction, play and social skills, toileting and building self-esteem. All See-n-Speak photographic visuals were

created by a mother and grandmother of a beautiful little boy with special needs. Through visuals he was encouraged to make his own choices, communicate, interact, build his self-esteem, relieve his anxiety with schedules and routines, and to expand his expressive and receptive language. Now the company is dedicated to helping other children benefit from visual communication.

Think In Pictures
PO Box 3087
Rouse Hill NSW 2155
02 8824 3917
www.thinkinpictures.com.au
Think In Pictures provides visual resources for schools, child care centres and families. The visual resources are designed for all children but with a focus on children with ASD, Attention Deficit Disorder, anxiety and impaired communication. The visual packages are designed to assist the children by providing structure and routine, supporting transitional times, providing forewarning of any changes, alleviating anxiety, increasing independence and reducing inappropriate and challenging behaviours. All visual products are designed and created by a special education teacher. Packages include timetables, calendars, choice boards and basic visual signs. Think In Pictures also offers custom made visual packages to meet individual needs.

Tiptoe Educational Products
www.tiptoeep.com.au
Reinforcer charts and weekly planners are available from this Adelaide-based website.

MLAK — Keys for Public Toilets
The MLAK is a scheme that provides a universal lock and key to allow people with disabilities 24-hour access to public facilities. Accessible facilities should be open during the day, but it is sometimes necessary to lock them after hours. The MLAK is designed to increase access to these facilities.

People with a disability can purchase their own universal key from their local Master Locksmith. Contact the Master Locksmiths Association on 1800 810 698 or www.masterlocksmiths.com.au. Availability is restricted to people who have a mobility difficulty OR who have written authority from a doctor or an organisation.

The scheme started in NSW and is rolling out across the states. Find more information on toilet locations at: www.scia.org.au.

Therapy Dogs

Righteous Pups

Bendigo

www.righteouspups.org.au

They provide trained therapy dogs to assist children with ASD.

See also:

www.humananimalinteraction.org.au

General Educational Resources Educational Experience

www.edex.com.au

Modern Teaching Aids

www.teaching.com.au

Australia-wide Training – For Parents and Professionals

Most **state autism associations** offer training; check your local state for details.

Many **early intervention providers** and multidisciplinary centres also offer training, see state listings.

See **ASD Consultancy and Support Service** on p. 250

See **Autism Essentials** above

See **Education Events** on p. 270

Autism Pro

www.autismpro.com.au

Autism Pro is an online autism therapy support system for families, educators and clinicians.

Finding Professionals

Most of the state autism associations can point you in the direction of professionals with experience and interest in ASD. Other parents can provide their own lists of favourite and not-so-favourite professionals: please bear in mind that whilst one family might get on well with a certain professional another family might not. You can also find professionals through their state and federal professional organisations.

Speech Pathologists
www.speechpathologyaustralia.org.au
Click on the *Public Information* link
The Speech Pathology Australia website includes private speech pathologist directories for some of the larger Australian states.

Occupational Therapists
www.ausot.com.au
The OT Australia website has a *Find an OT* link which clicks through to state directories of private occupational therapists.

Psychologists
www.psychology.org.au
Click on *Find A Psychologist*
The Australian Psychological Society (APS) is the largest professional association for psychologists with over 15,000 members.

Paediatricians, Developmental Paediatricians, Child Psychiatrists and Neurologists
It is important to find medical specialists who have a lot of experience with ASD. Again a good place to start is by calling your state autism association. Your GP may also be able to help.

ACT

State Autism Association

Autism Asperger ACT
c/- SHOUT (Self Help Organisations United Together)
PO Box 717
Mawson ACT 2607
02 6290 1984
http://autism.anu.edu.au
Autism Asperger ACT Inc is a non-profit, non-political community organisation, run by parents and other interested people. The association works to improve the lives of children and adults who have an ASD. Autism Asperger ACT is committed to raising the understanding of ASD in the ACT community. Membership is open to any one who has an interest in ASD. There is no membership fee.

Autism Asperger ACT activities are focused on exchanging information, developing support networks and assisting people to learn new skills. The Association holds monthly meetings, support groups and games sessions for people who have Asperger's syndrome. In addition, the association holds occasional workshops and seminars, and distributes a newsletter six times a year. A small group of siblings (7 to 12 years of age) also meets monthly to have fun and support one another.

State Disability Department

Therapy ACT and Disability ACT

ACT Department of Disability, Housing and Community
Nature Conservation House
153 Emu Bank
Belconnen ACT 2617
02 6207 1086
Intake 02 6205 1246
www.dhcs.act.gov.au/therapyact

Therapy ACT offers multi-disciplinary therapy and family support for children from birth to eight years of age and children, young people and adults with developmental disabilities from birth to 65 years of age who are residents of the ACT.

Therapy and support services are available for physiotherapy, occupational therapy, speech pathology, social work and psychology. Therapy ACT provides single and multi-disciplinary assessments and intervention services.

Therapy ACT provides a 'Drop-In' service for ACT residents. This service allows parents or caregivers with concerns about their child's development to attend a 'drop in' clinic to see a speech pathologist or physiotherapist without an appointment.

THERAPY ACT DIAGNOSTIC ASSESSMENT SERVICES

Therapy ACT provides a comprehensive multi-disciplinary diagnostic assessment for ASD. The assessment is carried by a team of psychologists, speech therapists and occupational therapists and is provided free of charge to ACT residents.

DISABILITY ACT INFORMATION SERVICE

The Information Service provides a centralised contact point for people with disabilities, their families and carers, and other members of the community seeking information about disability matters within the ACT. The service also provides information on respite options and disability services in the ACT.

The Information Service is also a point of application for Disability ACT's funding packages.

DISABILITY ACT RESPITE PROGRAM

Respite homes provide a supported environment that endeavours to make each person's stay as comfortable as possible to enable the primary carers to take a well-earned break. Disability ACT operates four respite houses. There are two houses for children (for children aged 5–12 years and young people

13–18 years) and two for adults. All ACT residents who support a person with a diagnosed intellectual disability or other significant developmental delay are eligible to access this service.

AFFIRM

A Family-centred Flexible Intensive Response Model (AFFIRM) is designed to respond to families of children and young people with a disability who have high and complex needs. The service is intended to address situations where ongoing family-based care is unlikely to be maintained in the absence of a specialised and/or intensive intervention. Referral and further information can be obtained through phoning (02) 6207 1086.

State Health Department

ACT Health

GPO Box 825
Canberra City ACT 2601
13 22 81
Community Health Intake 02 6207 9977
www.health.act.gov.au

CHILD HEALTH MEDICAL OFFICERS — offer services to children less than 18 years of age where there are medical or developmental concerns. A referral is required from other health or education professionals, or community workers.

COMMUNITY PAEDIATRICS AND CHILD HEALTH SERVICE — offer specialised secondary medical services to children and adolescents under 18 where there are medical or developmental concerns. The service provides medical and/or developmental assessment and case management. This service is not an acute response service. In order to access the service, the child must have been seen by primary assessment services such as other health or education professionals, or community workers, who will provide a written referral.

MATERNAL AND CHILD HEALTH NURSES — provided by Community Health Intake, they cover: postnatal and early childhood parenting support, lactation advice, home visiting, immunisation, asthma education, health checks and referral to multi-disciplinary professional services to children, youth and families.

Your Local Council

Many local councils around Australia have a Disability Information Officer or Community Care Officer. It is well worth getting in touch with your local council to ask about local services and assistance that may be available.

Early Intervention — General

ACT Department of Education and Training

220 Northbourne Avenue
Braddon ACT 2612
02 6207 5111
www.decs.act.gov.au
DECS offers a range of Early Childhood Programs:

PLAYGROUP EARLY INTERVENTION PROGRAM
For children 2–3 years. There are three general playgroup early intervention programs in the ACT. They focus on: communication and social awareness, and therapy/education.

GENERAL DEVELOPMENTAL PLAYGROUPS
Children attend one session a week: there are six children in each group. Programs focus on early developmental skills in the areas of joint-attention turn-taking, attending and communication. These playgroups are for children aged 2–3 years who have needs in two or more areas of development, or significant needs in one area of development, or who are experiencing social and emotional difficulties.

COMMUNICATION AND SOCIAL AWARENESS PLAYGROUPS (CASA)
Children attend twice weekly: there are six children in each group with a teacher and two assistants. CASA playgroups are designed to specifically address the needs of children aged 2–3 years who have significant needs in communication and social skills development.

THERAPY AND EDUCATION PLAYGROUPS
Children attend one session a fortnight. Teachers and Therapy ACT therapists work collaboratively to plan and run the program. There are eight children in each group. This playgroup is for children aged 18 months to 3 years with significant or multiple physical disabilities. The multi-disciplinary team approach allows for the overall management of complex issues. This program is resourced at one teacher and assistant to eight children.

EARLY INTERVENTION UNITS (EIU)

EIUs provide four hours (2 x 2 hours) of educational programs per week for groups of 12 children. Programs focus on attending skills, social interaction and independence and are held in preschool classrooms.

AUTISM INTERVENTION UNITS (AIU)

A small group program for children with a diagnosis of ASD. There are four children per group. Two four-hour sessions are provided weekly, staffed by a teacher and assistant. Children also attending preschool may receive support from AIU staff.

EARLY CHILDHOOD CENTRES (ECC)

These provide a small group setting within a regular preschool environment for children who have a mild to moderate delay and additional special needs. There are eight children in each group, with one teacher and assistant. These centres are administered by the primary special schools: Cranleigh, Malkara and Turner. Groups for three year olds operate for up to eight hours per week and 12 hours per week for four year olds. There are four early childhood centres in the ACT.

EARLY CHILDHOOD UNITS (ECU)

ECUs are for children with higher needs than Early Childhood Centres. There are two early childhood units in the ACT. ECUs are small part-time classes for children with moderate to profound intellectual or multiple disabilities in special school settings. Children are aged 3–5 years with moderate to severe cognitive delay. ASD eligibility follows a diagnosis and an adaptive behaviour test. There are six children in each group, with one teacher and assistant. Students in these programs are under school age.

INCLUSION SUPPORT IN PRESCHOOL

This is for students in mainstream preschools who meet the criteria for preschool support in the areas of: developmental delay, physical, ASD and chronic medical inclusion support.

Early Intervention — ASD Specific

Gay Von Ess
0413 776 922
www.gvoness.com
Gay Von Ess is an experienced early childhood and primary school teacher who works with children with ASD and their families. Her approach is a

developmental one aimed at helping each child develop age-appropriate functional skills and behaviours. The child's strengths and interests are incorporated into an individualised program which focuses on communication, play and socialisation.

Services are predominantly delivered in the home and include informally assessing the child's educational needs and providing a detailed individualised home program for the parents/carers to implement. See also **RDI®** in this section.

See **Therapy ACT** above

Early Intervention — ABA

Early Autism Intervention
PO Box 3774
Manuka ACT 2603
0402 280707

Early Autism Intervention is a modern ABA service provider based in Canberra, offering home-based early intensive intervention to teach language, communication and cognitive skills to children with autism and related disorders. EAI has a focus on teaching meaningful play and social skills and an emphasis on delivering fun, exciting sessions. A combination of structured and incidental teaching is used, with generalisation incorporated early to ensure new skills are used in a natural and functional way across everyday situations. All treatment planning is individualised according to each child's specific needs in order to help your child reach their full potential. Non-intensive treatment and Positive Behaviour Support consultancy are also available.

RDI®

There are several RDI® consultants in Australia. The Connections Center in Houston, Texas trains and certifies all RDI® consultants and their website has a comprehensive list: www.rdiconnect.com
There is also an Australian RDI® Yahoo group at:
http://health.groups.yahoo.com/group/RDIsupportgroup/
If you join this group, you can access a file which also lists RDI® consultants in training, who may be starting to work with families already. It also lists consultants from the US who come to Australia to work with families. This is a useful egroup for getting in touch with other families doing RDI® in your area.

Speech Pathologists, Occupational Therapists and Psychologists

Get in touch with Autism Asperger ACT to ask for recommendations. See p. 239 for details on how to get in touch with these professionals through their national and state organisations.

Schools

ACT Department of Education and Training

220 Northbourne Avenue
Braddon ACT 2612
02 6207 5111
www.decs.act.gov.au

The Student Support Section of DECS has a model of service delivery that is based on collaborative practice. The aim is to create more responsive, flexible and integrated services that are proactive and targeted to meet the needs of students in schools. The goal is to locate services more closely to schools and to increase the capacity of schools to provide individualised, engaging, educational programs that will improve the learning outcomes for students with diverse needs.

SCHOOL PROGRAMS

LEARNING SUPPORT UNITS (LSU)

There are nine primary school Learning Support Units and four high school/ college Learning Support Units. Students are eligible if they meet the ACT Student Disability Criteria for intellectual disability or ASD. Classes are located in regular primary schools. There are up to eight students in an LSU class. According to individual school approaches students can be partially integrated with the regular school program.

LEARNING SUPPORT UNIT — AUTISM (LSUA)

There are 16 primary school Learning Support Units and five high school Learning Support Centres for students who meet the ACT Student Disability Criteria for ASD. LSUAs are small classes of six students with a teacher and assistant in primary and high schools. According to individual school approaches students can be partially integrated with the regular school program.

LEARNING SUPPORT CENTRE (LSC)

There are 22 primary school Learning Support Centres and about 12 high school Learning Support centres. Students are eligible who meet the criteria for a borderline or mild intellectual disability or a significant learning difficulty.

There are 14 students with one teacher and an assistant in primary classes, and 16 students with a teacher and assistant in high school and college. According to individual school approaches students can be fully or partially integrated with the regular school program.

SPECIAL SCHOOL PROGRAMS
Several special school programs provide education for children with moderate to severe disabilities.

INCLUSION SUPPORT PROGRAM
Students are eligible to apply for additional support to attend mainstream classes if they meet the ACT Student Disability Criteria for:
- intellectual disability
- physical disability
- language disorder
- pervasive developmental disorder
- mental health disorder
- chronic medical condition
- hearing impairment or deafness
- vision impairment or blindness.

Schools are allocated resources to support Individual Learning Plans of eligible students.

COUNSELLING SERVICES
A team of school counsellors provide targeted and individual counselling to support students from preschool to college. In addition they provide proactive and preventative programs for school communities.

SUPPORT TEACHER SERVICES
Support teachers and consultants provide consultancy support through Integrated Service Delivery Teams to school communities to support the Individual Learning Plan process for high and complex needs students and for students who meet ACT Student Disability Criteria.

STUDENT MANAGEMENT CONSULTANTS
A team of student management consultants work to build teacher and system capacity to support learning outcomes for students with challenging behaviours. They work collaboratively with schools to assist in the development of Individual Learning Plans and base their work on data collection, analysis and effective pedagogical practice.

COMPLEX NEEDS TEAM
The Complex Needs Team consists of three student management consultants who work with young people with high needs. They provide immediate, short-term response to escalated or critical situations in primary and secondary schools.

SUPPORT TEACHERS — INCLUSION
This is a team of teachers that build teacher, school, and system skills, and the capacity to support the Individual Learning Plan Process for students with disabilities in mainstream classes. The team works collaboratively with other student support staff and with school-based teams to assess, analyse, plan and evaluate strategies that aim to maximise student access, engagement and participation.

INCLUSIVE TECHNOLOGY SUPPORT
A cross-disciplinary team providing technical support, professional learning, specialised advice and assistance for a range of technologies to address pedagogy and the needs of students with disabilities in schools. School staff are supported to implement government and departmental policies related to the provision of assistive technologies and to investigate, consider, trial and select from a range of assistive technologies for students with disabilities.

Archdiocese of Canberra and Goulburn Education Office
52–54 Franklin St
Manuka ACT 2603
02 6234 5455
www.ceo.cg.catholic.edu.au
In the ACT all Catholic schools are mainstream schools, there are no Catholic special school or special needs units. Call and ask to speak to the special needs co-ordinator.

Association of Independent Schools of the ACT Inc
12 Thesiger Court
Deakin ACT 2600
02 6162 0834
aisact@ais.act.edu.au
www.ais.act.edu.au
AIS ACT manages federal funding for students with special needs. Call the co-ordinator of student programs for information and advice.

Therapy Services for School-Aged Children

ASD Consultancy and Support Service

Deanne Michaels
45 Carter Crescent
Calwell ACT, 2905.
0429 983 936
02 6291 0425
www.programs4asd.com

Deanne Michaels offers consultancy and training to schools, community, government and non-government organisations, also providing assistance to individuals with ASD and their families through advocacy, education, support and individual programs.

Topics include but are not limited to:
- What is Autism Spectrum Disorder?
- Asperger's Syndrome Discovered
- Communication and Visual Strategies
- Sensory Issues
- Understanding Behaviour
- Social and Friendship Skills
- Developing Positive Profiles
- Work Issues
- Siblings and Family Support
- other topics developed to meet specific requirements.

Fun and interactive workshops allow participants to 'walk in the shoes' of someone with ASD, albeit briefly. This experience is guaranteed to increase knowledge and understanding, provide practical strategies that are easy to implement and energise participants.

Deanne is the author of *The Social and Friendship Skills Program* designed to assist children with social challenges achieve socially in their mainstream communities.

Bobbi Cook Behaviour Management

13 Jalanga Cres
Aranda ACT 2614
02 6253 3116
0408 405 684
www.bcbm.com.au

BCBM offers anger management, counselling and behaviour management to young children, adolescents and families. Bobbi is a registered Clinical member of the Australian Counselling Association.

See also **Early Intervention — ASD Specific** above

See also **Gay Von Ess** above

Inclusion

Optimal Inclusion
02 6291 0425
0429 983 936
www.programs4asd.com
Optimal Inclusion works with schools and communities to build optimal inclusion for all people with or without disabilities. Optimal Inclusion believes that everyone can be included in community regardless of difference.

Circles of Friends is a program that assists children with disabilities and/or social isolation to be included in their classroom, school and recreational settings. Students are asked to join together to develop friendships with the focus child. Circles of Friends can also be used as a way of developing optimal inclusion for adults in work, leisure and neighbourhood activities.

Respite and Carer Info

Carers ACT

Churches Centre
54 Benjamin Way
Belconnen ACT 2617
02 6296 9900
www.carersact.asn.au/
For details see p. 225.

Commonwealth Carer Respite Centres

1800 059 059
For details see p. 225.

FaBRiC — Family Based Respite Care Inc

The Grant Cameron Community Centre
27 Mulley Street
Holder, ACT 2913
02 6287 2870
www.fabricinc.com.au

FaBRiC provides respite and social support to families living in the ACT who have a child or young person with a disability aged 0-20 years. FaBRiC also provides intensive support through the AFFIRM Program.

Home and Community Care (HACC) Program
Call your council and/or state disability department about this program.

Adult Services
See **Bobbi Cook Behaviour Management**

Community Connections
Kambah Professional Centre
51 Jenke Circuit
Kambah ACT 2902
02 6296 1133
www.comcons.org.au
Community Connections assists people with disabilities through a variety of programs.

Community Options Inc
115 Canberra Ave
Griffith ACT 2603
02 6295 8800
www.communityoptions.com.au
Community Options assists people with disabilities through a variety of programs.

See **Disability ACT** above

Optimal Outcomes
45 Carter Crescent
Calwell ACT 2905.
0429 983 936
02 6291 0425
www.programs4asd.com
Optimal Outcomes helps people to develop ideas and solutions for better life outcomes using person-centred planning. Person-centred Planning uses tools such as PATH, MAPS and Personal Profiles to assist in the development of ideas and solutions for building a positive and possible future for an individual with a disability.

Training for Parents and Professionals

See **ASD Consultancy and Support Service** above

Parent Support Groups

Autism Asperger ACT runs several meetings and support groups.

Libraries & Resources

Autism Asperger ACT has a library.

When You Really Need To Talk to Somebody

Parentline
02 6287 3833 (cost of a local call)
Parentline is a free, confidential telephone counselling, referral, information and support service for parents, grandparents and carers in the ACT and surrounding districts.

Lifeline
13 11 14
www.lifeline.org.au
Lifeline offers telephone counselling throughout Australia — 24 hours a day, seven days a week.

NSW

First Things First

Autism Information Line
02 8977 8377
Autism Spectrum Australia (Aspect) provides practical support and advice to families, professionals and service providers.

Building Foundations
DVD and manual for all families of children newly diagnosed with an ASD, see Aspect listing below.

Through The Maze
PO Box 141
Northmead NSW 2152
Phone: 02 94891321
www.acdnsw.org.au
Through The Maze is a handbook for parents and carers of children with all sorts of disabilities. It is produced by the Association of Children with a Disability NSW. The handbook aims to help families navigate the complex maze of professionals and services. Topics covered include: medical issues, early intervention, schools, teenagers, post-school options, holidays, counselling, sports and respite. The handbook can be downloaded from the website.

State Autism Association

Autism Spectrum Australia (Aspect)
41 Cook Street
Forestville NSW 2087
02 8977 8300
www.aspect.org.au

ASPECT FAR NORTH COAST CENTRE FOR AUTISM
1/106 Main Street
Alstonville NSW 2477
02 6628 3660
Aspect is the major provider of services to the ASD community in NSW.

DIAGNOSTIC ASSESSMENT SERVICE
Aspect offers comprehensive diagnostic assessments of children suspected of
having an ASD. In addition, Aspect has been specifically funded by DADHC
to assess children aged younger than five in rural and regional areas.

BUILDING FOUNDATIONS
Aspect has produced a DADHC-funded information pack with a manual and
DVD specifically for families of children newly diagnosed with ASD. This
features four young children and their families and explains simple initial
steps that all families can take to assist their child. Building Foundations is
available in seven languages.

EARLY INTERVENTION
The Building Blocks Program includes family consultations, parent
information and support, and preschool consultations. There is a home-based
program (Early Play Program) involving fortnightly home visits and centre-
based service (Starting Blocks) in five locations around Sydney and at the Far
North Coast Autism Centre. Aspect receives some government funding for its
EI services and parents also pay fees by the term. Centre-based programs vary
in length from half day to a full day.

SCHOOLS
Aspect operates six schools in NSW: three in Sydney and one each in the
Hunter, Central Coast and South Coast. Each school has a base school and
a range of satellite classes based in either NSW Department of Education
or Catholic schools. There are also regional groups of satellite classes in the
Riverina and Far North Coast regions. Aspect has around 500 school-aged

students in its schools and classes.

SCHOOLS OUTREACH SERVICE
The School Outreach Service (SOS) is a multi-disciplinary team which supports children, families and schools using visits, school in-services, courses, workshops and social skills programs. SOS offers a series of training courses for parents and carers, teachers, special support personnel and other professionals. This service operates throughout NSW.

PARENT TRAINING
Recipe for Success is a parent-training workshop, aimed at parents and carers of children with an ASD from 3–16 years. This course is provided throughout the state and runs for three days.

PARENT SUPPORT
'Someone to turn to...'™ trains parents to act as volunteers who are then linked to other families, matched according to the age of their child.

SIBLING SUPPORT
'A' Kids Camp is run annually for sibling of children with an ASD.

TRAINING COURSES
Various training courses are offered throughout the year all over NSW.

BEHAVIOUR INTERVENTION SERVICE
Positive behaviour support programs are available to children and adolescents who have emerging or current challenging behaviour.

ADULT SERVICES
Suite 2, Macquarie House
32 Church Street
Ryde NSW 2112
02 8878 1806
For adults with an ASD, Aspect has an Adults and Behaviour Support Group. There are accommodation, employment and recreational services. An Adult Outreach and Training program works with funded adults with ASD who display challenging behaviour, their families and staff in group houses.

PUBLICATIONS
Aspect publishes several information kits and manuals which can be purchased via the website. There are also many useful leaflets and brochures available.

State Disability Department

Department of Ageing, Disability and Home Care (DADHC)

Level 5, 83 Clarence Street
Sydney NSW 2000
02 8270 2000
www.dadhc.nsw.gov.au

The DADHC provides and funds a range of supports and services for children and adults with a disability, their families and carers. These include services for people with a wide range of disabilities, such as supported accommodation, respite, therapy, day programs and post-school programs.

The department also funds an increasing number of programs and supports that are designed specifically for children and young people with ASD, in areas such as early childhood intervention. These services are provided directly to families and also by funding non-government and community organisations.

DADHC is working in partnership with organisations specialising in the ASD area on several pilot programs and initiatives. It has funded Autism Spectrum Australia (Aspect) for a pilot project entitled Co-ordinated Access to Services and Support. In conjunction with NSW Health and the Department of Education and Training, this service will provide information about the nature of case management and brokerage services that will best meet the needs of adolescents with ASD who are at high risk of early exit from school.

Other initiatives include:

- support to develop the Building Foundations kit for families with a child with ASD (see above)
- support to Autism Behaviour Intervention NSW (ABI) for a two-year demonstration project (commencing 2006) to provide behaviour support programs to families with young children with autism
- support to the University of Newcastle to provide professional training for front line workers in implementing positive behaviour supports and developing functional communication skills in young children with a disability, including autism

There is also a Family Assistance Fund, see www.dadhc.nsw.gov.au/dadhc/People+with+a+disabilityServices+for+ families.htm

Small amounts of discretionary funding are provided directly to families to help them address needs that cannot be met through the standard range of services or other funding. The primary purpose of this fund is to support the work that case managers are doing to assist families.

Contact the Department's Community Access Branch on 8270 2193 or visit its website, www.dadhc.nsw.gov.au.

State Health Department

NSW Health
73 Miller Street
North Sydney NSW 2060
02 9391 9000
www.health.nsw.gov.au

NSW

NSW Health provides a population health approach to screening and early detection of developmental delay or disability for children under five years of age. Developmental surveillance and monitoring is provided by a range of health providers such as general practitioners and clinicians based in child health centres.

DIAGNOSIS
NSW Health provides some specialist assessment services mostly located in metropolitan areas. Child and Family Health Services are provided in each Area Health Service. If a disability such as ASD is identified through the screening process, referral is made to the appropriate specialist agency such as DADHC or the Autism Association for appropriate assessment and treatment.

SPEECH PATHOLOGY AND OCCUPATIONAL THERAPY
NSW Health can provide limited speech therapy and occupational therapy to children with mild ASD upon referral through Child and Family Health Centres. Children with higher needs receive services from specialist services such as DADHC or non-government funded specialist paediatric services. Further details can be provided by general practitioners or local child and family health nurses.

PAEDIATRICIANS, SOCIAL WORKERS AND PSYCHOLOGISTS
Families can access a limited number of visits to these professionals through NSW Health, again further details can be provided by general practitioners or local child and family health nurse.

CHILD AND ADOLESCENT MENTAL HEALTH SERVICES (CAMHS)
Each of the eight geographic Area Health Services managed by NSW Health as well as Children's Hospital Westmead Department of Psychological Medicine and Justice Health provide Child and Adolescent Mental Health Services. Children and adolescents up to the age of 18 are eligible and the focus is on the range of psychiatric diagnoses within a developmental and family context. Generally those with moderate to severe difficulties tend

to be seen for assessment and treatment. Whilst fewer very young children with ASD are referred, there are clinics and centres where there is a focus on developmental disabilities. There is a mix of inpatient and community services with different arrangements across the Areas and variable capacity to assess and treat children and adolescents presenting with ASD. There is also variability in local partnerships with paediatric services and other key agencies. The multi-disciplinary approach lends itself to addressing the range and severity of presentations including the co-morbidities associated with ASD. CAMHS staff are also able to offer consultation to staff working in a range of other community-based services.

You can find your local heath services at www.health.nsw.gov.au/services/index.html. Search for child and adolescent mental health.

Different services are provided throughout the state so families need to find out what is provided in their local area first and foremost. The services offered by NSW Health, like all of the publicly-funded services, tend to be very heavily subscribed, so you may find there are long waiting lists.

Your Local Council

Many local councils around Australia have a Disability Information Officer or Community Care Officer. It is well worth getting in touch with your local council to ask about local services and assistance that may be available.

Early Intervention — General

See **Department of Education and Training** below

Early Childhood Intervention Infoline
Early Childhood Intervention Australia
1300 65 68 65
For the cost of a local phone call, the Infoline provides information about early childhood intervention services across NSW.

Lifestart Co-operative
78c Charles Street
Putney NSW 2112
02 9807 9700
www.lifestart.org.au
Lifestart is one of the largest early intervention organisations in Sydney, with centres at Baulkham Hills, Eastwood, Frenchs Forest, Hornsby, Lewisham, Maroubra and St Mary's. There is also a smaller school-aged services branch.

Lifestart is a parent co-operative providing a family-centred approach to the needs of children with disabilities and their families. Services include:

- open playgroup
- play-based learning groups
- individual sessions
- home visits
- educational workshops
- resource assistance

Hanen courses are run regularly (see p. 80) and Lifestart runs Hanen training workshops for speech pathologists.

Early Intervention — ASD specific

Autism Central

9 Oaklands Avenue
Beecroft NSW 2119
www.innovativeprogramming.net.au

Autism Central is a group of parents and professionals who work together to offer an integrated service to people on the autism spectrum and their families. Services include speech therapy, occupational therapy with a focus on sensory processing and an ongoing tutoring service. They offer support for some well-known programs such as Intensive Intervention, PECS, social interaction training, conversational skills training and RDI®. Autism Central aims to be a 'one stop shop'; the whole team is able to work together to understand and plan a way forward with the family and educational facility.

Connect Therapy

Suite 1, 9–11 Beaumond Ave
Maroubra NSW 2035
02 9460 9838
0402 119 319
www.connecttherapy.com

Connect Therapy is a Sydney based, in-home speech and occupational therapy program that empowers parents with the knowledge and skills they need to really 'connect' with their child with a child-centred and practical teaching approach.

Connect Therapy believes that when treating children with ASD it is fundamentally important to go back and develop the skills that should often have been learnt in the first 18 months of life. They prioritise treating these 'foundation' skills so that the child can then go on to learn as quickly and effectively as possible.

The program has a strong emphasis on parent education and empowerment and prioritises the following goals in the initial stages of intervention:

- getting to know the unique strengths, weaknesses and motivations of the child
- social and emotional development
- increasing the child's desire to interact and learn
- having the child in a calm and organised state for learning through sensory integration therapy as well as other techniques
- increasing the child's desire to communicate and building effective communication and language skills.

Giant Steps has an Early Learning component, see below.

Kaleidoscope Network
47 Juliet Street
Enmore NSW 2042
02 80016128
0411 848 137

Kaleidoscope Network offers a range of services for children with ASD and their families. Services include early intervention programs that are ABA and play-based, finding the approach that is best suited for the child and family. They also work with parents on managing their child's behaviour and assisting in functional communication.

There are groups for children with autism, programs for parents and in-service for preschools to assist teachers in managing and teaching students with ASD. Home visits are also an essential part of Kaleidoscope services.

NETwork Interventions
0400 308 099
www.networkinterventions.com

NETwork Interventions is a behavioural consultation company which provides services to learners with autism and development disabilities. The aim is to use the most recent advances in research (including AVB — Applied Verbal Behaviour) to equip parents and schools with the tools to enable their children to become conversational and socially integrated. NETwork Interventions teach learners of all ages, from three month olds with the initial signs, through to adults.

As well as single or ongoing consultations, NETwork Interventions provides hands-on workshops specific to each learner level. NETwork Interventions is dedicated to keeping costs as low as possible, to facilitate more frequent contact and quicker progress.

Early Intervention — ABA

See **Annie's Centre** below

NSW

Aspire Early Intervention

PO Box 811
Kings Langley NSW 2147
0433 999889
www.aspireearlyintervention.com

Aspire is an early intervention service that provides contemporary ABA services, based around a verbal behaviour framework. Teaching techniques used include natural environment teaching, precision teaching and discrete trial training. Aspire provides individual programs based around the family and the child's needs, addressing developmental areas such as communication, social skills, engagement, executive functioning, play and theory of mind skills. Comprehensive training and support is given to parents.

Autism Behavioural Intervention NSW

38B Langston Place
Epping NSW 2121
02 9869 2110
www.abinsw.org.au

ABINSW Family Support Services (FSS), established in 2006, is a pilot project evaluating the effectiveness of a 20-week model of early intervention for children with autism and their families. The program offers families 40 hours of service over a 20-week period, is home-based and has a strong focus on family training and supervision in the principles of ABA. ABI Behaviour Support Educators work in partnership with the family to create the optimal learning environment for their child in the family home and wider community.

DADHC Eligibility Criteria

- formal diagnosis of an ASD
- child must be under six years of age
- child must not be attending school

Referrals can be made to DADHC.

Information, Referral and Intake:

Metro South — 02 9334 3700
Metro North — 02 8855 4200

ABI also offers private consultation services for families, carers and centres. ABINSW can provide a variety of workshops and trainings for parents and professionals working with children with special needs.

Centre for Autism and Related Disorders (CARD)

Suite 45, 11–21 Underwood Road
Homebush NSW 2140
02 97635466
www.centerforautism.com.au

CARD is amongst the world's largest organisations treating children and young adults with ASD. Following the principles of ABA, CARD implements a customised curriculum for each client, teaching language and communication, play, adaptive, motor and school skills. Building on this foundation, CARD teaches advanced skills such as executive functions, cognition and social skills.

CARD II is a program designed for students from 8–21 years. As a flexible program tailored to individuals with different needs, it can assist families who may require support managing challenging behaviours, teaching basic communication and adaptive skills or teaching more complex social skills. The goal of CARD II is for individuals to live as independently as possible, participate in enjoyable and appropriate leisure activities, gain and maintain successful employment, have meaningful relationships and attend educational facilities where possible.

See **Lizard Children's Centre** below

Staff for ABA Programs

ABALink

P.O. Box 1738
Lane Cove NSW 1595
02 9411 4618
www.abalink.com.au

ABALink can provide fully trained ABA therapists, and preschool and school shadows for parents running ABA programs. After-school carers and babysitters with experience of children with ASD and with the use of positive ABA methods can also be provided.

Floortime™

Kids World: Paediatric OT — Floortime

469 Mowbray Rd
Lane Cove, NSW, 2066
02 9418 9995, 02 9418 9990 (fax)
www.kidsworldtherapy.com.au

Kids World: Paediatric OT is a private paediatric OT service focussed on working with children and their families who have disorders and difficulties with relating and communicating including ASD, sensory processing disorders, regulatory issues, dyspraxia, and developmental delays.

The practice incorporates the DIR® Model (Floortime™) and has a specialist understanding of the impact of sensory processing difficulties, regulatory issues and motor development and how these difficulties impact a child's ability to relate and interact with others.

Quickstepz Paediatric Therapy

Suite 203,
156 Pacific Highway (Cnr Greenwich Rd)
St Leonards NSW 2065
02 9460 6552
www.quickstepz.com.au

Quickstepz Paediatric Therapy is an early intervention service that provides children presenting with developmental difficulties with a comprehensive intervention program. Intervention for children and their families is based on the Developmental, Individual-Difference, Relationship-Based (DIR®)/ 'Floortime' Model™. Kate Boland is a Paediatric Occupational Therapist and DIR®/'Floortime'™ therapist who has trained with the Interdisciplinary Council on Developmental and Learning Disorders (ICDL) in the US. Kate specialises in working with toddlers and children from 0–5 years who have a diagnosis of ASD or early signs of ASD.

The Sensory Gym

8/28 Laurence Street
Hobartville NSW 2753
02 4578 9799

Colleen Hacker is an occupational therapist who has a DIR® Certificate, Level III.

RDI®

There are several RDI® consultants in Australia. The Connections Center in Houston, Texas trains and certifies all RDI® consultants and their website has a comprehensive list: www.rdiconnect.com

There is also an Australian RDI® Yahoo group at:
http://health.groups.yahoo.com/group/RDIsupportgroup/

If you join this group, you can access a file which also lists RDI® consultants in training, who may be starting to work with families already. It also lists consultants from the US who come to Australia to work with families. This is a useful egroup for getting in touch with other families doing RDI® in your area.

Speech Pathologists, Occupational Therapists and Psychologists

Aspect Infoline may be able to assist with recommendations. See p. 239 for details on how to get in touch with these professionals through their national and state organisations.

Multi-disciplinary Centres

Annie's Centre
Suite 2, 122a Belmore Rd
Randwick NSW
02 9314 5793
www.anniescentre.com

Annie's Centre is an independent Child and Family Health Centre in Sydney. It offers multi-disciplinary assessment, diagnosis and therapy services including:

- Clinical Psychology
- Speech Pathology
- Occupational Therapy
- Applied Behaviour Analysis (ABA)
- School Based Learning Support
- Parenting advice and behaviour management groups for parents
- Anxiety and depression management
- Social skills training
- many other specialist group programs relevant to ASD.

School observations and consultations are available, as well as in-service on issues relating to ASDs and their management. The School Learning Support Services Program includes the offer of teacher's aide and/or behaviour therapy support within schools, extra tutoring and learning support groups.

All the health professionals at Annie's Centre have extensive knowledge and skills in the assessment, diagnosis and treatment of ASDs or related pervasive developmental disorders.

Lizard Children's Centre

Level 3, 126 Greville Street
Chatswood NSW 2067
02 9904 8130
www.lizardcentre.com

Lizard Children's Centre is a private clinic in Sydney which provides a range of specialised paediatric services. Lizard is a rapidly expanding clinic with a range of staff providing services to children with autism and/or with speech, learning, behavioural or social difficulties, as well as being a training centre for ABA therapists and school or preschool aides.

Services include:

- Applied Behaviour Analysis (ABA)
- Speech pathology
- Educational Solutions remedial academic program
- Play and social skills training
- Behaviour management
- Diagnostic and intervention assessment
- School-based support
- Parenting advice and behaviour management groups for parents

The Lizard Training Centre also trains people interested in working as therapists for home-based ABA programs, as 'shadows' in preschool or school settings or as specialised nannies or babysitters for children with autism. They also run training for parents, and for teachers who work with children with autism.

Schools

Department of Education and Training (DET)
GPO Box 33
Sydney NSW 2000
02 9561 8000
    Hunter/Central Coast 4924 9999
    Illawarra and South Coast 4222 2929
    New England 6755 5934
    North Coast 6652 0500
    Northern Sydney 9886 7690
    Riverina 6937 3871
    South Western Sydney 9796 5446
    Sydney 9217 4877
    Western NSW 6841 2110
    Western Sydney 9208 9359
www.det.nsw.edu.au

DET provides a range of services to support students with disabilities, including ASD. Students with ASD can be enrolled in regular classes with additional support, in support classes in a regular school, or in a special school. The decision on where to enrol a student with a disability and with what level of support will depend on a number of factors. There are over 60 ASD support classes across NSW.

Who's Going to Teach My Child? provides information for parents about the way children with special learning needs are supported in government schools, and can be downloaded from the website.

Decisions about the most appropriate placement for children with disabilities and other additional support needs are made in consultation with parents/carers, the school principal, and regional support personnel. The regional Student Support Co-ordinator, Disability Programs is available to assist parents/carers with decision-making and can provide additional information about the support available in the local area. The Student Support Co-ordinator can be contacted at your local regional office by using 131 536.

The NSW Department of Education and Training operates 100 preschools across the state. Children with disabilities can attend the Department's preschools. Programs for children with disabilities are also available in 50 early intervention support classes across the state.

Information about enrolling in a NSW government school can also be accessed at: www.schools.nsw.edu.au/schoolfind/enrolment/index.php

Catholic Education Commission NSW
Polding Centre
Level 9, 133 Liverpool St
NSW 2000
02 9287 1555
www.cecnsw.catholic.edu.au

Within the Catholic Education system, a range of options for children with special needs is available. These options vary across local areas, known as Dioceses. Resources for children with special needs are primarily available to support children integrated into regular classes. Support in the implementation of individual planning is provided by special education teachers and by itinerant specialist teachers. Many Aspect satellite classes are based in Catholic schools.

There are a small number of special schools for children with a range of disabilities: St Lucy's, St Dominic's Centre for Hearing impaired children, St Edmund's school for children with special needs, St Gabriel's school for students with hearing impairment and Mater Dei school for children with an intellectual disability.

All Dioceses have Education Officers, guidance officers and/or itinerant support services. For further information contact the State Co-ordinator; Special Learning Needs at Catholic Education Commission New South Wales.

The Association of Independent Schools of NSW

Level 4, 99 York Street
NSW 2000
02 9299 2845
www.aisnsw.edu.au

AISNSW can provide information about independent schools to families of children with ASD including special schools and mainstream schools. The AISNSW administers federal funding for children with special needs to schools and can provide training and support to schools.

Giant Steps Sydney

'Step House'
23 Punt Road
Gladesville NSW 2111
02 9879 4971
www.giantsteps.net.au

Giant Steps is an independent school in Sydney which caters to students from ages 2–18 years who have a primary diagnosis of ASD and associated developmental delay. There is a high student–teacher/aide ratio and an emphasis on speech, occupational and music therapies.

Woodbury Autism Education and Research

Building 11
Balcombe Heights Estate
92 Seven Hills Road
Baulkham Hills NSW 2153
02 9639 6152
www.woodbury.org.au

Woodbury is the first school in Australia that follows the principles of ABA in educating children with autism. Woodbury was founded in 2006 and teaches students aged from 4.5 to 16 years. The school has a graduated approach to ABA with students initially receiving teaching in a staff–student ratio of 1:1, in both individual and small group programs. The children gradually progress to an staff–student ratio of 1:2, with a maximum of 1:4 for those in a transition class preparing for integration into another school setting. Programs are individualised and are driven by the analysis of continuously collected data.

The school day is highly structured with defined and measured objectives and a program covering motor skills, academics/pre-academics, play and leisure skills, daily living skills, social skills and communication skills. For older students a post-school program is under development.

Therapy Services for School-Aged Children

See **Annie's Centre** above
See **Autism Central** above
See **Autism Spectrum Australia (Aspect)** above
See **CARD** above

Innovative Communication Programming

9 Oaklands Avenue
Beecroft NSW 2119
www.innovativeprogramming.net.au

Innovative Communication Programming (ICP) was established in 1996, in response to the need for a planned approach towards creating communication opportunities for people with complex communication needs associated with developmental disability. ICP provides provide assessment, intervention ideas and ongoing consultation services to establish, train, problem solve and manage issues relating to communication. ICP has published a number of resources that are useful for anyone working with individuals with disabilities and they include a picture library program, books and training manuals to provide communication, literacy and positive behaviour support. (See p. 232)

Learning Links

www.learninglinks.com.au

Learning Links is a non-profit organisation which assists children who have learning disabilities, difficulties and developmental delays and their families. A school-aged service is available in several locations around Sydney.

See **NETwork Interventions** above

Respite and Carer Info

Carers NSW
Roden Cutler House
Level 18, 24 Campbell St
Sydney NSW 2000
02 9280 4744
Freecall: 1800 242 636
www.carersnsw.asn.au
For information see p. 225

Commonwealth Carer Respite Centres
1800 059 059
For details see p. 225

Home and Community Care (HACC) Program
Call your council and/or your state disability department about this program.
For details see p. 226

See **ABALink** above

Adult Services
See **Autism Central** above
See **Autism Spectrum Australia (Aspect)** above
See **CARD** above
See **DADHC** above
See **NETwork Interventions** above

Training for Parents and Professionals
See **Annie's Centre** above
See **Autism Spectrum Australia Aspect** above

Education Events
Sue Larkey
PO Box 20
Artarmon NSW 2064
0433 660 379

NSW

www.suelarkey.com
Sue Larkey runs workshops on practical strategies for ASD. Sue has taught both as a primary school teacher and at a Specialist Autism School, she has a Masters in Special Education and is undertaking a Doctorate in Education. Sue's workshops are aimed at parents and at teachers and other professionals who deal with children with ASD. A list of her speaking engagements is available on her website. Sue sends free newsletter packed with practical tips.

Support Groups

One of the best places to start looking for a support group is the Aspect website: click on *Links, Support Groups*.

Here is a list of other support groups not on the Aspect website at the time of writing or which have their own websites:

ASPIA Inc — Asperger's Syndrome Partner Information Australia

PO Box 57
Macarthur Square LPO
Macarthur NSW 2560
0408 817 828
www.aspia.org.au
ASPIA provides support and information to partners of adults with Asperger's syndrome. There are regular meetings in Sydney and a very useful website.

ASPIRE — Autism Spectrum Parents Information and Resources East

www.asdsupport.org
This parent support group has evening and daytime meetings in the eastern suburbs of Sydney.

AASS — Autism Advisory and Support Services

88 Memorial Ave
Liverpool NSW 2170
0432327096
www.aass.org.au
AASS was founded in 2007. The aim of AASS is to empower families through knowledge and support. The group operates mainly in South Western Sydney.

Autism and Asperger's Support Group
www.autismsupport.org.au
Richmond and Burwood (Sydney region).

Biomed
http://au.groups.yahoo.com/group/biomedicalautismgroup/
This biomedical interest group meets monthly in Sydney. Join the Yahoo group to find out details.

Coffs Coast ASD Parent Support Group
PO Box 1722
Coffs Harbour NSW 2450
02 6658 8330
www.coffscoastautism.org.au
This group has a useful website, holds monthly meetings and has produced a resource directory for the Coffs Coast.

Cooinda Family Support Services
www.cooinda.org.au
General disability support for families in the Albury Wodonga area.

Hills Support Group (NW Sydney)
02 9659 4960
elena.b@optusnet.com.au
The support group meets monthly for informal morning teas. Members also receive newsletters, and email alerts of any relevant news relating to autism.

L2L – Learning to Learn
http://health.groups.yahoo.com/group/learningtolearnsydney
L2L is a Sydney-based ABA interest and support egroup.

Luke Priddis Foundation
Po Box 1132
Penrith BC
NSW 2751
www.lukepriddisfoundation.com
The Luke Priddis Foundation works to improve awareness and services in Western Sydney. It also runs workshops and plans in the future to operate an early intervention centre.

Southern Suburbs Autism Support

c/- Sutherland Shire Learning Difficulties Support Group Inc.
PO Box 580, Sutherland NSW 1499
Meetings and members library is located at
Multi Purpose Centre for the Disabled
123 Flora Street
Sutherland
02 9545 1505
The group has been running for over 15 years. It meets on the first Tuesday
evening of each month for guest speakers, informal chats and resource library
borrowings. The office is open weekdays from 10am to 2pm.

Hornsby/Ku-ring-gai Asperger's/HF Autism Support Group

HKH Child Adolescent and Family Team
Hillview Community Health Centre
1334 Pacific Hwy
Turramurra NSW 2074
02 9024 9000
www.caft.notlong.com
Open to residents of Hornsby and Ku-ring-gai council areas, this group meets
monthly.

Libraries & Resources

Each Aspect school has a library for the use of pupils' families and teachers.

Aspect Far North Coast Centre for Autism has a small but growing
library.

Several of the support groups have their own library.

Advocacy

Family Advocacy

305/16–18 Cambridge Street
Epping NSW 2121
02 9869 0866
Freecall (non-metropolitan NSW callers only)
1800 620 588
www.family-advocacy.com
Family Advocacy is an independent, community-based social advocacy
organisation which works across New South Wales.

When You Really Need To Talk to Somebody

Parentline
1300 301300
www.parentline.com.au

Parentline is a 24-hour telephone help line for all parents of children 0–18 years of age living in NSW.

Lifeline
13 11 14
www.lifeline.org.au
Lifeline offers telephone counselling throughout Australia — 24 hours a day, seven days a week.

NT

First Things First

Call Autism NT on 08 8948 4424 or visit the office in Darwin.

State Autism Association

Autism Northern Territory Inc

Shop 19
Nightcliff Shopping Centre
Coconut Grove NT 0821
08 8948 4424
www.autismnt.com.au

Autism Northern Territory Inc is the key agency representing the Northern Territory at national levels, and families and individuals at the local level. Founded by parents, Autism NT acts as an information provider for parents and professionals throughout the Northern Territory. Autism NT operates on a 'shop front' and 'drop in' style. Recent funding has allowed Autism NT to employ two staff, one full time and one part time, who work with the public to actively promote the understanding and acceptance of people with ASD to enable them and their families to be an integral part of the community.

Information sessions, seminars and workshops are organised and facilitated across a wide range of ASD related topics. Autism NT is proactive in bringing professional development opportunities to the NT for families, individuals with an ASD, educators and other professional or individuals with an interest in ASD.

Autism NT has a comprehensive library of books and resources which are available for loan to members. This resource is based at the Darwin office and includes an informal quarterly mobile access to the Darwin/Palmerston rural area. Some of these resources are based in Alice Springs on a rotational basis.

Committee Meetings are held monthly the first Tuesday of each month in Darwin and the third Wednesday of each month in Alice Springs where they are organised by a voluntary Alice Springs coordinator.

Territory Health and Disability Department

Department of Health and Community Services

Health House
87 Mitchell Street
Darwin, NT
08 8999 2400
www.health.nt.gov.au

In both Darwin and Alice Springs, Children's Development Teams provide OT, speech pathology, social worker (family support) and physiotherapy. The Teams recognise early intervention as a valuable strategy to optimise a child's developmental potential and maximise their physical, intellectual, social and emotional well-being.

If the diagnosis is significant and is impacting on family dynamics, a referral can be made to the Child and Adolescent Team at Mental Health Services who have access to a child psychiatrist. Children with ASDs can also be referred to psychologists, behaviour educators and/or Local Area Co-ordinators. Funding may be available for respite and other support services.

Therapists provide home visits, school visits, and support for children, family and carers. For example, in Alice Springs they provide teachers with one to one 'modelling' to assist them in dealing with children with ASD in the classroom.

A new centralised access process is being developed for implementation across all NT disability services in 2008. This will include families with children with ASD and will ensure that clients are directed to the best service available for their needs. In the remote areas a trans-disciplinary approach is being developed to ensure families are provided with a range of therapeutic support while the specialised professional is planning their visit.

Your Local Council

Many local councils around Australia have a Disability Information Officer or Community Care Officer. It is well worth getting in touch with your local council to ask about local services and assistance that may be available.

Early Intervention — General

See **Department of Health and Community Services**

Department of Employment, Education and Training
PO Box 4821
Darwin NT 0801
08 8999 5659
www.deet.nt.gov.au/education
Regional Offices

Darwin/Palmerston	08 8999 8787
Alice Springs	08 8951 7100
Katherine:	08 8973 8914
Nhulunbuy:	08 8987 0451

EARLY INTERVENTION SERVICES (BIRTH – 6 YEARS)
DEET operates two generic intensive Early Childhood Intervention programs for children aged 3–5 years (Alice Springs and Darwin).

Student Services ECI Advisory Teachers work in collaboration with government and non-government community-based agencies and services. An holistic and family-centred best practice model of service delivery is used to ensure best educational outcomes for the child and family.

Collaboration may occur with:
- allied health therapists and regional aged and disability teams
- Carpentaria Disability Services Early Intervention Services (Darwin and Palmerston)
- Guidance Officers and other Student Services Advisory Teachers
- preschools, schools and child care centres.

Services include:
- targeted screening and assessment
- targeted interventions/strategies
- input into the diagnostic process
- consultancy support to preschools, specialist intervention groups and

families
- referral to other services, agencies and specialists
- information to families in relation to accessing services, preschool and school options, and transition planning
- facilitating entry into child care, preschool and full-time school
- assistance in planning, monitoring and reviewing the school's educational adjustments for the student.

Access to services is by parental self-referral or referral from allied health professionals, therapists, community health nurses, paediatricians and other specialists.

Carpentaria Disability Services Inc
37 Henbury Avenue
Tiwi NT 0810
08 8945 4977
www.carpentaria.org.au
Carpentaria Disability Services Inc provides generic early intervention services from the Palmerston office.

Play Therapy NT
2/5 Gardens Hill Cres
The Gardens, Darwin NT 0820
0411 118 620
www.playtherapy.com.au
Josephine Martin is a trained play therapist working in private practice.

Early Intervention — ASD specific

At the time of writing, there is no ASD-specific early intervention available in the Northern Territory. Some families do access EI providers based in other states.

Speech Pathologists, Occupational Therapists and Psychologists

Autism NT may be able to assist with recommendations. See p. 239 for details on how to get in touch with these professionals through their national and state organisations.

Schools

Department of Employment, Education and Training

PO Box 4821
Darwin NT 0801
08 8999 5659
www.deet.nt.gov.au/education
Regional Offices

Darwin/Palmerston	08 8999 8787
Alice Springs	08 8951 7100
Katherine:	08 8973 8914
Nhulunbuy:	08 8987 0451

DEET provides developmentally appropriate curriculum for its students as articulated in the NT Curriculum Framework. For students with special needs DEET has two key service delivery areas that support schools to assist the student in need: Student Services and Teaching, Learning and Standards.

Student Services is the principal provider of support for students with disabilities. Student Services personnel are located in Darwin and the major regional centres of Alice Springs, Katherine and Nhulunbuy. Advisory Teacher specialisations include:

- Early Childhood Intervention (ECI)
- Behaviour
- Transition from school
- Vision
- Hearing
- Gifted children
- Special Education Consultant Teachers
- Guidance Officers (School Psychologists).

In accordance with its Students with Disabilities Policy DEET operates an Inclusion Model. This involves supporting students with disabilities in mainstream classes, in annexes to mainstream schools, or in special schools, with the parents having the choice. All requests for service from Student Services are initiated by the school in consultation with the family and the Special Education Consultant Teachers.

SCHOOL AGED SERVICES (YEARS 1–12: PRIMARY, MIDDLE AND SENIOR SECONDARY)
DEET is presently operating a trial alternative specialised program at Malak Primary School in Darwin for up to five students. The aim of the program is to provide short-term, intensive crisis intervention for students with High-Functioning ASD/Asperger's syndrome and challenging behaviours. It is

designed to teach these students appropriate coping strategies in response to stressful situations with the view to returning to their home school. Professional learning is also provided for home school staff to be in a better position to accommodate the specific learning needs of the student and to support a smooth transition back to the mainstream.

Services available from Student Services for school-aged students include:

- assisting schools with the completion of the Request for Service, and identifying the schools' needs
- assisting schools with the development, planning, implementation and evaluation of educational programs
- assisting schools with the development of Educational Adjustment Plans
- academic assessments
- involvement in case conference and review meetings
- providing advice in relation to specific resources and strategies
- assisting schools with the acquisition of work experience opportunities for the student and in the development of individual Transition Plans.

NT Catholic Education Office

Cnr of Hidden Valley Rd and Beatons Rds
Berrimah NT 0828
08 8984 1400
www.ceo.nt.catholic.edu.au
Call for information on special needs enrolment and assistance.

Association of Independent Schools NT Inc

GPO Box 2085
Darwin NT 0801
08 8981 8668
www.aisnt.asn.au
AISNT works with schools to support children with special needs and manages federal funding to support their needs.

RDI®

There are several RDI® consultants in Australia. The Connections Center in Houston, Texas trains and certifies all RDI® consultants and their website has a comprehensive list: www.rdiconnect.com
There is also an Australian RDI® Yahoo group at:
http://health.groups.yahoo.com/group/RDIsupportgroup/
If you join this group, you can access a file which also lists RDI® consultants

in training, who may be starting to work with families already. It also lists consultants from the US who come to Australia to work with families. This is a useful egroup for getting in touch with other families doing RDI® in your area.

Therapy Services for School-Aged Children
See **Department of Health and Community Services** above

Inclusion — Support for Child Care Providers

Children's Services Support Program (Central Australia) Inc
1st Floor Eurilpa House
25 Todd Mall
08 8953 4059
www.childrenservices.com.au
CSSP is a non-profit community based organisation that provides support and advice, resources and educational training for the Children's Services sector to the southern region of the Northern Territory. The role of CSSP is to develop the capacity of the service to include all children. CSSP does not work with the child/family.

Early Childhood Australia (ECA) NT
71 Coonawarra Rd
Winnellie NT 0821
08 8947 4776
www.earlychildhoodaustralia.org.au/state_territory_branches/northern_territory_branch.html
ECA NT is a branch of Early Childhood Australia, which is a national non-government, non-profit advocacy organisation that speaks out on behalf of all young children from birth to eight years of age. The branch is also funded to provide the Inclusion Support Agency for the Top End of the NT. This service is provided by the Children's Inclusion Support Service, which supports inclusion of children with additional needs into their programs.

Respite and Carers

Carers NT
Boulter Road
Berrimah NT 0828
08 8948 4877
Unit 1, 17 First Street
Katherine NT 0851
08 8971 2766

Westpac Breezeway
Todd Mall
Alice Springs NT 0870
08 8953 1669
www.ntcarers.asn.au
See p. 225 for details

Commonwealth Carer Resource and Respite Centres
1800 059 059
For details see p. 225

Home and Community Care (HACC) Program
Call your council and/or your state disability department about this program.
For details see p. 226

Parent Support Groups
Autism NT holds meetings and information nights in Darwin, Katherine and
Alice Springs monthly. Call the office for current details.

Libraries & Resources
See **Autism NT** above

Darwin Toy Library
Marrara Neighbourhood Centre
McMillans Road
MOIL NT 0810
08 8927 9077
www.darwintoylibrary.org
Darwin Toy Library aims to provide services to children who are disadvantaged

in the community.

Central Australian Community Toy Library
Shop 8, Diarama Village
Larapinta Drive
Alice Springs NT 0870
08 8952 6720
The Central Australian Community Toy Library is a community-based Early Childhood Centre providing programs, resources, community information and links to other early childhood services for families with children from babies up to eight years.

When You Really Need To Talk to Somebody

Parentline
1300 30 1300 (cost of a local call)
8am to 10pm, seven days a week
www.parentline.com.au
Parentline is a confidential telephone counselling service aimed at providing professional counselling and support for parents.

Lifeline
13 11 14
www.lifeline.org.au
Lifeline offers telephone counselling throughout Australia — 24 hours a day, seven days a week.

QLD

First Things First

Autism Queensland 07 3273 0000

The Family Support Team and Outreach Team can be contacted during business hours.

State Autism Association

Autism Queensland

437 Hellawell Road

Sunnybank Hills Qld, 4109

07 3273 0000

www.autismqld.com.au/

Autism Queensland celebrated its 40th anniversary in 2007. With over 150 staff in centres in Brisbane, Rockhampton and Cairns, Autism Queensland is the largest ASD service provider in the state.

EARLY INTERVENTION

Early Intervention Group Placement — Brisbane

Autism Queensland runs two Early Intervention groups in the Brisbane Metropolitan area These run for one year and comprise a 2-day per week attendance. Autism Queensland staff also make regular visits to each child's home and other educational settings (eg SEDU, child care centres, preschools).

Early Intervention Outreach Support — Statewide Advisory Visits and Programs
Autism Queensland consultants are able to provide visits to the educational placement (eg kindy, preschool, SEDU) of a young child with ASD to observe and provide information, advice, support and individualised strategies to parents, staff and other personnel. This service is available as an individual advisory visit, or as a short-term program consisting of 3–6 sessions. Teams consist of teachers, OTs and speech pathologists.

Central Queensland Early AQtion Programs
Breakspeare St
Gracemere, Qld, 4702
07 4921 1788
07 4927 4706
This service provides specialist early intervention to children under six years of age, with a diagnosis of ASD in Rockhampton and surrounding towns and areas. A range of program options are available including intensive group placement programs (3–5 days per week), playgroups, individual programs and outreach support.

Far North Queensland Early AQtion Programs
15 Marr St
Edmonton, Queensland, 4869
1800 657 077
This service provides specialist early intervention to children under six years of age, with a diagnosis of ASD and their families in Cairns and surrounding towns and areas. A range of program options are available including intensive group placement programs (3–5 days per week), playgroups, individual programs and outreach support.

Individual Programs (unsubsidised)
The content format and duration of these programs are flexible and able to be tailored to the needs of the child with ASD. Programs are available in Brisbane and regional Queensland in a variety of settings.

Autism Spectrum Disorder Therapy Clinic (unsubsidised)
Occupational therapy and Speech Pathology services are available through the ASD Therapy clinic.

SCHOOLS AND SCHOOL-AGED SUPPORT
Group Placement Programs
Autism Queensland has two Education and Therapy Centres, in Brighton and Sunnybank, which operate as accredited Independent Schools. Students attend Group Placement part-time for a period of 12 months to 2 years. They attend one of the Centres for 1–3 days per week whilst continuing to attend their local school. Students are grouped according to age, ability and needs, with a maximum of six per group.

Each group is staffed by a Group Teacher and Teacher Aide. Speech Pathology, Occupational Therapy and Physiotherapy are provided for two- and three-day group placements. One-day group placements are intensive and targeted programs which focus on specific areas of need including social skills, communication, self-management, school issues, organisational skills, assignment and homework.

Home AQtion Programs
This is a short-term program which focusses on home-based issues affecting school performance and participation, facilitated by a Group Teacher.

School Outreach Support — Statewide Advisory Visits
Autism Queensland's Outreach Services Team visit children with ASD in their educational settings throughout Queensland. The visiting team (which usually consist of two staff from a team of teachers, occupational therapists and speech pathologists) work with the child's school support team and family to identify strategies to improve educational outcomes.

Individual Programs (unsubsidised)
The content, format and duration of these programs are flexible and able to be tailored to the needs of the child. Programs are available in Brisbane and regional Queensland in a variety of settings.

Autism Spectrum Disorder Therapy Clinic (unsubsidised)
See above

TRAINING FOR PARENTS AND PROFESSIONALS
Workshops
Workshops are conducted in both metropolitan and regional centres throughout the year. An annual training and consultancy booklet can be downloaded from the AQ website, www.autismqld.com.au/resources/workshops.php

Individualised Training Modules
Autism Queensland is also able to tailor individual modules to suit the needs

QLD

of the organisation or agency requesting the training. Content, format and location are flexible.

Extended Consultations
Consultations may be arranged by families, schools or other agencies to provide an opportunity for provision of information, development of strategies, program planning, etc for a child or adult with ASD.

Nationally Accredited Training
Autism Queensland is a Registered Training Organisation. Programs being developed include: Teacher Aide, Teacher, Support Worker and Respite Carer.

FAMILY SUPPORT SERVICES
Counselling and Information Services
Counselling, support and information regarding family issues, advocacy, respite, access to other services/agencies and employment issues are available.

Support Groups
Autism Queensland Support Groups are established to provide support in coping as parents or other primary caregivers of a person with ASD. There are currently support groups in the following locations: Adults with ASD (Brisbane), Bowen, Brighton, Bundaberg, Cairns, Childers, Emerald, Gold Coast. Gladstone, Mackay, Maryborough, North Queensland, Redlands, Rockhampton, South Burnett, Sunnybank Hills, Sunshine Coast, Toowoomba.

For current details and to download newsletters from some groups. check Family Support Services on the AQ website.

Parent Programs
Parent Programs are held at the Brisbane, Rockhampton and Cairns campuses. These programs are based on the 'Care for Caring Parents' program. This program aims to encourage parents to make full use of all areas of support and to build on existing strengths.

Sibling Groups
Autism Queensland runs two sibling programs — younger sibling group and teenage sibling group. The aim of these programs is to provide opportunities for siblings of children with ASD to meet other children. This helps to alleviate the sense of isolation and allows the children to discuss their feelings and any issues that may be of relevance in a non-threatening and non-judgmental environment.

Sibling Camps
Two camps are held each year: one group specifically caters for teenagers.

Mother's Time Out Camps
Two mothers' camps are held per year.

Respite Services for Children

RESPITE AND FAMILY SUPPORT SERVICE — OXLEY
Oxley Respite and Family Support is a multi-dimensional and innovative service which caters for families who have the demanding role of caring for someone with a disability and complex, challenging behaviours. The clients may be of any age, have any number of disabilities and must live within the Brisbane City Council area.

OVERNIGHT AND WEEKEND RESPITE BIRRALEE
Birralee is a centre-based respite service which operates from Friday to Sunday and provides overnight and weekend respite to children and adolescents. The residence is a light, open-plan house that is spacious and welcoming, and has been modified to safely accommodate children and adolescents with ASD. The residence is also conveniently located next door to Sunnybank Therapy Centre, and provides access to a safe and secure playground with bikes, a trampoline and a large swimming pool.

DAY RESPITE PROGRAMS
Autism Queensland offers day respite holiday programs during the school holidays (excluding Easter).

ADULT SERVICES
RESPITE AND FAMILY SUPPORT SERVICE — OXLEY
See above.

SUPPORTED ACCOMMODATION
Autism Queensland provides two kinds of supported accommodation, both of which are only available to members of Autism Queensland who are currently in receipt of an Adult Lifestyle Support Package (ALSP).

24-HOUR SUPPORTED ACCOMMODATION
Autism Queensland provides 24-hour supported accommodation to individuals who are in receipt of an ALSP. This service is conducted within houses in the community (which are either owned or leased by Autism Queensland) ranging from the Ipswich region, Brisbane south and the Bay area.

IN-HOME SUPPORT
Accommodation support can also be provided to individuals who are in receipt of an ALSP and are living in their own home. This type of support can vary from a couple of hours a week to 35 hours per week, and can vary according to the individual's skills, abilities and future plans.

QLD

ADULT REC GROUP

This group for young adults with ASD meets on a fortnightly basis. Activities include various outings to a range of venues appropriate to the group as well as regular meetings at Autism Queensland.

RESOURCE CENTRE

The Autism Queensland Resource Centre contains books, magazines, journals, and other material on issues related to ASD. Financial members of Autism Queensland are able to access this library during office hours. Books may be borrowed and posted out on request.

State Disability Department

Disability Services Queensland
Level 3A, Neville Bonner Building
75 William Street
Brisbane Qld 4000
1800 177 120
www.disability.qld.gov.au

Disability Services Queensland (DSQ) provides a range of services for people with disabilities under the Commonwealth-State/Territory Disability Agreement. Whilst specific access criteria and prioritisation processes exist for many of the programs, persons with autism and their families are encouraged to enquire about the following direct and funded service options:

Direct services include:
- Family and Early Childhood Services
- Child Behaviour Support Teams
- Local Area Coordination
- Adult and Community Support Services
- Intensive Behaviour Support Teams
- Friendship Program

Family and Early Childhood Services and the Child Safety and Behaviour Support Teams provide a family and child-centred service to children aged 0–6 years who have, or are at risk of, a significant developmental delay. This may include children with ASD.

Local Area Coordination supports people with a disability to access the support they need and build informal and community networks. The program operates in rural and remote locations.

Adult and Community Services support adults who have an intellectual disability and high support needs. Services include case management, information and referral and skill development. The program also supports school aged children with an intellectual disability to access respite.

Intensive Behaviour Support Teams assist families, carers and service providers to meet the needs of adults with a disability who have complex and challenging behaviour support needs.

The Friendship Program supports adults with a disability who are socially isolated to develop friendships. The program also works to raise community awareness of disability and increase the involvement of people with a disability in the community.

Funded services include:

- Lifelong planning
- Post-School Services
- Adult Lifestyle Support Program
- Family Support Program — children and adults
- Accommodation support services for adults
- Respite Services
- Advocacy Support
- Autism Early Intervention Initiative for children under six years

Lifelong Planning is an early intervention strategy to strengthen the ability of community service organisations to provide support and information to all people with a disability.

Based upon assessment and prioritisation of needs, individual funding packages are provided under Post-School Services, the Adult Lifestyle Support Program and the Family Support Program for approved service providers to respond to the needs of people with disabilities, including those with autism. DSQ also funds service providers to provide respite services to children and adults.

Autism Queensland Inc receives specific funding to provide respite and accommodation support programs for children and adults with ASD.

Under DSQ's Autism Early Intervention Strategy, Autism Queensland and the Autism Early Intervention Outcomes Unit (AEIOU) operate Early Intervention Centres in Brisbane and regional Queensland. This strategy aims to strengthen family capacity and reduce the long-term care and support costs for families.

State Health Department

Queensland Health
147-163 Charlotte Street
Brisbane Qld 4000
07 3234 0111
www.health.qld.gov.au

Queensland Health strives to provide quality early intervention services for children with developmental disorders and developmental delay including assessment and multi-disciplinary treatment for children diagnosed with autism.

Across Queensland, 17 Children's Developmental Services deliver standardised assessments and integration of information, including specialist developmental assessment by a developmental paediatrician, and/or multiple assessments conducted by allied health professionals.

Differing levels of individual and family intervention services may be offered depending upon resource allocation and the type of intervention, including individual therapy, home programs, group therapy, advocacy and a consultation-liaison response with other service providers such as education services, general paediatricians and other disability services.

The services providing assessment for moderate to severe developmental problems will usually offer a combined medical and allied health multi-disciplinary approach delivering diagnostic and intervention services for children with autism and other developmental delays or disabilities. In some instances, there are cross-agency service arrangements to ensure that children receive the most appropriate service. QH may, by default, become the provider for groups who do not qualify for services from Disability Services Queensland (DSQ), Education Queensland (EQ) or non-government organisations.

The practice of diagnosis and assessment of ASD in Queensland Health Developmental Services will usually involve the completion of standardised assessments in the area of cognition and communication, sensori-motor functioning and a comprehensive developmental review by a developmental paediatrician or general paediatrician. The collection of additional information from other sources such as day-care, education providers, primary health nurses etc allows integration of information about a child's functioning across a number of settings.

Parents and carers are considered important collaborators in the assessment and treatment process. They provide useful observational and factual information about their child's development, engage with health professionals to set priorities for their child's skill acquisition and work collaboratively through clinic and home-based intervention to promote their child's ongoing learning and developmental needs.

MEDICAL AIDS SUBSIDY SCHEME
www.health.qld.gov.au/mass
This scheme subsidises some equipment eg communication devices and continence aids which are useful for those at the more severe end of the spectrum.

Your Local Council

Many local councils around Australia have a Disability Information Officer or Community Care Officer. It is well worth getting in touch with your local council to ask about local services and assistance that may be available.

Early Intervention — General

See **Department of Education, Training and the Arts DETA** below

Early Childhood Intervention Australia (ECIA)

www.ecia.org.au

ECIA is a national organisation which promotes the public profile of Early Childhood Intervention, facilitates effective liaison and advocacy in the community, and fosters quality information and service provision.

Early Intervention — ASD Specific

See **Autism Queensland** above

QLD

AEIOU

PO Box 806

Nundah Qld 4012

07 3849 6100

www.aeiou.org.au

AEIOU is a not-for-profit charity providing full-time early education programs for children with ASD, aged two and a half to five years of age. AEIOU's mission is to provide a placement to every child with ASD, from the time of diagnosis, to facilitate their transition to mainstream education and to continue to support the child and their family through the child's schooling years.

The program at AEIOU is based on an intensive, functional, task-orientated approach that includes activities for cognitive development, daily living skills, play skills, and communication skills. The program is tailored to meet the specific needs of each child and family. Comprehensive assessments and weekly reviews are essential elements.

Specialist practitioners — early childhood teachers, OTs, speech pathologists — are involved in every child's program. Staff work with families to ensure that learning is carried from the educational setting into the home environment. The children participate in a combination of small group activities and one-on-one time with staff. The small groups join together for meal times, and some free play.

Families pay fees equivalent to private child care costs. As the centres are registered as Long Day Care there may be access to the Child Care Benefit.

AEIOU operates centres at Moorooka, Bray Park, Toowoomba, Townsville and Park Ridge and in 2009 will open in Brisbane's western suburbs, and on the Sunshine Coast and Gold Coast.

An additional teacher supports the transition of children to school and provides ongoing follow-up of the child, the child's family and teachers through the schooling years.

Early Intervention — ABA

Autism Behavioural Intervention Queensland (ABIQ)
PO Box 7053
Brendale Qld 4500
Office Address (Please use postal address for mailing)
Unit 13, 357 Gympie Road
Strathpine
07 3881 1868
www.abiq.org

ABIQ is a volunteer organisation promoting effective early intervention for children with autism, including the use of ABA. ABIQ offers education, resources and a support network for families of children with autism, living in Queensland.

ABIQ services for members include:

* affordably priced education events organised regularly for parents and professionals, covering ABA and other approaches to autism
* resource collections containing therapy materials for children undergoing home-based intervention and a reference library suitable for parents and professionals (loans are mailed to members in regional areas)
* parent-to-parent support and advice via telephone, email, support groups and social activities
* quarterly newsletter to members and frequent updates from the autism community via email
* maintaining a register of teaching assistants interested in working within home-based programs.

ABAQ — Applied Behaviour Analysis Queensland
111 Jospeh Ave
Moggill Qld 4070
07 3202 7305

0417 520 523

ABAQ offers a comprehensive, multi-disciplinary behavioural and educational service for families with young children with ASD. This family-centred practice provides in-home and school based services:

- parent workshops
- Hanen programs, Applied Verbal Behaviour
- naturalistic, activity-based learning through play and daily routines
- mobile speech pathology service (PECS, Makaton, PROMPT)
- PRT
- Positive Behavioural Support programming.

ABA International Inc.

Southport
Gold Coast, Qld
07 5528 3478

ABA International provides educational assessments, intensive early intervention programs and behavioural intervention programs for children with autism through the application of behaviour analysis. Verbal behaviour assessment and intervention is also available. Behaviour programs address common issues associated with autism, including, but not limited to: eating, sleep, toileting, frustration, self-injury and self-stimulation. All programs are empirically based. Ongoing education requirements assure that new developments within the field of autism are incorporated into assessments and programs.

Autism Partnership

P.O. Box 1198
Robina DC Qld 4226
07 5535 9182
0409 013 709
www.autismpartnership.com/aus.htm

Autism Partnership is a private agency specialising in behavioural intervention programs for children with autism and related disorders. Providing services to children and families throughout Queensland, Autism Partnership believes in comprehensive intervention designed to meet the individual needs of each child.

Bayside Psychology and Health Services

Shop 4 Dean Building
Crn Bloomfield & Queen Streets
Cleveland Qld 4163

07 3488 0483

Bayside Psychology and Health Services is a local practice with a psychologist who specialises in working with children who have special needs including those with ASD. Services include:

- Diagnosis and Assessment
- Applied Behaviour Analysis Developmental Autism Programs
- Play Therapy
- Expressive Therapies
- Medical/Legal Assessments
- Applied Behaviour Analysis Assessments and Positive Behavioural Support Planning for challenging behaviour
- Counselling for families
- Parenting Programs

Little Souls Taking Big Steps

1 Allied Drive
Arundel Qld 4214
07 5563 1490
www.littlesouls.com.au

Little Souls Taking Big Steps is a child care centre catering for children aged two to six with a diagnosis of ASD and for typically developing children. The centre has a series of one-on-one therapy rooms so that children with ASD/PDD are able to access ABA therapy on a one to one basis throughout the day.

Children with a diagnosis of ASD or PDD attend the centre five days a week, and receive 1:1 instruction for a portion of the day as well as having the opportunity to integrate with their typically developing peers in a classroom setting. The amount of time spent in each setting is dependent on the skill level and needs of the individual child. Little Souls is a not-for-profit organisation, registered as a charity, and provides some scholarships for those children whose parents are unable to meet the full cost of tuition.

Victorian ABA Providers Pty Ltd

Queensland office
07 5485-2036
0407407936

Victorian ABA Providers is a company that specialises in teaching preschool children with autism, pervasive developmental disorders, and related developmental disabilities using ABA methodology. Victorian ABA Providers services clients in both Victoria and Queensland. The company has strong links with the Lovaas Institute at the Psychology Department at UCLA; twice yearly visits are made by its director to Australia.

RDI®

There are several RDI® consultants in Australia. The Connections Center in Houston, Texas trains and certifies all RDI® consultants and their website has a comprehensive list: www.rdiconnect.com
There is also an Australian RDI® Yahoo group at:
http://health.groups.yahoo.com/group/RDIsupportgroup/
If you join this group, you can access a file which also lists RDI® consultants in training, who may be starting to work with families already. It also lists consultants from the US who come to Australia to work with families. This is a useful egroup for getting in touch with other families doing RDI® in your area.

Speech Pathologists, Occupational Therapists and Psychologists

Autism Queensland may be able to assist with recommendations. See p. 239 for details on how to get in touch with these professionals through their national and state organisations.

Multi-disciplinary Services

Child Development Network

3/30 Annerley Road
South Brisbane Qld 4101
07 3010 3366
www.cd.net.au
The Child Development Network is a private, multi-disciplinary service for children (and their families) who have problems of development and behaviour, including ASD. The team comprises specialist paediatricians, psychologists, educators and therapists. The emphasis is support and management over time, beyond initial diagnosis and treatment.

Minds and Hearts Clinic

6/88 Boundary Street
West End Qu 4101
07 3844 9466
www.mindsandhearts.net
Minds and Hearts is a unique clinic specialising in Asperger's syndrome and autism. Minds and Hearts was conceived to meet the enormous need

for specialist services for children and adults with ASD. Minds and Hearts was designed to provide specialised knowledge and assistance from a multi-disciplinary team of experienced professionals. Minds and Hearts can assist with assessment, individual and group therapy, problem-solving sessions and also provide workshops. Medicare and private health insurance rebates are also available.

Schools

Department of Education, Training and the Arts (DETA)
Mary Street
Brisbane Qld 4000
07 3237 0111
www.education.qld.gov.au
The Inclusive Education Policy of DETA reflects the values and culture of an education system committed to enhancing equitable educational opportunities and improved outcomes for all students, including students with disabilities. More information on Inclusive Education in the Queensland state schooling context is available at: http://education.qld.gov.au/strategic/eppr/curriculum/crppr009/

There is an array of programs and services to support students with ASD attending Queensland state schools (prep to year 12). Support is provided through school-based and or visiting specialist support staff. Early childhood development programs and services are also available for children under school age.

Partnerships with community agencies supporting students with ASDs is also valued, and facilitated where appropriate. To access information on the programs and services available in schools in the local area contact the local school principal and or the Principal Education Officer (Student Services) based in the local education district office. Further information on schools and education districts within Queensland can be found at: http://education.qld.gov.au/parents/

The Education Adjustment Program (EAP) is the process used for identifying and responding to the educational support needs of students with disabilities: http://education.qld.gov.au/students/disabilities/adjustment/

Online resources and more information relating to students with ASD is accessible on the Autism Spectrum Disorder Professional Learning Community managed by Disability Services Support Unit, Student Services Division, DETA: www.learningplace.com.au/en/dssulc/asd

Queensland Catholic Education Commission

143 Edward Street
Brisbane Qld 4000
07 3336 9306
www.qcec.qld.catholic.edu.au
There are five dioceses in Queensland. Click on Links to find contact details
for your local diocese.

Independent Schools Queensland

First Floor, 96 Warren Street
Spring Hill Qld 4000
07 3228 1515
www.aisq.qld.edu.au
ISQ manages federal funding for children with special needs in independent
schools and has a special needs adviser who supports school staff.

Therapy Services for School-Aged Children

See **Department of Education, Training and the Arts (DETA)**

SchoolLinks

Child Development Network
Suite 3, Mater Community Services Building,
39 Annerley Road
South Brisbane Qld 4101
07 3010 3366
www.cd.net.au
schoollinks.cd.net.au
SchoolLinks fills a gap in services available to families, schools and health
professionals. The team brings together a broad range of skills and strategies
to help you understand and manage children whose difficulties impact on life
at school. SchoolLinks is a new program developed by the Child Development
Network.
See **Minds and Hearts Clinic** above
See **Child Development Network**

Respite and Carer Support

Carers Queensland

15 Abbott St

Camp Hill Qld 4121
07 3843 1401
www.carersqld.asn.au
See p. 225 for details
Carers Queensland's library contains over 1,500 books, videos, CDs, audios and reports on carer-related topics. Carers Queensland's library is located with the Commonwealth Carer Resource Centre at 972 Logan Road, Holland Park, Brisbane. Opening hours are Monday to Friday, 8am to 2pm. For members of the Association who are unable to visit the library in person, material can be posted out free of charge.

Commonwealth Carer Respite Centres
1800 059 059
For details see p. 225

Home and Community Care (HACC) Program
Call your council and/or your state disability department about this program.
For details see p. 226

Adult Services
See **Autism Queensland** above
See **Disability Services Queensland** above

Training for Parents and Professionals
See **Autism Queensland** above
See **EI and School-Ages Service Providers** above

Support Groups
See **Autism Queensland** above

Asperger Services Australia (ASA)
Shop 4 7 5,
235 Zillmere Road
Zillmere Qld 4034
07 3865 2911
www.asperger.asn.au

ASA provides support to families, carers, and siblings as well as to children, adolescents and adults with Asperger's syndrome. The office is generally open during the mornings in school terms but it is best to call ahead to check. ASA runs support groups and conferences. It has a newsletter, a resource library and has a forum on its website.

Autism Regional Education (ARE) Inc
P.O. Box 2059
Aitkenvale BC Qld 4814.
0418 186 294
07 4723 9650
www.autismgroup.com
ARE aims to raise awareness of ASD and to provide support to families.

See also **Professor Tony Atwood's** website www.tonyattwood.com.au

QLD

Libraries & Resources
See **Autism Behavioural Intervention Queensland (ABIQ)** above
See **Aspergers Services Australia (ASA)** above
See **Autism Queensland** above
See **Carers Queensland** above

When You Really Need To Talk to Somebody

Parentline
1300 30 1300 (cost of a local call)
8am to 10pm, seven days a week
www.parentline.com.au
Parentline is a confidential telephone counselling service which provides professional counselling and support.

Lifeline
13 11 14
www.lifeline.org.au
Lifeline offers telephone counselling throughout Australia — 24 hours a day, seven days a week.

SA

First Things First

Autism SA Infoline

1300 288 476

The Info line provides non-clinical information about ASD and offers referrals. It is available 9am-4pm Monday-Friday.

State Autism Association

Autism SA

3 Fisher Street

Myrtle Bank SA 5064

08 8379 6976

www.autismsa.org.au

Autism SA was founded by a group of parents in 1964 and has grown to become the largest provider of services to people with an ASD and their families in the state.

DIAGNOSTIC SERVICES

Autism SA is one of the major centres for diagnosis of ASD in South

Australia. Assessments can be made for both children and adults, meeting the international recommendations for best practice adopted by the Office of Disability and Client Services and the Board of Management of Autism SA.

EARLY DEVELOPMENT PROGRAM

In the metropolitan area, early intervention services are provided through group and consultancy programs, staffed by multi-disciplinary teams including speech pathologists, occupational therapists and education staff. Consultancy programs are available in the home, kindergarten and/or child care.

For preschool children who live outside the metropolitan area, services are offered through Autism SA's School Program. Children outside the metropolitan area are also eligible for services through the Early Development Group Program. However, it is the responsibility of parents to transport their child to centre-based programs.

SCHOOL PROGRAM

This is a multi-disciplinary program which provides support to students and schools, primarily in the metropolitan region. Assistance can include transition support, social skills training, professional development, or attendance at review meetings. Fee for service support is available as are one-to-one short-term programs. Support to country schools/preschools is limited. Visits to country areas occur twice a year for individual schools and training and development opportunities.

FAMILY AND INFORMATION SERVICES

Autism SA runs a very wide variety of Family and Information Services including:

- Post Diagnostic Appointments: providing additional information about ASD, relevant services, intervention and treatment programs.
- Training and Development: Family and Information Services: providing workshops for families, and information sessions for the public and for other agencies.
- The Mentoring Program: assisting people between the ages of 12 and 25 by providing trained peer mentors — the mentors and mentees meet fortnightly for social activities supervised by the co-ordinator.
- Parent Support Networks: 'Someone to turn to...'™ provides one-on-one telephone support to parents who are dealing with new a diagnosis, family issues or emotional stress. Autism SA also supports the development of parent support groups across the metropolitan area.
- Social Development Programs: ALPHA provides community-based outings for people with autism and Triple A is an arts-focused group

SA

for people with Asperger's syndrome.
- Brief Clinical Support: offering a time-limited number of sessions to families to assist them with self-management.

RESOURCES, TRAINING AND DEVELOPMENT
Autism SA provides a range of training options including scheduled training for parents and professionals and flexible fee-for-service workshops. A training schedule is available from Autism SA or you can discuss your needs with the Co-ordinator Family and Information Services. Training topics include:
- information sessions for new families
- introduction to ASDs
- working through difficult behaviours
- facilitating social skills
- sensory issues
- communication
- teaching strategies
- behaviour management.

COMMUNITY SERVICES
The Kandu (Clovelly Park) and Kandu II (Craigmore) programs are specialised day options services tailored to meet the needs of young people and adults with an ASD who no longer attend school. The aim is to enhance lifestyles by providing support in a range of recreational and prevocational experiences and opportunities.

RESPITE SERVICES
Weekend respite is available at two houses, one in Craigmore and one in the southern suburbs. Priority is given to children with challenging behaviours.

EMPLOYMENT SERVICES
Towards a Skilled Crew (TASC) provides supported employment in jobs such as cleaning, car detailing, enclave at the Institute of Medical and Veterinary Science and the assembly and packaging of various medical and laboratory kits. Support includes the development of social and vocational skills, counselling and guidance, enhancing awareness of work opportunities and other vocational services. There are also limited unpaid work experience placements available for students who are transitioning from school to work.

Worklink is an open employment service that assists clients to find work within the field that best suits their skills and support needs. Once participants find a job or work place training, time-limited support can be provided at the worksite whilst the worker learns about their new job.

SA

ASPITECH

www.aspitech.org.au

ASPITECH is a not-for-profit organisation owned by Autism SA. Based in Bedford Park, ASPITECH sells, repairs and recycles computers and associated hardware.

MAGAZINE — THE AUTISER

The Autiser is Autism SA's quarterly newsletter that aims to keep members up-to-date with local events, training and development and new resources. An electronic version is available for download.

State Disability Department

Disability SA

103 Fisher Street

Fullarton SA 5063 SA

08 8272 1988

1300 786 117 Eligibilty and Intake

www.disability.sa.gov.au

Disability SA Child and Youth Service provide support and services to children and young people, from birth until transition to post school options. An Early Childhood Program provides support to young children until the transition to school and the School-Age and Youth Programs provides services to older children and youth.

The metropolitan teams include service coordinators, social workers, speech pathologists, physiotherapists, OTs, developmental educators and psychologists who work in partnership with families and ensure a co-ordinated approach.

The country teams are smaller and located in all regional areas throughout South Australia providing developmental and behavioural services and support for families where there are high and complex needs. Senior Developmental Programmers provide specialist interventions and case management for children 0–8 years of age.

Aims:

- to enhance the development of individuals and their participation in community life.
- to strengthen and support families in their caring role.

Services:

- developmental assessments and recommendations to promote learning and functional skills for children and youth
- assessment of need and identification of goals and priority areas

SA

- information to assist understanding of developmental disabilities and the effect that particular diagnostic conditions may have
- family support
- parent/carer education
- support at key transitions
- developmental groups
- assistance with emerging behavioural issues and challenging behaviours
- sibling support
- opportunities for parents and carers to meet other parents and carers
- equipment prescription — assessment and recommendations
- opportunities for inclusion and participation within the community
- service co-ordination
- planning for pathways beyond school
- planning for transition from care for children under the guardianship of the Minister
- access to intensive intervention programs

Asperger's syndrome and Higher Functioning Autism
Disability SA provides intervention and case management for Asperger's syndrome and high functioning autism, offering individual and family support and information services.

Referrals can be made by contacting Disability SA Intake on 1300 786 117 (local call cost for country callers). Referrals can also be made in person at your local Disability SA Office.

State Health Department

SA Health strives to provide quality early intervention services for children with developmental disorders and developmental delay including assessment and multi-disciplinary treatment for children diagnosed with autism. The aim of the assessment process is to develop an understanding of a child's developmental profile focusing on where the child's abilities are across areas of self-care, motor coordination and mobility, communication, cognition, learning, emotion and behaviour.

Child Development Units
A range of assessments may be undertaken as part of an autism diagnostic process. Parents and carers are an essential part of the assessment process.

Other assessments may focus on the area of cognition and communication, sensori-motor functioning and/or a comprehensive developmental review by a paediatrician. The collection of additional information from other sources such as day-care, education providers, general practitioners, primary health nurses, is usual as the integration of information about a child's functioning across a number of settings is helpful to enhance the accuracy of diagnostic formulation.

The location of key contacts for diagnostic services for children with autism are listed in the table below.

Organisation	Address	Unit	Contact
Lyell McEwen Hospital	Haydown Road Elizabeth Vale SA 5112	Child Development Unit	Unit Coordinator 08 8182 9379 (referral required)
Women's and Children's Hospital Outpatients	72 King William Road North Adelaide SA 5006	Paediatric Outpatients Department	08 8161 6644 (referral required)
Women's and Children's Hospital	72 King William Road North Adelaide SA 5006	Child Development Unit	Unit Coordinator 08 8161 6176 08 8161 8011 (referral required)
Flinders Medical Centre	Flinders Drive Bedford Park SA 5042	Children's Assessment Team	Unit Coordinator 08 8204 4433 (referral required)

SA

Child and Adolescent Mental Health Services (CAMHS)

Child and Adolescent Mental Health Services in South Australia have community based clinics across South Australia. CAMHS provides counselling to children and young people with autism who also have mental health issues.

The location of key contacts for counselling services for children with autism who also have mental health issues are listed in the table below.

Organisation	Address	Unit	Contact
SAHS-CAMHS Southern Mental Health Service	c/- Block E The Flats Flinders Drive Bedford Park SA 5042	SAHS-CAMHS Southern Mental Health Service	08 8204 5412
Women's and Children's Hospital	72 King William Road North Adelaide SA 5006	CAMHS	08 8161 7389

Child and Family Health

Child and Family Health Services provide Maternal and Child Health nursing services for all children in South Australia. These services cover postnatal and early childhood parenting support, breastfeeding advice, home visiting, immunisation, health checks and referral to multi-disciplinary professional services to children and families. For further information contact Children, Youth and Women's Health Services on telephone 1300 733 606.

Intervention services are also provided by **Autism SA** and **Disability SA**.

Your Local Council

Many local councils around Australia have a Disability Information Officer or Community Care Officer. It is well worth getting in touch with your local council to ask about local services and assistance that may be available.

Early Intervention — General

Early Childhood Intervention Australia (ECIA)

www.ecia.org.au

ECIA is a national organisation which promotes the public profile of Early Childhood Intervention, facilitates effective liaison and advocacy in the community, and fosters quality information and service provision. It has a South Australian chapter.

Department of Education and Children's Services (DECS)

Disability and Statewide Programs
Level 5 Education Centre
31 Flinders Street
Adelaide SA 5000
08 8226 0546
www.decs.sa.gov.au/speced/pages/specialneeds/Earlychildhood/

INCLUSIVE PRESCHOOL PROGRAMS

IPPs support children with disabilities and high support needs to optimise their learning outcomes within a localised preschool setting. IPPs operate as centres with expertise, supporting educators within the network of local preschool services to develop skills and expertise. This is achieved through a range of staff training and mentoring strategies. Staffing consists of a 0.5 teacher and 0.5 early childhood worker for a group of up to six children per program aged from 4 years. There are seven IPPs located across metropolitan and country districts.

SA

THE PRESCHOOL SUPPORT PROGRAM

The Preschool Support Program supports the inclusion of children with additional needs and provides expertise to preschool teams. It aims to maximise the child's learning by minimising the impact the disability and/or developmental delay has on the child's development. The target group is children aged 4–5 years. (Early Entry at 3.5 years and extension of time for one term may occur with approval).

Children with a range of needs including autism, global developmental delay, severe multiple disabilities, delayed communication (either speech and/or language) can be supported through the Preschool Support Program. Some of these children can be referred to intensive programs such as the Speech and Language Program, the Inclusive Preschool Program, the Learning Links Program or the Briars Special Early Learning Centre.

THE BRIARS SPECIAL EARLY LEARNING CENTRE

The Briars is a specifically designed facility and a stand-alone preschool for young children with significant developmental delay and/or disability. It provides a specialised program for children aged 3.5–6 years who have an intellectual disability, significant developmental delay and/or multiple physical disabilities. The Briars also provides a peer-based training and development program for community preschools and mentoring to the Inclusive Preschool Program staff teams.

Children who are eligible may attend one full day per week (two sessions) from age three increasing to two full days per week (four sessions) at age four. In addition to a range of developmentally appropriate preschool activities, staff implement structured programs to assist children's independence with toileting/self-care and eating/drinking.

Early Intervention — ASD specific

See **Autism SA Early Development Program** above

Headstart Intervention Services

69 Goodwood Road
Wayville SA 5034
08 83734531

Headstart Intervention Services specialises in psychological services for children, adolescents and young adults. Headstart can develop and introduce a tailored program to meet the learning needs of children with developmental disorders and/or delays. For younger children, considerable time is dedicated to developing home-based intervention packages based on applied behavioural techniques. Hands-on therapy sessions can also be arranged. Clients may also wish to engage in one of Headstart's social skills training groups directed at children, adolescents and parents.

The psychologists provide services relating to school difficulties, anxiety and depression, as well as eating, sleeping and conduct disturbances. Parent education, training and support is also offered.

Early Intervention — ABA
ISADD — Intervention Service for Autism and Developmental Delay
PO Box 2076
Magill North SA 5073
0419 857 417
www.isadd.org
See ISADD description in WA listings on p. 349

Key Early Years
19 Charles Street
Norwood SA 5067
08 83632969
0400 240 345
www.keyearlyyears.com
KEYS provides a special education service to schools, offering:
- observations
- training in behaviour management of challenging behaviours
- effective teaching strategies for children with autism including Asperger's syndrome
- social skills training
- counselling
- assessments

KEYS also acts as a parent advocate in schools and provides information for parents on choosing schools.

Early Intervention Research Program (EIRP)
Flinders University EIRP
School of Psychology
Flinders University

GPO Box 2100
SA 5001
08 8201 5261
www.socsci.flinders.edu.au/psyc/research/autism/about.php
EIRP is an intensive intervention program specifically designed to work with young children and their parents. It is currently offered as a free service to families. Once diagnosed, children and their families begin immediate intensive intervention based on the techniques of ABA. Intensive training is provided for parents and volunteers to target and modify the early behaviours considered to be linked to core neurological deficits of ASD.

This program is based on the Clinical Practice Guidelines recommended by the New York State Department of Health and is being continually evaluated to ensure the best possible outcomes for the children. To be eligible, children must be under the age of five and be diagnosed with autism or as 'at risk' of developing autism. Families must also commit to conduct therapy for a minimum of 15 hours per week for 18 weeks and agree not to begin new interventions over the course of the 20-week program.

The objectives of the EIRP are:
- to identify children with autism as early as possible, preferably before the age of two
- to start immediate intensive early intervention with the EIRP
- to help children reach their full potential both academically and in each of the three areas associated with autism:
- social
- communication
- stereotypical/ritualistic behaviours
- to increase children's play abilities, eye contact and general enjoyment of social activities and play with peers
- to increase the children's ability to communicate verbally or through alternate means (PECS, sign)
- to decrease and prevent stereotypical, repetitive and ritualistic behaviours
- to educate and empower parents in the education of their children

RDI®

There are several RDI® consultants in Australia. The Connections Center in Houston, Texas trains and certifies all RDI® consultants and their website has a comprehensive list: www.rdiconnect.com
There is also an Australian RDI® Yahoo group at:
http://health.groups.yahoo.com/group/RDIsupportgroup/
If you join this group, you can access a file which also lists RDI® consultants

SA

in training, who may be starting to work with families already. It also lists consultants from the US who come to Australia to work with families. This is a useful egroup for getting in touch with other families doing RDI® in your area.

Speech Pathologists, Occupational Therapists and Psychologists

Get in touch with Autism SA to ask for recommendations in SA. See p. 239 for details on how to get in touch with these professionals through their national and state organisations.

Schools

Department of Education and Children's Services (DECS)
Disability and Statewide Programs
Level 5 Education Centre
31 Flinders Street SA 5000
08 82261000
www.decs.sa.gov.au
DECS provides a range of services and programs to support students with disabilities, including those with autism.

Students with autism in regular classes may receive support from the Disability Support Program. Special classes in regular schools provide a special placement option for students with a range of disabilities including autism. Special schools provide an option for students with autism and high needs. The decision on where to enrol a student with a disability, appropriate program options and their level of support is part of a negotiated education planning process involving DECS teachers, district services staff, parents and, where appropriate, other agencies.

Information for parents can be accessed on: www.decs.sa.gov.au/speced/pages/specialneeds/intro

The Manager, Student Support and Disability, is available to assist parents/carers with this decision-making and can provide additional information about the support available in the district. A list of district offices can be found at:
www.decs.sa.gov.au/custserve/pages/default/districtoffices

Association of Independent Schools of SA (AISSA)
301 Unley Road
Malvern SA 5061

08 8179 1400
www.ais.sa.edu.au
AIS manages federal funding for special needs children in independent schools.
Contact the special education adviser for advice on school enrolment.

Catholic Education Office
116 George Street
Thebarton SA 5031
08 8301 6600
www.cesa.catholic.edu.au
Within Catholic Education SA, a range of support options exist for students with special needs. This includes mainstream schooling, units and special schools. A team of Special Education Consultants assist families and schools during the enrolment process. Schools receive some resources to assist in the inclusion of students with disabilities.

Therapy Services for School-Aged Children
See **Autism SA** above
See **Headstart Internention Services** above

Adult Services
See **Autism SA** above
See **Disability SA** above

SA

Swimming
SASRAPID Inc — South Australian Sport and Recreation Association for People with Integration Difficulties Inc
Level 2, Station Arcade
52–54 Hindley Street
Adelaide SA 5000
08 8410 6999
www.sasrapid.com.au
SASRAPID provides Aquatic Therapy for Children with Autism, a specialised program within Rapid Swim which is for children diagnosed with ASD.

Aquatic Therapy for Children with Autism is a specialised service for children with autism aged 1–12 years. Programs run in blocks of eight weeks, during school terms only. Each child receives a 1:1, 30-minute session per week. Sessions combine OT and speech pathology with the many benefits of an aquatic environment. Therapists use sensory integration techniques. Rapid Swim provides 1:1 water awareness, confidence and swimming lessons to people of all ages who have integration difficulties. Costs are kept as low as possible.

Inclusion

Inclusive Directions
5–7 Rasheed Ave
Newton SA 5074
08 8165 2900
www.directions.org.au
Inclusive Directions works with child care, out of school hours care and vacation care services to support the inclusion of children with special needs. Training, support and advocacy are offered. Inclusive Directions allocates the Inclusion Support Subsidy.

Respite and Carer Info

Carers SA
58 King William Road
Goodwood SA 5034
08 8271 6288
1800 815 549 Toll Free
www.carers-sa.asn.au
For information see p. 225

Commonwealth Carer Respite Centres
1800 059 059
For details see p. 225

Home and Community Care (HACC) Program
Call your council and/or your state disability department about this program.
For details see p. 226

Parent Support Groups
Autism SA website has a regularly updated list of family support groups.

Beyond the Square

www.beyondthesquare.org.au

Beyond the Square provides support to parents, families, carers and siblings as well as to female children, adolescents and adults with Asperger's syndrome.

Training for Parents and Professionals

See **Autism SA** above

Libraries & Resources

See **Autism SA Resource Centre** above

Disability Information & Resource Centre Inc (DIRC)

195 Gilles Street

Adelaide SA 5000

08 8236 0555

1300 305 558 SA only

www.dircsa.org.au

DIRC provides information and referral services for all sorts of disabilities. DIRC has a library which is open Monday – Friday, 9am – 5pm.

When You Really Need To Talk to Somebody

Parent Helpline SA

1300 364 100 (cost of a local call)

24 hours a day, seven days a week

www.parenting.sa.gov.au

The Parent Helpline is a service of Children, Youth and Women's Health Service and provides telephone information, counselling and support.

Lifeline

13 11 14

www.lifeline.org.au

Lifeline offers telephone counselling throughout Australia — 24 hours a day, seven days a week.

TAS

First Things First
Autism Tasmania — Family Support
03 6423 2288 or 0407 320 048

Through The Maze
Association for Children with Disability (Tas) Inc
202 Liverpool Street
Hobart
Tas 7000
03 6231 2466
www.acdtas.com.au
Through the Maze is a comprehensive guide to services for parents of children with a disability in Tasmania. It is produced by the Association for Children with Disability (Tas) Inc and can be downloaded from their website.

State Autism Association

Autism Tasmania
PO Box 1552
Launceston Tas 7250
General Enquiries & Library
03 6362 4755
Family Support Service, Information and Training
03 6423 2288 or 0407 320 048
www.autismtas.org.au

Autism Tasmania provides support and information to families of children who may be undergoing investigation or who have a diagnosis of ASD. Ongoing support and advice is continued to families both on a personal basis and through regular regional Parent Support get-togethers.

Support and information is also available to families who have older people in their families with ASD. Autism Tasmania's library is available to members. Social functions for parents, families, carers and professionals are held as are seminars, conferences and workshops. At the time of writing, Autism Tasmania receives no public funding and relies upon donations, grants and its tireless voluntary workers.

State Disability and Health Department

Department of Health and Human Services (DHHS)
GPO Box 125
Hobart Tas 7001
03 6233 3185
www.dhhs.tas.gov.au

TAS

DIAGNOSIS AND HEALTH

In the south, diagnosis and assessments for children under six years are made by paediatricians in collaboration with relevant therapists through DHHS Children's Therapy Services, Calvary Hospital, Tasmania. Private paediatricians also provide this service.

In the north and north west, staff of DHHS Child Development Unit, Child Health and Parenting Services provide multi-disciplinary diagnosis and assessment. Private paediatricians also provide this service.

DHHS Child and Adolescent Mental Health Services (CAMHS) assist in the assessment of ASD in school-aged children and adolescents. Assessment is multi-disciplinary and multi-modal including a mental health, cognitive and academic, and occupational therapy assessments (play, motor skills, sensory processing and self-care skills).

Families also have access to a range of specialist and specific health services that are provided by DHHS Primary Health to the wider Tasmanian community.

DISABILITY SERVICES

Disability Services are provided through Area Offices in Launceston, Burnie and Hobart. Disability Services also funds community-based organisations to provide a wide range of disability services.

- Service Coordination — ensures that services are directed at meeting client needs and are delivered in a way that best suits each individual.
- Resource Team — provides specialist advice, assessment, intervention and education including speech pathology, psychology, occupational therapy, social work and nursing.
- Respite Services — available through a respite centre, in a person's home, or through other flexible options. Respite may be available for a couple of hours, a few days, or a longer period.
- Day Options — provides many different activities for people with a disability during the day. Activities are selected based on the needs of the person and may include work, education, skills development and community access.
- Short Term Support — accessed through the Service Co-ordination Team, this program provides short-term support packages, usually focusing on building new skills to achieve specific goals.
- Residential Services — provides longer-term supported accommodation in the community. Most of these services are shared accommodation, managed by community-based organisations.
- Individual Funding — provides funding packages on an individual basis. Supports may include direct support, respite or equipment, and depend on individual needs and goals. Packages may also offer supports to families and carers.
- Supporting Individual Pathways Program — provides assistance to young adults with disabilities as they make the transition from school to adult life.

Disability Services' Area Offices are the first point of contact for all services.

Disability Services does not duplicate services offered by other agencies, and may refer people to services that are more appropriate to meet their needs.

TAS

North
John L Grove Centre
33–39 Howick Street
Launceston Tas 7250
03 6336 4130

South
Woodhouse Building, St John's Park
New Town Tas 7008
03 6230 7600

North West
2nd Floor, Parkside, Brickwell Street
Burnie Tas 7320
03 6434 4103

State Office
Gellibrand House
St John's Park
New Town Tas 7008
03 6230 7525

Your Local Council

Many local councils around Australia have a Disability Information Officer or Community Care Officer. It is well worth getting in touch with your local council to ask about local services and assistance that may be available.

Early Intervention — General

Early Childhood Intervention Service (ECIS)

Department of Education, Community and Cultural Development
116 Bathurst Street
Hobart Tas 7000
1300 135 513
www.education.tas.gov.au/early-learning
ECIS is a statewide service providing family-centred intervention services to families and young children, from birth to kindergarten. ECIS employs early childhood intervention teachers and teachers' assistants, and has consultative support from speech pathologists, occupational therapists, physiotherapists and psychologists.

ECIS runs autism-specific early intervention programs. These start with individualised programs to help families and children communicate, play and

TAS

interact, then move on to small group programs. Family support programs are also run, and children are supported as they transition into other community settings.

With parental consent, anyone who has a concern about a young child's development may make a referral.

State Coordinator
Early Childhood Intervention Service
174 Brooker Avenue
Hobart Tas 7000
03 6234 8238

Early Childhood Intervention Service Burnie
Beaufort Street
Somerset Tas 7322
03 6435 2021

Early Childhood Intervention Service Hobart
174 Brooker Avenue
Hobart Tas 7000
03 6231 1625

Early Childhood Intervention Service Devonport
51 Steele Street
Devonport Tas 7310
03 6424 3111

Early Childhood Intervention Service Launceston
11a Munford Street
Kings Meadows Tas 7249
03 6344 1729

Kidscode®
0418 316 754
www.parentswantinghelp.com
Kidscode® offers intensive practical early intervention in your own home for the whole family over five days to improve independence in the following areas:
- calming behaviour
- managing sleep, eating and toileting difficulties
- developing communication and understanding
- creating an easier way to function as a family unit.
Kidscode® continues family support with pre-care and after-care and transition into school.

Early Intervention — ASD Specific

Giant Steps Tasmania
35 West Church Street
Deloraine Tas 7304
03 6362 2522
www.giantsteps.tas.edu.au

Giant Steps is an independent special school focusing on students with moderate to severe autism. Students range in age from 4-18 years. Staff include teachers, a speech pathologist and OT, and a team of therapy assistants. A typical group of six students will have five staff working with them at any time.

The program is eclectic, drawing on elements of structured teaching, PECS, visual scheduling, sensory integration, and Makaton®, among other influences.

Early Intervention — ABA

ISADD provides services in Tasmania. For information see WA listings p. 349

RDI®

There are several RDI® consultants in Australia. The Connections Center in Houston, Texas trains and certifies all RDI® consultants and their website has a comprehensive list: www.rdiconnect.com

There is also an Australian RDI® Yahoo group at:
http://health.groups.yahoo.com/group/RDIsupportgroup/
If you join this group, you can access a file which also lists RDI® consultants in training, who may be starting to work with families already. It also lists consultants from the US who come to Australia to work with families. This is a useful egroup for getting in touch with other families doing RDI® in your area.

TAS

Speech Pathologists, Occupational Therapists and Psychologists

Autism Tasmania may be able to assist with recommendations. See p. 239 for details on how to get in touch with these professionals through their national and state organisations.

Schools — General

Department of Education, Community and Cultural Development

116 Bathurst Street
Hobart Tas 7000
1300 135 513
www.education.tas.gov.au

In Tasmania students with ASD may be eligible for placement on the Register of Students with Severe Disabilities. Such students must have:

- a confirmed diagnosis of autism in the upper moderate/severe range
- demonstrated functional abilities consistent with this diagnosis, particularly in relation to DSM-IV-TR criteria and associated educational implications

It is recognised that ASD forms a continuum from mild to severe and from low to high functioning. The social and functional implications and the educational impact of ASD varies depending on the relationship between these two dimensions. A diagnosis of ASD alone is not sufficient to ensure eligibility for the Register. The Register identifies students for whom the learning/educational implications resulting from ASD are the most severe.

For those students that meet the criteria per capita funding is available directly to schools; such funding is usually spent on additional teacher aide resourcing. In addition, support from other personnel is made to each cluster of schools for speech and language pathology, school psychologists, social workers and support teachers to assist with student programs, and professional learning and staff support.

There are also six positions across the state filled by Autism Consultants working in either Early Intervention programs or with the school-age population. These staff work collaboratively with families, school personnel and other support staff on specific programs, development of IEPs and professional learning.

The Early Intervention program for very young children with ASD (prior to formal schooling) operates through the Early Childhood Intervention Service across the state within a family partnership model of practice and offers:

- individual 1:1 centre-based sessions
- home or community-based programs
- therapy provision with occupational, physiotherapy and speech and language pathology
- family support programs.

Students who do not meet the eligibility criteria for the Register but are on the autism spectrum receive support at the school cluster level through Additional

Needs funding support as well as access to the services of cluster support staff.

The Department of Education has recognised the need for increased professional learning for teachers and teacher aides within the autism field and to this end established a graduate certificate in ASD in conjunction with the Institute of Inclusive Learning Communities at the University of Tasmania, with 220 participants enrolled.

Catholic Education Office

5 Emmett Place
New Town Tas 7008
03 6210 8888
www.ceo.hobart.catholic.edu.au

Approximately 60 students with the diagnosis of ASD are currently included in Catholic schools in Tasmania. Support is provided at individual, class and whole school level. This includes:

- school-based case manager/support teacher
- collaborative development of IEP
- provision of teacher aide time
- allocation of funds for resources to support both students and teachers
- professional learning (social stories, visual schedules, etc)
- speech pathology
- occupational therapy
- behaviour support
- Commonwealth funding (if eligible)
- state support service funding (if appropriate)

The Association of Independent Schools of Tasmania (AIST)

Level 3 'The Galleria'
33 Salamanca Place Tas 7000
03 6224 0125
www.aist.tas.edu.au

AIST supports schools through federal special needs funding, specialist support and professional training.

Schools — Autism Specific

Giant Steps Tasmania

35 West Church Street

Deloraine Tas 7304
03 6362 2522
www.giantsteps.tas.edu.au
Giant Steps is an independent special school focussing on students with moderate to severe autism. Students range in age from 4–18 years. Staff include teachers, a speech pathologist and OT, and a team of therapy assistants. A typical group of six students will have five staff working with them at any time.

The program is eclectic, drawing on elements of structured teaching, PECS, visual scheduling, sensory integration, and Makaton®, among other influences.

Therapy Services for School-Aged Children
See **Department of Education, Community and Cultural Development** above

Respite and Carer Info
Through the Maze — see **First Things First** above — has a useful section on Respite.

Carers Tasmania
'Westella'
181 Elizabeth Street
Hobart
Tasmania 7000
03 6231 5507

Shop 8 Jimmys Shopping Complex
216 Charles Street
Launceston
Tasmania 7250
03 6334 9917
www.carerstas.org
For information on services see p. 225

Commonwealth Carer Respite Centres
1800 059 059
For details see p. 225

TAS

Home and Community Care (HACC) Program

Call your council and/or your state disability department about this program. See p. 226

Parent Support Groups

Contact Autism Tasmania for information about current groups. Groups usually include an Adult Asperger's Support Group.

Libraries & Resources

Autism Tasmania has a library — see contact details above.

Toy Town

1 Tower Road
New Town Tas 7008
03 6228 4196

Toy Town lends toys and equipment to families, schools and institutions. It aims to help meet the special needs of people with disabilities of all ages in the areas of education, recreation and therapy. Families pay an annual membership fee and a very small fee to borrow each item. There is indoor and outdoor equipment for loan, and advice and help can be given by staff. Call ahead to check current opening days and hours.

When You Really Need To Talk to Somebody

Parenting Line

1300 808 178 (cost of a local call)
The Parenting Line is available at any time to assist parents with stressful parenting issues or concerns.

Lifeline

13 11 14
www.lifeline.org.au
Lifeline offers telephone counselling throughout Australia — 24 hours a day, seven days a week.

TAS

VIC

First Things First
Autism Victoria Infoline
03 9885 0533
1300 308 699 (rural and regional callers)

Through the Maze
Association for Children with a Disability
Suite 2, 98 Morang Road
Hawthorn Vic 3122
03 9818 2000, 1800 654 013 (rural callers)
www.acd.org.au/
Through the Maze is a resource booklet with information about services for families of children with a disability in all regions of Victoria. It can be downloaded from the Information and Support for Families section of the ACD website. ACD is an information, support and advocacy organisation for children with a disability and their families.

State Autism Association

Autism Victoria

35 High Street
Glen Iris VIC 3146
PO Box 235
Ashburton VIC 3147
03 9885 0533
1300 308 699 (rural and regional callers)
www.autismvictoria.org.au

Autism Victoria is the state peak body for ASD. It is first and foremost an information provider rather than a service provider. This can be clearly seen in the quality of its website which is an excellent and comprehensive information source.

FOR PARENTS AND FAMILIES
- answer general queries by phone, mail or email
- guide families through the maze of services and options
- provide information materials in print or electronic format
- Library and Resource Centre (for Autism Victoria members)
- Autism Alert Cards

FOR PROFESSIONALS
- specialist information packages
- Integration Aide Register
- Annual Research Forum
- help with sourcing appropriate professional development
- Library and Resource Centre (for Autism Victoria members)

FOR INDIVIDUALS WITH ASD
- answer general queries about ASD by phone, mail or email
- information about services for adults
- Library and Resource Centre (for Autism Victoria members)

VIC

FOR OTHER INTERESTED PEOPLE
- information for students at primary, secondary and tertiary level
- information for people who wish to volunteer
- information and comment to the media
- information and speakers to help the general community learn more about ASDs

State Disability and Health Departments

Department of Human Services (DHS)

50 Lonsdale Street
Melbourne Vic 3000
1300 650 172 freecall inside Victoria
03 9096 0000
www.dhs.vic.gov.au
www.health.vic.gov.au

The DHS is responsible for providing general health and support services to all Victorians.

ASD specific responses include:

- Child and Adolescent Mental Health teams — undertake complex ASD diagnostic services. Both CAMHS and adult mental health services are available for people with an ASD who also have a mental health condition.
- Disability Services — provide a wide range of specialist services to eligible people including support, therapy, accommodation and individually designed service packages.
- Home and Community Care Program — provides support and respite services.

A range of community service organisations are funded by DHS to provide information and advocacy services to particular groups of Victorians, including Autism Victoria. DHS has close links to Autism Victoria. For information on Victoria' Autism State Plan visit http://autismstateplan.dhs.vic.gov.au

Your Local Council

Many local councils around Australia have a Disability Information Officer or Community Care Officer. It is well worth getting in touch with your local council to ask about local services and assistance that may be available.

Early Intervention — General

Early Childhood Intervention Services (ECIS)

Department of Education and Early Childhood Development
2 Treasury Place
East Melbourne Vic 3001
03 9637 2000
Information and Referral Service

VIC

03 9637 2222 or 1800 809 834

www.office-for-children.vic.gov.au/ecis

Victoria's Department of Education and Early Childhood Development (DEECD) is responsible for providing public education and early childhood services to all Victorians. ECIS is therefore a part of DEECD. The Early Childhood Intervention Services are provided by DEECD employees and by funded community services organisations to provide services to children who are assessed with a developmental delay, including children with an ASD. Kindergarten services and preschool field officers are also managed through DEECD.

ECIS has a close relationship with Autism Victoria and up-to-date information on services can be found on Autism Victoria's website.

Early Childhood Intervention Australia (Victorian Chapter)

www.eciavic.org.au

ECIA is the Victorian peak body for early intervention and can provide information on local early intervention services.

Early Intervention — ASD Specific

Irabina Childhood Autism Services

193 Bayswater Rd

Bayswater Vic 3153

03 9720 1118

www.irabina.com

Irabina Childhood Autism Services provides programs for children diagnosed with ASD aged from birth to school age, and their families, who live in the Eastern region of Melbourne. Programs include individual therapy, targeted small groups, inclusion support, parent education, transition to school support, family counselling, assessment and sibling programs. Irabina is funded to provide services to 146 families per year, and there is usually a waiting list for services.

Noah's Ark West — Autism Early Childhood Intervention

Main office at Highpoint Shopping Centre

Programs operating at Werribee and Albanvale sites

03 9304 7400

www.noahsarkinc.org.au

Noah's Ark West provides services for families with children with a diagnosis of an ASD (or awaiting an assessment), under six years of age. It covers families living in the Western metropolitan region of Melbourne; mainly in Brimbank, Hobsons Bay or Wyndhamvale.

All referrals are held and co-ordinated through Western Region Central Intake. Parents or professionals can find out more, or make a referral by telephoning Central Intake on 1800 783 783.

Staff are from a range of disciplines, all with in-depth experience in ASDs. The service works in collaboration with families to develop an individual and flexible program to meet the differing needs of each child and family. Services provided include:

- home visits to support parents with information
- strategies and skills to support their child's development
- visits to child care and or kindergarten to consult with staff
- group programs to address specific goals
- parent information and education sessions
- transition to school support.

Northern Autism Outreach Service

1 Kalparrin Avenue
Greensborough
03 9435 8311

The Northern Autism Outreach Service, a joint partnership between Specialist Children's Services and Kalparrin Early Intervention Program, is an interim service for children and their families residing in the local government areas of Banyule, Nillumbick, Darebin, Whittlesea, Yarra, Moreland and Hume who a) have a diagnosis of an ASD, OR b) are on the waiting list for ASD assessment, OR c) parents and professionals have raised concerns about the possibility of ASD AND d) the child/family is not receiving early intervention services through Specialist Children's Services of Early Intervention Agencies AND e) the child is 0–6 and not attending school.

The type and duration of service provision is based on the individual needs of the child and family and includes:

- individual and group information
- home, kindergarten and child care programs focussing on communication, socialisation and academic skills
- advice and support for behaviour management.

Referrals can be made by parents or professionals. Contact the intake worker at Specialist Children's Services on 9479 0121.

utistic School Early Education Program

St

Vic 3165

8139

Southern Autistic School provides educational programs to suit the special learning requirements of children with autism. It is a regional school and covers the Southern Metropolitan Region.

Southern Autistic School enrols students from three years of age into Early Education, a three days a week program. This is usually complemented with the student attending their local kindergarten. Early Education in a Department of Education school is defined as: *An educational program specifically designed for preschool children who are within the severe range of ASD aged between two years eight months and four years eight months as at 1st January at age of entry.*

Early Education classes have eight students (but five on any one day) with a teacher and an assistant. They access the same curriculum as the rest of the school (literacy, maths, topic development, library, art, PE, swimming) with each child having an individual program. The school employs two speech pathologists and two occupational therapists to assist with implementing these programs

Early Childhood Autism Service — North (ECAS-N)

Yooralla Society of Victoria
48-50 Box Forest Road
Glenroy Vic 3046
03 9359 9366
www.yooralla.com.au

Early Childhood Autism Service — North (ECAS-N) offers an holistic service to families, comprising home visits, centre-based therapy, support to child care and preschool and support for families in accessing their local community. ECAS-N employs an occupational therapist, a speech pathologist, and special education teacher. ECAS-N offers services to children who display more severe characteristics of autism in the years before school. Eligibility criteria include severe language delay and challenging behaviours which impact on the child's ability to function in everyday environments. ECAS-N is funded through DHS and client families must reside in the northern metropolitan area of Melbourne. Intake is managed through the Northern Early Childhood Intervention Services — Central Intake: 03 9479 0121.

VIC

Early Intervention — ABA

Autism Behavioural Intervention Association (ABIA)
PO Box 239
Canterbury Vic 3126
03 9830 0677
www.abia.net.au
ABIA is the peak body representing ABA providers and families using ABA in Victoria. ABIA runs workshops and training courses and has a library for the use of members. A counselling service has been set up. A regular newsletter is sent out to members and support groups are run. ABIA shares office space with the Learning for Life Centre and visitors are welcome, please call to make an appointment first.

ABAcus Learning Centre
5/30 Robertson Drive
Mornington Vic 3931
www.mpas.net.au
ABAcus provides centre-based ABA therapy for children with ASD aged 2–13 years. It has been developed by Mornington Peninsula Autism School Ltd a not-for-profit organisation. Children can attend the Centre full-time or part-time.

Autism Partnership
3/115 Victoria Road
Northcote Vic 3070
03 9481 2611
ausadmin@autpar.com
Autism Partnership is a private agency specialising in behavioural intervention programs for children with autism and related disorders. It provides services to children and families throughout Victoria and Queensland. The agency is overseen by Karen McKinnon, who is a registered psychologist.

Autism Partnership believes in comprehensive intervention designed to meet the individual needs of each child. The agency is devoted to enhancing overall quality of life through treatment focused upon the development of improved social interaction, play and leisure skills, meaningful communication, classroom readiness, peer relationships and improved independence. It provides families with program supervision for their behavioural intervention program, which includes running regular team meetings, staff training, and liaising with school staff.

VIC

IEC — Integrated Education and Communication
182 Canterbury Rd
Blackburn Vic 3130
03 9893 5547
www.abaservicesaustralia.com.au

IEC offers specialised educational and behavioural support services for children who have ASD. IEC provides individual educational and behavioural programs, specifically designed to meet, challenge, strengthen, and optimise a child's education and inclusion. The intervention approach adopted by IEC utilises the core principles of ABA.

IEC offer highly-structured teaching programs where skills are broken down into their simplest most manageable form, a process guided by the child's learning pattern and current level of functioning. Success is achieved through consistency, prompting, repetition and reinforcement techniques. IEC aim to provide children with the skills necessary to utilise the educational and social opportunities available in their family and community.

Services:
- Psychologist — assessments, programs and recommendations
- Therapists — implementing programs and recommendations
- Playdaze — social skills groups
- Workshops — ABA Workshops and autism specialist workshops

ISADD – Intervention Services for Autism and Developmental Delay
www.isadd.org

This WA-based group offers services in Victoria, see p. 349

The Learning for Life Autism Centre
276 Canterbury Road
Surrey Hills Vic 3127
03 9836 0422
www.learningforlife.com.au

Learning for Life Autism Centre provides subsidised, intensive, early intervention programs to preschool children. It is a not-for-profit, incorporated association dedicated to making these programs accessible to families who might not otherwise be able to afford them.

The Centre's objective is to increase the number of subsidised ABA therapy programs to meet the increased prevalence of ASD, through fundraising and donations. The Centre aims to establish an enduring professional career path for therapist staff and collect data for research that demonstrates the efficacy of ABA therapy.

VIC

Therapists work with children in their own homes and each child has a tailored program overseen by a program supervisor.

Victorian ABA Providers Pty Ltd

PO Box 255
Balwyn North Vic 3104
0407 660 882
Victorian ABA Providers is a company that specialises in teaching preschool children with autism, pervasive developmental disorders, and related developmental disabilities using ABA methodology. Victorian ABA Providers services clients in both Victoria and Queensland. The company has strong links with the Lovaas Institute of Early Intervention in the US.

RDI®

There are several RDI® consultants in Australia. The Connections Center in Houston, Texas trains and certifies all RDI® consultants and their website has a comprehensive list: www.rdiconnect.com
There is also an Australian RDI® Yahoo group at:
http://health.groups.yahoo.com/group/RDIsupportgroup/
If you join this group, you can access a file which also lists RDI® consultants in training, who may be starting to work with families already. It also lists consultants from the US who come to Australia to work with families. This is a useful egroup for getting in touch with other families doing RDI® in your area.

Speech Pathologists, Occupational Therapists and Psychologists

Autism Victoria may be able to assist with recommendations. See p. 239 for details on how to get in touch with these professionals through their national and state organisations.

Multi-disciplinary Services

Time for a Future — Centre for Child Development

56 High Street
Woodend
Vic 3442
03 5427 4052
www.timeforafuture.com.au

Time For A Future was established in 2007 by child psychiatrist Prof Bruce Tonge, special education consultant Dr Avril Brereton, special education consultant Kerry Bull and educational psychologist Melissa Kiomall. This multi-disciplinary team provides a range of professional services to children and adolescents with special needs: assessment, diagnosis, therapy, parent education and professional development programs. Courses offered include the comprehensive 'Pre-Schoolers with Autism' parent education program and a short 'Understanding Autism' course for professionals (see **ACT-NOW** below).

School

Department of Education and Early Childhood Development (DEECD)

2 Treasury Place
East Melbourne.
Vic 3001
03 9637 2000
Information and Referral Service
03 9637 2222 or 1800 809 834
www.education.vic.gov.au

DEECD recognises the complexity of ASD and the need for parents, teachers and school leaders to work together to support students with ASD to achieve their potential, and to focus on the teaching-learning relationship to meet the individual needs of all students.

Students with ASD can be supported in different school settings including integration into mainstream schools, enrolment in special schools and enrolment in schools for students with ASD.

DEECD has established and resources five schools that specialise in the support of students with ASD: Bulleen Heights Special School, Wantirna Heights School, Northern Autistic School, Western Autistic School and Southern Autistic School. These schools also provide outreach services and support to other schools to ensure that students with ASD benefit from the expertise of these specialised settings. Some of the schools have websites:
www.westernautisticschool.vic.edu.au
www.bulleenheights.vic.edu.au

A range of additional supports is available in special and mainstream schools. In 2007 over $50 million is being allocated to a range of support services including psychologists, social workers, youth workers, speech pathologists, occupational therapists, visiting teachers and curriculum consultants who are available to assist all Victorian government schools.

VIC

A Student Support Group is required for every student receiving support through the Program for Students with Disabilities, and every Victorian government school is encouraged to establish a Student Support Group for any individual student with additional learning needs. A Student Support Group is a co-operative partnership involving parents, school representatives and professionals that ensures co-ordinated support for each student's educational needs through the development of specific educational goals and a tailored educational program. The Student Support Group will develop an Individual Learning Plan which sets educational goals, both short and long-term. This process focuses on the student taking an active role in the school and wider community into the future. Further information is available at: www.sofweb. vic.edu.au/wellbeing/disabil/index.htm

DEECD is committed to increasing the capacity of schools and teachers to cater for the diverse needs of the student population in Government schools. Work is underway to ensure that the expertise of specialist autism schools is made available to support students with ASD in all government schools. In 2006 the Department established the Autism Teaching Institute based at Western Autistic School. The institute provides training courses accredited by the Victorian Qualifications Authority to build teacher capacity and knowledge regarding teaching students with ASD. Professional development opportunities are also provided to schools to assist them in supporting the needs of students with ASD. More information is available at: www. autismteachinginstitute.org.au

Autism Victoria is funded by DEECD to provide ASD information and advocacy services including an Infoline.

Further information about the range of supports available for students with ASDs is available from regional Disabilities Coordinators by contacting the relevant Department of Education and Early Childhood Development regional office. Contact details are available at: www.education.vic.gov.au/ about/structure/regions.htm

The Catholic Education Commission of Victoria (CECV)
James Goold House
228 Victoria Parade
East Melbourne Vic 3002
03 9267 0228
www.cecv.vic.catholic.edu.au
Call and ask to speak to the student services manager.

Association of Independent Schools of Victoria
20 Garden Street

South Yarra Vic 3141
03 9825 7200
www.ais.vic.edu.au
Call and ask to speak to the student services manager.

Mansfield Autism Statewide Services
81 Highett Street
Mansfield
03 5775 2876
Mansfield is a DHS-funded program which has an Early Intervention service and its unique travelling teacher service. Families in regional areas can request that a teacher visit them at home and provide assistance with their child. If the teacher thinks it appropriate, children can attend the Mansfield short-term placement residential school for one term. There are very long waiting lists for this service at the time of writing.

Therapy Services for School-Aged Children
See **Autism Partnership** above
See **Time For A Future — Centre for Child Development** above
Some other early intervention providers also provide services to school-aged children.

Respite and Carer Support

Carers Victoria
Level 1 37 Albert Street
Footscray Vic 3011
03 9396 9500
1800 242 636
www.carersvic.org.au
For details see p. 225

Commonwealth Carer Respite Centres
1800 059 059
For details see p. 225

Home and Community Care (HACC) Program
Call your council about this program. For details see p. 226

Adult Services

Alpha Autism Inc (AAI)

1939 Malvern Rd
Malvern East Vic 3145
03 9885 2777
www.alpha-autism.org.au

Alpha Autism Inc is a specialist support service assisting adults, 18 years and over, with ASD to meet the challenges of daily life and participate as a valued member of the community. AAI provides a wide range of services including day centres, employment support, respite and recreation and a social club for adults with ASD or people with similar needs. These services are primarily located in the Melbourne metropolitan area but can be extended to rural and regional areas through partnerships with local providers.

See **Autism Plus** below
See **Department of Human Services (DHS)** above

Mansfield Adult Autistic Services (MAACRO)

8 Highett Street
Mansfield Vic 3724
03 5775 1904

MAACRO offers supported accommodation and a day program with educational and vocational opportunities.

Statewide Autistic Services Inc

7 Apsley Place
Seaford Vic 3198
03 9773 6044
www.sasi.org.au

SASI runs adult day programs, full-time accommodation, recreation programs, children's respite and holiday care. SASI offers most services in the Southern and Eastern Metropolitan Regions and Gippsland, but offers respite and community education to people from all regions.

Training — for parents and professionals

See **Autism Victoria** above
See **Autism Plus** below

VIC

See **Autism Teaching Institute** in DEECD
See **Autism Behavioural Intervention Association** above
See **Time For A Future** above

ACT-NOW

Centre for Developmental
Psychiatry and Psychology
Faculty of Medicine, Nursing and Health Sciences
Monash University
Victoria 3800
03 54273 852 / 9905 1442
www.med.monash.edu.au/spppm/research/devpsych/actnow/project.html

The Autism Secondary Consultation and Training Strategy is funded by DHS (Victoria). The project aims to build skills and capacity across each DHS region in the area of Early Childhood (0–6 years) to enable regional service providers to:

- identify Pervasive Developmental Disorders (PDD) and promote understanding of PDD in the wider community and strategies for working effectively with these children and their families
- provide a more integrated range of evidence based early interventions for young children with autism and their families that will complement and interface with other agencies and services
- improve links between service providers and strengthen partnerships between services and families

Initially, the ACT-NOW project was funded from July 2004–June 2007. The strategy impacted on parents, early years service providers and the community. The development of nine Regional Autism Coordination Teams (ReACTs) to facilitate cross-program partnerships successfully harnessed the good will and interest of a range of individuals focussed on a common goal. Non-recurrent funds were recently allocated to continue the ACT-NOW strategy from July 2007– December 2008.

Stage two provides an opportunity to respond to the needs identified by the ReACTs. In particular, this includes providing support, supervision, mentoring and consultation for professionals working with young children with autism and their families. Each ReACT meets regularly with the ACT-NOW team to identify and respond to autism-specific training and consultation needs. Sub-groups work on specific issues (eg transition to school) and have begun to develop regional training materials. ReACTs have also developed regional action plans that look at a range of broader issues such as developing service directories, links with paediatricians and information for GPs.

The ACT-NOW team is based at the Centre for Developmental Psychiatry

VIC

and Psychology at Monash University. The members of the team have experience and expertise in specialist service provision, community and professional education, service development, support and consultation, and family advocacy. The team is internationally recognised for its research in the field of PDD. Ongoing evaluation and review of the ACT-NOW program is conducted through a reference group made up of professional, consumer and parent representatives. This group is convened and chaired by the DHS to offer support and advice to the ACT-NOW team.

One of the many programs delivered by the ReACTs is the parent training program 'Preschoolers with Autism'. This is an evidence-based, best practice manualised parent education program that was developed as a response to concern that parents and carers of young children with autism can easily be left out of the learning loop. Families benefit enormously when parents are trained in what autism is and how it affects their child's development, play and behaviour, communication skills and ability to socialise with others.

The 'Preschoolers with Autism' program was designed for children with autistic disorder diagnosed using DSM-IV criteria, aged 3–5 years and diagnosed within the previous 12 months. It is a 20-week program with ten group sessions (90 minutes) and ten individual sessions (60 minutes). The groups have a maximum of five families. It is recommended that the program be delivered by an experienced clinician with a strong background in child development, experience working with children who have autism and their families, and experience in counselling or group work. The program manual can be purchased via the ACT-NOW website. Quarterly newsletters from the ACT-NOW team and fact sheets are available on the ACT-NOW website.

Directors Prof. Bruce Tonge Child Psychiatrist; Dr Avril Brereton Special Educator, Early Childhood. Manager Ms Kerry Bull Special Educator, Early Childhood; *Staff* Mr Paul Bower Research Assistant

ASD — Trained Staff

Autism Plus
PO Box 2047
Seaford Vic 3198
03 9782 1843
www.autismplus.com.au
Autism Plus is a service focussing on staff placement (agency and individual supports), training and case management. Autism Plus is also a training agency and can provide case management and behavioural intervention.

Support Groups

Autism Victoria's Information Officer can provide current contacts for family support groups.

ABIA organises family support groups.

The Asperger Syndrome Support Network (Vic) Inc (ASSN)

54 Railway Rd
Blackburn Vic 3130
03 9845 2766
assnvic@mssociety.com.au
http://home.vicnet.net.au/~asperger
ASSN holds regular coffee mornings and evenings, information sessions and seminars. Volunteers check the phone messages regularly. The following items are available on request:

- quarterly newsletter *ASSN Vic Inc Update* — available to all members
- directory of the Asperger's syndrome and Autism Support Groups in Victoria
- list of books/videos/DVDs & CDs to borrow from the library
- ASSN Information Kit.

Autistic Family Support Association (AFSA)

PO Box 235
Ashburton Vic 3147
03 9885 8777
http://home.vicnet.net.au/~afsainc
AFSA is a parent self-help group based in Melbourne; it is the Autism Victoria parent voice.

Ballarat Autism Network

www.ballaratautism.com
Ballarat Autism Network is a group of parents and professionals in the Ballarat area. The Network's main function is to connect the autism community, and to educate and raise awareness. It offers support, monthly meetings, advocacy and information.

Libraries & Resources

Autism Victoria's library has over 1,700 books, videos and newsletters about ASD available to Autism Victoria members. Items can be posted.
ABIA has a members library
ASSN (Vic) Inc has a members' library
Ballarat Autism Network has a book and toy library.

Toy Libraries
www.toylibraries.org.au
The 150 toy libraries in Victoria are listed on this website.

When You Really Need To Talk to Somebody

Parentline
13 22 89 (cost of a local call)
www.parentline.vic.gov.au
8am – 12am Monday to Friday, 10am – 10pm weekends.
Parentline Vic is a statewide telephone counselling, information and referral service for parents and carers with children from birth to 18 years. It is a confidential and anonymous service.

Lifeline
13 11 14
www.lifeline.org.au
Lifeline offers telephone counselling throughout Australia — 24 hours a day, seven days a week.

WA

First Things First
The Autism Association of Western Australia (Inc)
See below
08 9489 8900

Autism Services Directory
Therapy Focus Inc
Ground Floor, 2 Hawthorne Place
Burswood WA 6100
08 9478 9500
www.therapyfocus.org.au
This directory is compiled each year. It can be downloaded from the website's *Resources* section. Call the office for a copy if the website version is not up to date. This directory is a terrific resource, with lots of practical information and an excellent section on things to think about when choosing services.

Autism: Where To Start
This DVD and Parent Resource Package is provided to newly diagnosed families by the Disabilities Service Commission — see below.

WA

State Autism Association

The Autism Association of Western Australia (Inc))

37 Hay Street,
Subiaco WA 6008
08 9489 8900
www.autism.org.au

The AAWA was founded in 1967 and is the major service provider for children and adults with autism in Western Australia. The Association has also published a useful series of books including: *Good Nights: A manual for parents and carers who have a child experiencing sleep difficulties; Making Sense of the Senses in children with Autism: A workbook for teachers and parents; Everyone Dies One Day*, a booklet explaining the concept of death, loss and the grieving process; *Autism in the Classroom*, a resource kit for teachers; *Living with Autism: Practical Strategies for Supporting people with Autism*.

EARLY INTERVENTION SERVICES

The Association is an accredited and funded provider of Early Intervention Services (see **Disability Services Commission** entry below). Early intervention services are available to newly diagnosed children and their families. The service is based on the wide body of evidence-based research in autism and its implications for intervention. Each child's intervention plan is based on an individual assessment by a multi-disciplinary team. In addition, parent programs are provided to help families develop the skills necessary to optimise child development. Preparation for the transition to preschool and school is also included.

FAMILY CONSULTANCY

Families and individuals can access individual support and advice services. Training and information resources are also available to families and those who work with children with ASD.

SCHOOL CONSULTANCY

Support and advice services are available to schools, to assist in various areas eg curriculum modification and child management. Training/professional development can be provided to schools.

RESPITE AND SCHOOL HOLIDAY PROGRAMS

The AAWA runs respite homes in the metropolitan area, providing respite at weekends and in school holidays. Children aged 6–18 years can attend

WA

and suitable activities are organised such as trips to the beach, train rides, barbecues, outings and bush walks. School holiday programs for children and teenagers are run in most school holidays.

ALTERNATIVE TO EMPLOYMENT AND POST-SCHOOL OPTIONS PROGRAM

These programs offer daytime activities designed to assist people with ASD to maintain and develop their skills. All activities are community based and focus on providing the person with enjoyable opportunities to participate in community life. Each person's program is designed in consultation with them and/or their family. Activities include recreation, independent living skills, prevocational skills, social skills and community participation.

AIM EMPLOYMENT SERVICES

Individual support and training is provided by the Association's employment team, AIM Employment Services, to assist people with ASD to gain and maintain employment. The service includes matching individuals to jobs and marketing for job opportunities with employers, preparing the individual for work and placing the person in employment, providing on-the-job training together with the level of support required.

RESIDENTIAL SERVICES

Group homes are provided to individuals who require full-time care. All staff are trained in providing support to people with autism and are supported by an experienced residential team, including clinical staff. For those people who wish to live independently, support is provided through the Individual Options Program. Staff provide support and training to assist the person in all skill areas necessary to maintain their independent living eg budgeting, shopping, cooking, domestic tasks, personal care and making connections in the community.

TRAINING

The AAWA offers many training seminars throughout the year. A training calendar is available on the website. Topics usually include: Introduction to Autism, Teaching children with ASDs in mainstream schools, TEACCH, Managing difficult behaviour, Teaching children with autism in early childhood settings. Training courses can be specifically designed for schools and other organisations.

WA

State Disability Department

Disability Services Commission (DSC)

146 -160 Colin Street

West Perth WA 6005

08 9426 9200

1800 998 214 Freecall (country)

www.disability.wa.gov.au

DSC has a Metropolitan Autism Service which has diagnostic teams in Perth. The DSC Country Autism Team carries out assessments throughout the state.

Once assessments have been completed, DSC Eligibility Coordination will let families know what level of services they will receive. After diagnosis DSC sends out a DVD explaining what the diagnosis means and showing interviews with families who have a child with an ASD. A Parent Resource Package gives clear details on how to go about accessing DSC Early Intervention services as well as some helpful tips from parents.

A diagnosis of autism or PDD-NOS makes a child in WA eligible for ASD-specific Early Intervention services funding. There are three options for service provision in Perth: DSC Individual & Family Support (IFS) Mildred Creek Autism Team, Intervention Services for Autism and Developmental Disabilities Delay (ISADD) and the Autism Association of WA (AAWA).

Children who are at risk of intellectual delay are offered all three providers to choose from, other children get the choice of AAWA and ISAAD.

Each ASD funded provider has a specific number of funded places. If these are all taken up by, for example, April, then newly diagnosed children will not be allocated a place until further funding is made available, which is usually offered in August or September, or may have to wait until the next year (when school-age children leave the service) to gain a place.

Children with a diagnosis of ASD (with or without intellectual delay) may be able to access services provided by generic disability service providers, but these are not autism-specific.

Services for school-age children with ASD in the metropolitan area are provide by two agencies: Therapy Focus and Rocky Bay School Age Therapy Services. In the WA country areas, therapy services are generally provided by generic health department staff, with specialist support from DSC's Country Services Coordination staff.

There are no specific services for adults with autism. Generic services are provided by the health department and private practitioners. Information and some individual and group support is available through AAWA (eg employment support for people with autism).

WA

State Health Department

WA Health

189 Royal Street
East Perth WA 6004
Australia
08 9222 4222
www.health.wa.gov.au

WA Health provides multi-disciplinary diagnostic assessments for children and adolescents with possible ASD. Children and adolescents may receive some limited therapy services in the period prior to diagnosis, and immediately after diagnosis, but WA Health does not provide ongoing therapy services. Some paediatricians will continue to follow-up children and adolescents with ASD in order to provide medical and developmental review.

Your Local Council

Many local councils around Australia have a Disability Information Officer or Community Care Officer. It is well worth getting in touch with your local council to ask about local services and assistance that may be available.

Early Intervention — ASD Specific

Department of Education and Training (DET)

Hale House
Parliament Place
West Perth WA 6005
08 9426 7110
www.det.wa.edu.au/education

DET offers a wide range of services to young students with ASD. Services can be accessed at age four, in the Kindergarten year. Four Autism Units are run at the following schools:

Allenswood Primary School
Beckenham Community Kindergarten
Hillcrest Primary School
North Fremantle Community Kindergarten.

There is also a similar early intervention unit run in Bunbury.

To ensure quality control the Units are supported by a full time Program Co-ordinator. There are three children per class, with one teacher and two assistants. Children attend 12 hours a week over four half days. Each child has an Individual Education Plan. The educational programs are based on the

WA

principles of ABA. Parents are very much encouraged to support the program at home. Most children attend for two years and then have a transition program from the Unit to mainstream throughout the Pre-primary year. In Year 1 they attend their local primary school full-time.

The Department provides educational services for some Kindergarten and Pre-primary children with ASD through special education provision. A number of special schools offer preschool Early Intervention Programs; again using the principles of ABA. These special schools include Kim Beazley School, Sir David Brand School and Kenwick School. In the Pre-primary year children also attend their local primary school to ensure a smooth transition.

Some parents opt to enrol their Kindergarten or Pre-primary child with ASD at the local school. Additional support is available to the school in the form of an education assistant and teacher time, plus visiting teacher and school psychology services.

Kidscode®

0403 005 134

www.parentswantinghelp.com

Kidscode® offers intensive, live-in practical early intervention for the whole family over five days with the aim of creating independence in the following areas:-

- calming behaviour
- managing sleep, eating and toileting difficulties
- developing communication and understanding
- creating an easier way to function as a family unit.

This service is offered throughout Australia.

Early Intervention — ABA

Early Intervention WA (EIWA)

PO Box 4205

Mosman Park WA 6012

0411 130411

www.earlyinterventionwa.com

EIWA provides trained ABA therapists to home-based program working with the child's psychologist/paediatrician — client services include parent training and a parent support group.

WA

Early Intervention Centre (EIC)
Unit 6
205 Alexander Road
Belmont WA
08 9478 5191
www.interventioncentre.com

The Early Intervention Centre is a group of clinical and developmental psychologists who have extensive experience in learning and developmental disorders. EIC only uses methods that have scientific evidence supporting them and have been proven to work. EIC offers the following services:

DEVELOPMENTAL THERAPY PROGRAM: AGES 2 TO 12
This program uses principles from ABA: Discrete Trial Teaching, Fluency, Verbal Behaviour Analysis, Relational Frame Theory, Natural Environment Teaching, Pivotal Response Teaching and play-based methods. A focus is on teaching the child the most effective ways to learn to learn, to develop key adaptive cognitive abilities and functional and meaningful relationships via social skills and interpersonal development.

Programs can be delivered in three ways;
- parent lead
- home-based
- centre-based.

COURSES IN BEHAVIOUR MANAGEMENT AND DEVELOPMENT
Comprehensive training in ways to manage behaviour by promoting development are offered for professionals and families. The goal is to foster a sense of empowerment and confidence while giving a strong sense of where evidence based practice currently stands. A special topic for parents is how to distinguish well-researched proven methods from the fads and fashions.

ASSESSMENT
EIC offers Autism Assessments, Intellectual Disability Assessments, assistance with Differential Diagnosis in ADHD, ODD and Conduct Disorders. It also provides developmental assessments to assist with identifying current levels of functioning in Social Skills, Language Development, Theory of Mind and pivotal learning skills.

SCHOOL ASSISTANCE
EIC staff visit schools to assist with;
- planning for consistency across learning environments
- strategies for promoting development

- strategies for managing behaviour
- IEP plans

CLINICAL PSYCHOLOGY
- family and adult services
- child services

All psychologists at the centre are trained to assess and treat;
- behavioural problems
- obsessive and routine bound behaviours
- depression and anxiety

ISADD — Intervention Service for Autism and Developmental Delay

Office:
2 Butcher Road
Roleystone WA 6111
Meeting Rooms:
Suite 5, 324 Onslow Road
Shenton Park
08 9397 5970
www.isadd.org

ISADD is an ABA provider and one of the three DSC-approved Early Intervention Centres. DSC funded places provide a small number of hours of therapy a week and parents often fund more hours themselves.

ISADD supports a network of experienced and dedicated therapists. All programs are determined by individual assessment and conducted on a one-to-one basis. ISADD emphasises training in methodology and attention to detailed behaviour analysis in program implementation.

Programs are home-based and are also available in the child's day placement such as day care or kindy, where appropriate, teaching the skills in the environment in which they will be needed.

THERAPEUTIC APPROACH
ISADD follows the ABA/DTT approach as developed by Ivar Lovaas and adds extra components supported by more recent research. The directors of ISADD were trained by Lovass at UCLA and have extensive experience in the field.

PROGRAM
This includes individual assessment to determine program needs, parent training in ABA/DTT, and Case Management. The program developed is

comprehensive, addressing all aspects of the child's development including:

- ability to attend and cope with sensory information
- social behaviour
- language development
  receptive (understanding what is said)
  expressive (using a language code, eg pictographs, speech)
  articulation (speech, pronunciation and voice)
  communication ('talking' to people)
- cognitive/conceptual skills (the 'thinking' skills)
- visuo-spatial skills
- fine motor skills
- gross motor skills.

PARENT TRAINING

Parents are promoted as partners in the programs and supported in becoming effective therapists and long-term advocates for their child. Parents may deliver therapy themselves, as well as purchase therapy from ISADD accredited therapists.

The Whole Behaviour Program

David J Leach
15 Hakea Plaza
Canning Vale
Perth WA 6155
0431 267 771
08 9456 2423

Associate Professor David Leach is an experienced clinical psychologist who works privately with a small number of families and their children with developmental disabilities as well as teaching and researching at Murdoch University. His publication of an Australian evaluation of a partial replication of Lovaas's Early Intervention Program (with Dr J. Birnbrauer) is widely quoted as part of the supportive evidence for the effectiveness of early, intensive, behavioural intervention. David has been developing and testing his own intervention package 'The Whole Behaviour Program (WBP)' for the last ten years. It has many curriculum strands that interlock to form efficient and effective teaching programs for children with ASDs in the 2–10 year age range at home or in school.

WA

Floortime™

Sensory Connections Occupational Therapy Services

3 Pearson Place
Floreat WA 6014
08 9387 8538
0424 288 779
www.sensoryconnections.com.au

Sensory Connections is a private practice providing assessment, intervention and consultation for families with children presenting with challenges associated with disorders of relating and communicating such as ASD.

The DIR®/Floortime™ model is used. This provides a comprehensive framework for understanding and supporting children's development. The method focuses on helping children master the building blocks of relating, communicating and thinking.

Director Kathy Walmsley has a DIR® certificate and is a Facilitator and Trainer for the DIR training body in the US and has worked and trained internationally. She provides long distance consultations for parents and supervision of other professionals using DIR/Floortime, within Australia and the Asian region.

All other staff employed by Sensory Connections are trained in DIR®/ Floortime™ and have extensive experience in their discipline specific areas. Services include clinic-based and home consultations, individual parent-child, peer and small group programs, and school visits. The client group is generally children from birth to 18 however consultative services can be provided for all age groups.

RDI®

There are several RDI® consultants in Australia. The Connections Center in Houston, Texas trains and certifies all RDI® consultants and their website has a comprehensive list: www.rdiconnect.com
There is also an Australian RDI® Yahoo group at:
http://health.groups.yahoo.com/group/RDIsupportgroup/
If you join this group, you can access a file which also lists RDI® consultants in training, who may be starting to work with families already. It also lists consultants from the US who come to Australia to work with families. This is a useful egroup for getting in touch with other families doing RDI® in your area.

Speech Pathologists, Occupational Therapists and Psychologists

Autism WA may be able to assist with recommendations. See p. 239 for details on how to get in touch with these professionals through their national and state organisations.

Schools

Department of Education and Training

Hale House
Parliament Place
West Perth WA 6005
08 9426 7110
www.cis.perthwa.net

DET's Centre for Inclusive Schooling provides visiting teachers to support teachers statewide. In relation to students with ASD and challenging behaviours there is an Autism Intervention Team which provides a statewide teacher consultancy, school support and professional learning program. The visiting teachers from the Team work in close collaboration with the school psychologist.

There are no autism units in primary or secondary schools. However DET is reviewing options for secondary aged students: Years 8 to 10. Parents also have access to the Education Support Centres (special education centres in mainstream schools). These programs are often accessed by students with ASD plus intellectual disability.

Canning Vale
Merriwa
South Ballajura
South Bunbury
Gwynne Park
Creaney

Catholic Education Office of WA

50 Ruislip Street
Leederville WA 6007
08 6380 5200
www.ceo.wa.edu.au

The CEO has a team of special learning consultants who provide support to schools.

WA

The Association of Independent Schools of WA
Suite 3/41 Walters Drive
Osborne Park WA 6017
08 9441 1600
www.ais.wa.edu.au
AISWA has Special Education Program Officers who consult with schools.

Therapy Services for School-Aged Children

See **Early Intervention Centre** above

PLEDG — Parent Learning and Educational Development Group

Darrell Wills BA/MEd
Principal — Educational Consultant
Director — Inclusion and Development Projects
08 0720 1054
0419 955 012
www.pledgonline.com
PLEDG provides families and teachers with training and support for the inclusion of children with special needs in mainstream schools. PLEDG is both an association of parents and a service instrument for those parents. It operates all over WA, including rural and some remote areas.

Services include assisting parents to understand the particular developmental 'package' of their child; assisting schools to accommodate and teach all children well, and together; and assisting systems to restructure so that parents can take a role.

Rocky Bay Peel SATS (School Aged Therapy Service)

60 McCabe Street
Mosman Park WA 6012
08 9383 5150
www.rockybay.org.au
This is a government-funded service, and children must be registered at Level 2/3 and registered in schools in the Peel Education District. Services are provided from centres in two schools, in Safety Bay and Mandurah. Physiotherapy, occupational therapy and speech pathology services are available at no cost.

WA

Social Skills Australia
08 9276 6769
www.socialskillsaustralia.com.au
Run by two psychologists, Social Skills Australia provides group sessions usually running for two hours weekly during school terms. Using research-based methods, the children are taught the core social skills necessary for everyday social development in a structured learning environment.

Therapy Focus
Level 2
161 Great Eastern Highway,
Belmont WA
08 9478 9500
www.therapyfocus.org.au
Therapy Focus is a non-profit organisation which provides services to children with special needs and their families. Services include speech pathology, occupational therapy and physiotherapy. Support and advice to schools is available and social skills groups are run. School-aged children with ASD are usually eligible for DSC-funded services. Families can also pay for some services.

Inclusion
See **PLEDG (Parent Learning and Educational Development Group)** above

Respite and Carer Information
See **Autism Association of WA** above
The **Autism Services Directory** from *Therapy Focus* has useful information on respite, see above.

Carers WA
255 Walcott Street
North Perth WA 6006
08 9444 5922
1300 227 377
24hr Carer Counselling Line
1800 007 332
www.carerswa.asn.au
For information on services see p. 225

WA

Commonwealth Carer Respite Centres
1800 059 059
For details see p. 225

Home and Community Care (HACC) Program
Call your council and/or your state disability department about this program.
For details see p. 226

Adult Services
See **Autism WA** above
See **Disability Services Commisssion** website

Training for Parents and Professionals
See **Autism WA** above

Medical & Research

Western Australia Autism Research Group
c/- 150A Drummond St
Bedford WA 6052
www.autismwa.org.au
The WA Autism Research Group is a not-for-profit organisation which raises money for autism research. The website has very readable reports on completed autism research projects done in WA and details of current research projects needing participants. On this site you can find the WA Autism Register, a database of all people in WA diagnosed with an ASD since 1999. Annual reports can be downloaded.

The Western Australian Autism Diagnosticians' Forum (WAADF)
http://waadf.org.au
WAADF meets quarterly to discuss standards, process, and clinical issues in the assessment and diagnosis of ASD in WA. Members include diagnosing clinicians across the disciplines of speech pathology, paediatrics, psychiatry, social work, clinical psychology and research working in the Health Department, DSC and in private practice.

Support Groups

Call the **Autism Association of Western Australia** to ask about current groups.

ADAPT Forum (Autism, Development and Parenting Therapies)

www.adapt.org.au
This is an online forum whose membership is free.

Western Australia Autism Support Group

www.waasupport.bravehost.com
This is an online support group run through Yahoo groups.

Autism Solutions Incorporated and JazLea Dancers

http://members.ozemail.com.au/~leannel/
Autism Solutions Incorporated is a not-for-profit organisation formed to provide services for families with children with ASD. Autism Solutions Incorporated also runs JazLea Dancers, a group specifically designed for children with ASD and their siblings. JazLea Dancers promotes balance, flexibility, rhythm, co-ordination, strength and artistic expression.

Libraries & Resources — for Families

Activ Library

41 Bishop Street
Jolimont WA 6014
08 9387 0458
www.activ.asn.au
The Activ Library opening hours are 9 am–3.30 pm on Monday, Wednesday, Thursday and Friday, and 9 am–5.00 pm on Tuesday. Activ is a not-for-profit foundation which provides services and information about all disabilities. It has a wide range of books and videos on ASD.

Noah's Ark Toy Library and Computer Club

73 Angove Street
North Perth WA 6006
08 9328 1598
www.natl.org.au
Noah's Ark offers specialised toys to the parents and therapists of children

WA

with special needs. There is a mobile service operating in outer metropolitan areas, and a country mobile service operating within a 350km radius of Perth. Toys can be posted out to more distant rural areas. A computer club runs on Saturdays and in school holidays for children aged five years and over.

WA Association of Toy Libraries
www.waatl.org.au
This website has a list of toy libraries in WA.

Libraries & Resources — for Child Care

RUCSN – Resource Unit for Children with Special Needs
5 Carson Road
Malaga WS 6090
08 9249 4333
www.rucsn.org.au

The inclusion of children with special needs in child care is the main thrust of RUCSN's work. RUCSN provides support, training and resources to the child care industry. The Resource Centre has over 4,000 items covering child development, child care and disability. This collection includes books, videos, journals and audio tapes and a comprehensive collection of toys and equipment suitable for children with disabilities. Brochures and information on other relevant agencies are also available.

When You Really Need To Talk to Somebody

Parenting Line
08 9272 1466
1800 654 432 (free for STD callers)
24 hours a day, 7 days a week

The Parenting Line is a free telephone service providing information and advice for people caring for children and teenagers up to 18 years of age.

Lifeline
13 11 14
www.lifeline.org.au
Lifeline offers telephone counselling throughout Australia — 24 hours a day, seven days a week.

WA

RECOMMENDED WEBSITES

A very small selection of the very large number of websites about ASD.

ASD General

www.autism-help.org
A comprehensive and reliable Australian website.

www.autisminfo.org.au
An Australian website with resources and a free downloadable magazine.

www.autismspeaks.org
The most comprehensive autism resource, based in the US with a UK offshoot. Has the most extensive information on current research.

www.google.com.au/alerts
Gives you news clipping from around the world — but beware, the standards of journalism are very often woefully low and many stories are simply wrong.

http://scholar.google.com.au
Searching Google using the Scholar function is a quick and easy way of finding scientific articles on ASD.

http://autism.about.com
Extensive information and a sensible, thought-provoking blog which reacts to news stories.

Asperger's syndrome
http://members.ozemail.com.au/~rbmitch/Asperger.htm
Asperger's syndrome Australian information centre.

www.tonyattwood.com.au
Prof Tony Atwood's own website has a huge amount of useful information.

Australian websites by and about people with an ASD
www.laserbeakman.com
Tim Sharp is a young artist from Queensland who has created the character Laser Beak Man.

www.pinglian.com
Ping Lian is a young artist based in Sydney.

www.autismadventure.com
One family shares their experiences of life with two young children with ASD.

www.mugsy.org/wendy
Wendy Lawson is author, consultant and international speaker about ASD.

www.donnawilliams.net
Donna Williams is author, consultant and international speaker about ASD.

www.banoncom.com/isa
A family describe therapy and life with their daughter.

Prayer Networks
www.childrenofdestiny.org
www.healingministrysydney.org
www.healingrooms.com.au

Research and Biomedical
Bear in mind that there are many, many websites with no credibility whatsoever. A good website to start with is:
www.abc.net.au/health/healthyliving/healthconsumer/default.htm
In the Consumer Guides section are sections on evidence-based medicine, *Making Sense of Health Information* and *Quacks*.

Beware the many websites which cite scientific research but then only have anecdotal evidence of effectiveness, and no promise that good quality evidence is being sought.

www.autism.com
US-based Autism Research Institute.

www.autism-unravelled.org
A UK-based group of parents and academics.

www.fabresearch.org
Food and Behaviour Research is a UK charity.

www.researchautism.net
Research Autism is an offshoot of the UK's National Autism Society.

RECOMMENDED READING LIST

If you're into reading you'll have heard of sci-fi, crime fiction and 'chick lit' but did you know there was also 'autism lit'? You'll be surprised just how many books have been written about ASD, although not all of equal quality.

So how do you know where to start? Here's one suggestion: start at the library, it's cheap. In the Resource Guide you can find out whether there is a specialist autism library near you. Your local library will also have some books on ASD. You can ask your library to buy in books, many libraries are very willing to help and actively seek book purchase ideas from users.

Here are some of our favourite books:

The Autism Sourcebook: Everything You Need to Know About Diagnosis, Treatment, Coping and Healing, Karen Siff Exkorn (Regan Books, HarperCollins, 2005). A very comprehensive, authoritative yet warm guide to all matters ASD.

Overcoming Autism: Finding the Answers, Strategies and Hope That Can Transform Your Child's Life, Lynn Kern Koegel and Clare LaZebnik (Viking Penguin, 2004) A family-friendly book written by an early intervention specialist and a mother.

Understanding Autism, Susan Dodd (Elsevier Australia, 2005). Written by a former Manager of Early Intervention Services at Aspect, this is a useful book for both parents and professionals.

Let Me Hear Your Voice: A Family's Triumph over Autism, Catherine Maurice (Ballantine Books, 1994). A beautifully written book about a family's struggle and success with two children diagnosed with ASD.

Thinking in Pictures and Other Reports from My Life with Autism, Temple Grandin (First Vintage Book, 1995). Temple Grandin is the best known of the authors who themselves have an ASD. Her earlier book: *Emergence: Labelled Autistic* is another good read.

Send in the Idiots: Stories from the Other Side of Autism, Kamran Nazeer (Bloomsbury, 2006). Find out what happens when the author, a university graduate and British civil servant, traces four of his former schoolmates from New York school for children with ASD — a warm, poignant and funny book.

The Curious Incident of the Dog in the Night-time, Mark Haddon (Doubleday, 2003). Award-winning novel about a 15-year old boy who likes computers, murder mysteries and maths but doesn't get jokes, hates touching and hugging and can't fathom the feelings of others.

Unstrange Minds: Remapping the World of Autism, Roy Richard Grinker (Basic Books, 2007). An anthropologist and father of a girl with autism travels to South Korea, South Africa, Peru, and India to explore the cultural differences in attitudes to autism.

Lessons From My Child, Cindy Dowling, Neil Nicoll and Bernadette Thomas (Finch, 2004). A wonderful collection of personal stories from Australian parents of children with many different disabilities.

Freeks, Geaks and Asperger Syndrome, Luke Jackson (Jessica Kingsley Publishers, 2002). An articulate British teenager with Asperger's gives advice on dealing with the teenage years.

Strange Son, Portia Iversen (Riverhead Books, Penguin, 2006). The founder of Cure Autism Now writes about how her severely autistic teenage son finally learned to communicate.

Asperger's and Girls, Tony Attwood et al (Future Horizons, 2006). At last! A collection of articles about girls and women with Asperger's.

Autism and Attention Deficit Disorders: Understanding and Managing Diet Therapy for your Child, Judith Salmon and Leanne Pearce (self-published, 2006). An Australian book about dietary intervention.

Changing the Course of Autism: A Scientific Approach for Parents and

Physicians, Bryan Jepson (Sentient Publications, 2007). The latest book from the US on biomedical treatments for ASD.

Can't Eat, Won't Eat: Dietary Difficulties and Autistic Spectrum Disorders, Brenda Legge (Jessica Kingsley, 2002). Practical advice on dealing with picky eating.

The Out-of-Sync Child has Fun: Activities for Kids with Sensory Processing Disorder, Carol Stock Kranowitz (Perigree, 2003). The second in her series on Out Of Sync kids has lots of ideas for games and play.

My Baby Can Dance: Stories of Autism, Asperger's and Success Through the Relationship Development Intervention® (RDI®) Program, Steven E Gustein (Connections Center Publishing, 2006). Families and consultants write about their personal experiences.

APPENDIX 1:
ASD Research

By Associate Professor Deb Keen MAPS

Deb Keen is an Associate Professor in the School of Education and Professional Studies at Griffith University and member of the Griffith Institute for Educational Research. She has been involved with individuals with autism and related disorders for over 25 years as a psychologist, educator, administrator and researcher. Her research interests are primarily in the areas of educational, communication and behavioural interventions for individuals with autism across the lifespan. Funded research projects include early intervention with families, and engagement and learning in children with autism.

Research undertaken in relation to ASD has resulted in the development of earlier and more accurate screening and diagnostic procedures, effective teaching approaches and ways to enhance communication skills.

However, controversial treatments for autism have proliferated over the years, often accompanied by claims of success and even cure, but with little in the way of evidence to support their effectiveness. It is not until these treatments are tested through well-structured research studies that these claims can really be evaluated.

One reason why research is so important is that unproven treatments have the potential to do harm and to take valuable time away from proven treatments that are known to improve outcomes for people with ASD. An excellent article by Richard Simpson about the current evidence base for various practices in relation to children with ASD is recommended reading.[1]

Research in the area of autism has a relatively brief history when compared to many other disorders and this reflects both the lack of a biological marker for the disorder and the relatively recent 'discovery' of autism in 1943 by Leo Kanner. Since this time, the funding for international autism research has increased, particularly in the US over the past decade. As a result, centres and networks for autism research have been established throughout the US and have contributed significantly to our increased knowledge and understanding about ASD. Research undertaken usually relates to one of the following broad areas: epidemiology, the characterisation of autism, the role of the environment, neuroscience, screening, early intervention, specific treatments, and school and community interventions.[2]

At the time of publication, and despite efforts to do so, no centres for autism research have been established in Australia and levels of funding are relatively small. Research is generally funded through institutional and/or government grants awarded to individuals based at one of the universities. The Apex Trust for Autism is the only autism-specific funding available in Australia on an annual basis: www.apexfoundation.org.au/Autism.htm.

Quality research does however occur throughout Australia and individuals with ASD, families, clinicians, educators and others can both benefit from and contribute to these research efforts. Research findings are usually published in scholarly journals but researchers are keen to ensure these findings are also made available more widely through conferences, seminars, workshops and newsletters produced by service providers and support groups.

Interested people can respond to invitations to participate in specific research projects or register interest through an autism register such as the one operated in Western Australia: www.autismwa.org.au/index.html.

There are many researchers interested in ASD; some Australian-based researchers, their institutional affiliations at the time of publication and key research areas are listed in Table 1. These researchers come from a variety of disciplines including medicine, education, psychology, speech pathology and occupational therapy. All have published in high quality peer-reviewed journals. Increasingly information is finding its way into the public domain and many universities are now making research available via their web sites. It is often worth searching these sites for recent publications and information. To locate any of the researchers listed, you can search the university web site with whom they are affiliated.

Table 1. Australian Researchers

RESEARCHER	INSTITUTION	RESEARCH AREA
Attwood, Tony	The Asperger's Syndrome Clinic	Asperger's syndrome, anxiety
Arthur-Kelly, Michael	Newcastle University	Multiple/severe disability, communication, positive behaviour support
Brock, Jon	Macquarie University	Language, memory, perception, cognitive and neural integration
Botroff, Verity	Flinders University	Social cognition, inclusion, friendship, bullying, challenging behaviours
Brereton, Avril	Monash University	Early intervention, parent education, emotional & behavioural problems
Dissanayake, Cheryl	LaTrobe University	Early detection, social-cognitive/emotional development, pretend play
Gray, Kylie	Monash University	Diagnosis, screening, behaviour/emotional problems, development
Keen, Deb	Griffith University	Communication, educational and behavioural interventions, families
Kilham, Chris	Canberra University	Early intervention, communication
Maybery, Murray	University of Western Australia	Cognitive and perceptual strengths and weaknesses
McGillivray, Jane	Deakin University	Mental health and wellbeing
Nielsen, Mark	University of Queensland	Social learning, social cognition, pretend play
Prior, Margot	Melbourne University	Broader Autism Phenotype, early intervention, repetitive behaviour
Richdale, Amanda	RMIT University	Sleep, intervention, language, social cognition
Rinehart, Nicole	Monash University	Neuromotor features of autism and Asperger's disorder
Roberts, Jacqueline	University of Sydney	Early intervention, education, communication
Rodger, Sylvia	University of Queensland	Early intervention, families, play, parent education, Asperger's syndrome
Sofronoff, Kate	University of Queensland	Asperger's syndrome, anxiety

RESEARCHER	INSTITUTION	RESEARCH AREA
Tonge, Bruce	Monash University	Psychiatry
Williams, Katrina	University of NSW	Early identification, prognosis, epidemiology, treatment
Woodyatt, Gail	University of Queensland	Asperger's syndrome, language
Wray, John	State Child Development Centre, Health Service, West Perth	Biology, epidemiology, alternative therapies
Young, Robyn	Flinders University	Early diagnosis and intervention

USEFUL RESEARCH WEB SITES

It is not possible to list every web site related to autism research but the sites listed below are reliable and reputable. Some provide links to other sites and researchers.

National Institutes of Health (NIH) has several autism research networks that can be accessed through the following web site: www.autismresearchnetwork.org/AN/default.aspx

Another NIH organisation is the Interagency Autism Coordinating Committee:www.nimh.nih.gov/research-funding/scientific-meetings/recurring-meetings/iacc/index.shtml

The International Society for Autism Research (INSAR) holds an annual conference called the International Meeting for Autism Research (IMFAR). Abstracts from the conference can be downloaded: http://autism-insar.org/index.php

Interactive Autism Network (IAN) is an online project to facilitate and accelerate autism research. The primary aim is to generate and maintain an online research data set on children with autism which will be made available to researchers: www.IANproject.org

Autism Speaks (www.autismspeaks.org/science/research/index.php) is a not-for-profit organisation that fundraises to promote research. Research grants are available through this organisation as is the Autism Treatment Network (ATN) that was designed to share evidence-based practices with a patient registry to inform treatment outcomes. www.cureautismnow.org/ATN

Up-to-date information on intervention research via a not-for-profit organisation in the UK: www.researchautism.net

AUSTRALIAN WEB SITES WITH INFORMATION AND LINKS TO RESEARCH

Autism Victoria has an active research group with information: www.autismvictoria.org.au/research/

Autism Spectrum Australia (ASPECT) lists current research projects: www.aspect.org.au/research/studies.asp

The Australian Advisory Board on ASD is the peak body for a number of autism associations around Australia and their web site has links to these associations and their national autism conference: http://autismaus.com.au/aca/

References
1. Simpson, R. (2005). Evidence-based practices and students with autism spectrum disorders. *Focus on Autism and Other Developmental Disabilities*, 20(3), 140–149.
2. Interagency Autism Coordinating Committee. (2006). *Evaluating progress on the IACC autism research matrix*. Bethesda, MD: Author.

APPENDIX 2:
Advocating for your child with ASD

By Bob Buckley

Bob Buckley is Convenor of A4, Autism and Aspergers Advocacy Australia, and a Director of the Australian Advisory Board on Autism Spectrum Disorders.

ACTING IN YOUR CHILD'S BEST INTERESTS

At times parents have to speak up for their children. At times they need to protect their child against moves to deprive them of an essential service or a critical resource ostensibly 'for the greater good'. This is especially true for children with ASD.

Children with autism are among the most vulnerable people in our community. They have limited abilities to defend their rights. Many of them have difficulty speaking for themselves even on simple issues. On complex issues, they may not even understand what is happening. Our community does not respect the rights of children with ASD to essential services, to choose differently from others and to have a valued place in the community. These things are basic human rights.

Parents and the families of children with ASD have a critical role in advocating, in vigorously defending and protecting the rights of children with ASD. Rarely does anyone understand the needs of a child with ASD as well as the family, and no one else has the same commitment.

At times, others will be involved in advocating for your child:

- The manager in a child care centre may ask a government department, or a school principal may ask the education department, for additional or specialist support for your child.
- A child's teacher will ask the school for resources and for special consideration for your child.
- Your child may have some support from a case manager or case worker.
- Your child's GP may help advocate for services through the health or social security systems.
- You may get an advocacy service provider involved.

These people may help with your advocacy. To keep their help and support going, you should recognise and express appreciation for their efforts and achievements in advocating for your child.

However, in the big battles, who will advocate for your child through to the end? No one else has the same commitment. No one else puts your child's interests ahead of everything else. Parents are usually a child's most committed, fervent and effective advocates.

WHAT IS ADVOCACY?

Advocacy is effective or successful negotiation. Advocacy for a child with ASD is getting what your child needs when they need it.

Advocacy is a process. Once you have worked out what is best for your child, you need to work out where you might get the things your child needs. Advocacy is the process of getting others to contribute to meeting your child's needs.

Advocacy is often easiest and most effective in relation to an individual, but some advocacy is best done in groups. When you know others with the same needs, you will generally be better off working as a group.

Advocacy is often divided into two types:

- Individual advocacy — the advocacy is meant to benefit a particular individual and may require an individual solution.
- Systemic advocacy — changing the systems to benefit people more generally.

Much of what follows relates to both individual advocacy and systemic (or group) advocacy.

WHAT TO ADVOCATE FOR

It is essential that you work out what you are advocating for. Try to express what it is you want in terms of outcomes rather than processes.

Imagine several quite different ways your goals can be achieved. You don't have to work out any details: that comes later, once there is agreement to go ahead. For example, you might want a situation for your child that protects them from bullying through lunch periods at school. There are a number of ways this could be achieved: support or closer supervision in the playground, inside activities in a smaller group, easy access to a refuge space or a mixture of approaches.

It is important to be sure that what you want is possible. Your advocacy goals have to be winnable targets. Ask yourself 'can I reasonably expect a politician would give me what I want?' If not, how can a government official say 'Yes' to your requests? Equally important is not to aim too low.

You may have a lot of targets. Try to sort out your priorities; which things are most important.

Making a case is easier when advocating for something that is a right. Children have the right, under the UN Convention on the Rights of the Child, to education, treatment and rehabilitation etc. The right to education does not mean your child is 'present' while other children are being educated, it means your child receives an education service that is effective for your child.

WHEN TO ADVOCATE

Start off choosing just a couple of things that are achievable and winnable targets and that are relatively high priority or urgent. Go after them first. Get some wins first.

It is important to get going. Do not put it off.

Keep focused on your first two or three goals.

HOW TO ADVOCATE

'How' to advocate for a child with autism is a pretty big subject. There are a lot of strategies and different things work best with different people in varied circumstances.

Letting people know what you want is essential. If you do not get it immediately, then write to service providers asking for services to meet specific needs. Specify the outcome you want.

In your communication, do **not** tell them:

- why you want it, or
- how it can be achieved.

Simply tell them you child has autism and needs the service or resource you are requesting.

In your letter, you can suggest a meeting or ask them to contact you. They may call you back to set up a meeting. If not, call them.

Go to meetings prepared. Have your own agenda. Write down the issues you want to discuss and what you expect the meeting to achieve. If you get to the meeting and there is no agenda, give people a copy of your agenda and try to keep the meeting on your agenda. Alternatively send yours before the meeting. If your agenda items are not covered in a meeting, then insist on a follow-up meeting to cover these items.

Always take notes; keep a record. Keep your notes together. Review your notes before meetings.

After a meeting, review your agenda and the notes. If they distracted or diverted you from your agenda, get back to them, preferably in writing, asking that your concerns be addressed promptly.

If you make any progress, ensure that it is documented. If you are negotiating with government, make sure they keep a record and that it records the things you regard as significant or important. If things are omitted, you can write to them after the meeting to confirm your understanding. Write a letter that says ...

> Dear Ms Smith
> I write to confirm that in our last meeting we agreed your goal is outcome X within the next three months. To this effect:
>
> - Service P would provide N hours of B, starting in two weeks;
> - You would ensure staff involved were trained effectively in B
> - etc

Leave them with the action items. Make sure they are not waiting for you. If they need you to do something (sign a form, make a decision etc) get it done at the meeting or immediately afterwards. And tell them it has been done.

Make sure the people you are working with are actually able to deliver what you need. If they do not have the authority to allocate resources then they cannot help you. Insist on meeting with people who can actually help.

When parents are advocating, they are asked a lot of questions. When asked 'What do you want?' or 'What do you need?' remember to tell them what you need, not how to go about it.

What you say next depends on the people in the meeting. Generally it is best to only give brief, non-specific answers at first; for example: 'To achieve outcome X, you could provide an autism-specific intervention or service that targets the specific challenge'. If you have spoken with a professional about your concerns, and they have provided you with advice, you can say 'I suggest you call Y. You can contact her on ....'.

Effective advocacy is about outcomes for your child, not whose idea it was or who has the best ideas. Harry S. Truman said:

> *It is amazing what you can accomplish if you do not care who gets the credit.*

Frequently, a teacher, case manager or service provider comes up with a fantastic idea which is something you have said before. The worst thing to say is 'that was my idea' or 'I suggested that weeks ago'. Instead, say 'what a brilliant idea'.

Successful advocacy involves getting people to devise and implement ideas that succeed. It is not about your own ideas. If B is the best approach sometimes it is best to get people to think of B for themselves. You can suggest they try either A or C, things on either side that are similar and let them come up with B. In some cases, you'll meet a team player; you can say directly 'I think B will work' and they'll agree.

Once they come up with the idea, encourage them. Then get the timeframes and resources agreed and documented. When will things be done? When should we see results?

This is even more crucial if they decide to do something that you doubt will work. Put in place a plan to review the result and move on if it does not work. They may suggest the same thing for you if you insist on your idea and they doubt it will work.

If your advocacy is not working, it might be best to try somewhere else. You can try several places at once. Try to keep moving forwards. Avoid delays and pauses in the process.

Finally, in advocating for services, continually review your actions. Are you using your effort in the best way? Your child's needs must be met. If you are spending more time on advocacy than on meeting your child's needs then advocacy may not be the best use of your energy, especially if it is unlikely to succeed.

WHO TO CONTACT

Choose your targets for advocacy. Where are you most likely to get what you want? Is a government agency or service provider more likely to give you what you need? Sometimes a charity may be the best source of help.

You should spend your efforts on people who make decisions. Do not waste your time with people who do not have the authority to make decisions. Thus, at schools, you will generally need to deal with the principal. No one else really has the authority.

Often the decision relates to policy or an interpretation of policy. When you encounter a policy barrier, go to the people who make the policy and get them to vary or reinterpret the policy for you. Do not argue with the people who are merely controlled by the policy.

If you cannot get a decision from someone, ask to meet or speak with their supervisor. Generally, you can take one or two steps up the organisation but if you still do not get a decision, go right to the top. As you progress through an organisation try to make friends rather than enemies: be polite and understanding.

If someone is blocking you, it is usually best to go around them rather than trying to knock them out of the way.

ALONE OR WITH HELP

Advocacy as a small group can be especially effective. You give each other energy and support. A group can be wiser and more informed than an individual. Make sure the group understands the goals. Make sure the group agrees to stick together because you are less likely to succeed if the group is divided.

Federal and state governments fund a number of advocacy services in Australia. You can approach these agencies for help. The main criticisms of government funded advocacy services are:

- they lack understanding of the specific needs of people with autism
- many have their own agenda which may not be consistent with the needs of people with ASD and their families
- they are often too thinly spread and do not have the capacity to support the high needs of people with ASD.

If you need help and support getting started, an advocacy service may be useful. They can help you prepare and may be able to organise or come with you to meetings so you are not alone. Sometimes it may be best to take a friend or relative to meetings. They can serve as a witness or they can just help you through some difficult situations.

ADVOCACY TOOLS

Advocacy is described above as successful negotiation. It is important to develop and improve negotiation skills. If you get a chance to learn negotiation techniques, do so. There are courses and books or you can just observe. Think about what it takes to get you to do things for others and what would motivate others to help you.

Effective advocacy makes everyone a winner. Try to see why someone would do something to help you and your child. How would they benefit, too? Many people want to help because it makes them feel good, so make them feel good about helping. Let them know they did a good thing.

Think about things that would prevent them helping you. Steer well clear of those barriers or remove them.

It's useful to know facts and to have good information but do not use it to tell people they are wrong. Instead, offer the information. Suggest there is a range of views on various issues. Always try to keep negotiations positive.

Do not attribute to malice anything that could be due to a lack of knowledge. Generally people get things wrong through not thinking things through sufficiently and not knowing enough. Quite often we need to give people information then give them time to understand what we have told them.

Do not make threats. Threats get you nowhere. If things go so badly that you feel you have to make a formal complaint, just do it without warning. Do not threaten or talk about it — there is no point. You may get yourself into trouble, damage your case or cloud the issues with emotion and angry interaction.

SYSTEMIC ADVOCACY
Systemic advocacy is advocacy directed at or about changing systems. Systemic advocacy for autism in Australia usually involves a high degree of political lobbying. Its goal is to try to get government and bureaucracies to recognise and address the needs of people with ASD.

There is a wide range of organisations involved in systemic advocacy. Most groups have a broad range of interests and systemic advocacy is just a part of what they do. They may focus on the needs of a sub-group such as people with Asperger's syndrome, or young children. Their goals may relate to a particular service, treatment or therapy. Or they may be interested in people with disabilities in general. They may have a particular ideology.

Other types of advocacy include:

- self-advocacy where the person involves advocates on his/her own behalf.
- group advocacy
- legal advocacy.

GETTING STARTED
Advocacy sounds complicated but it is simple.

The most important thing is to just do it. If your child needs services and resources that you cannot provide, or that the child care centre or school does not provide, then you need to ask for them. Do not worry too much about getting it right.

You do not have to follow all advice in this document; the above are merely some suggestions about advocacy. Plenty of people succeed without any advice or by using quite different methods. You will have more success with practice. Emphasise the benefits for your child. Focus on helping your child and how good outcomes will benefit everyone.

GLOSSARY

Adaptive Behaviour Assessment System (ABAS): Measure designed to assess adaptive living skills.

Adaptive living skills: Behaviours necessary for people to live independently and to function safely and appropriately in daily life, such as grooming, dressing, ability to work, social skills etc.

Adjustment: A measure or action taken to assist a student with a disability to participate in education and training on the same basis as other students.

Applied Behavioural Analysis (ABA): An intervention model based on Skinner's theory of operant conditioning, which reinforces wanted behaviours and reduces unwanted behaviours.

Asperger's disorder/syndrome: A form of ASD, characterised by normal IQ but impairments in social interaction and communication.

Attention deficit hyperactivity disorder (ADHD): Disorder in children associated with three main kinds of problems: overactive behaviour (hyperactivity), impulsive behaviour and difficulty in paying attention.

Atypical antipsychotic: A newer type of medicine, used to treat psychosis, which has a better side effect profile than older antipsychotic medications; sometimes used to treat some of the symptoms of autism.

Auditory Integration Therapy (AIT): Therapy in which a child with ASD listens to a selection of music which has been modified.

Augmentative communication: Use of sign language, picture communication symbols or speech generating devices to replace or augment the speech of a person with autism.

Autism: A condition characterised by impairments in social interactions, communication and behaviour.

Autism Detection in Early Childhood (ADEC): An ASD screening tool.

Autism Diagnostic Interview–Revised (ADI-R): A diagnostic interview for ASD.

Autism Diagnostic Observation Schedule (ADOS): A diagnostic tool for ASD.

Autism Spectrum Disorders (ASD): Umbrella term for a range of neurological disorders characterised by severe and pervasive impairment in several areas of development including social skills, communication and repetitive behaviour.

Autistic disorder: See autism.

Bayley's Scales of Infant Development: A developmental assessment.

Blind or blinded study: A study in which the researcher and/or the patients are unaware of whether they have been assigned to the group receiving the active treatment or to the control group

Blood brain barrier: A protective barrier which prevents some substances in the blood from entering brain tissue.

Central nervous system: The part of the nervous system that consists of the brain and spinal cord.

Checklist for Autism in Toddlers (CHAT): An ASD screening tool

Childhood Autism Rating Scale (CARS): A screening and diagnostic tool for ASD.

Childhood disintegrative disorder: An extremely rare pervasive developmental disorder in which a child appears to develop normally until the age of two and then regresses.

Clinical trial: A research study conducted with patients which tests out a drug or other intervention to assess its effectiveness and safety.

Cognitive: Pertaining to cognition, the process of being aware, knowing, thinking, learning and judging.

Conduct disorder: A disorder of children and adolescents involving persistent antisocial behaviour.

Control: In clinical trials comparing two or more interventions, a control is a person in the comparison group that receives a placebo, no intervention, usual care or another form of care.

Core stability: 'Core' muscles whose strength is vital as a base of support for efficient and effective limb movements; most commonly refers to the pelvic floor, deep abdominals and deep spinal muscles in the back.

Developmental disorder: A disorder that interrupts normal development in childhood. A developmental disorder may affect a single area of development (specific developmental disorder) or several (pervasive developmental disorder).

Diagnostic and Statistical Manual of Mental Disorders 4th edition, Text Revision: American Psychiatric Association's official manual used by most professionals for diagnosis of ASD. Sometimes the ICD 10 is used (see below).

Diagnostic Interview for Social and Communication Disorders (DISCO): A diagnostic interview for ASD.

DIR®/Floortime: A developmental early intervention model. DIR stands for Developmental Individual-Difference Relationship-Based Model.

Discrete Trial Training (DTT): An ABA method which requires the therapists to break down skills into small tasks that are achievable and taught in a very structured manner.

Dyspraxia: A disorder of motor planning.

Echolalia: Repeating words or phrases, often over and over, without necessarily understanding their meaning.

Endpoint: Overall outcome that the trial is designed to evaluate.

Epidemiology: The study of how often diseases occur in different groups of people and why.

Epilepsy: A brain disorder involving recurrent seizures; sudden changes in behaviour due to excessive electrical activity in the brain.

Evidence-based: Refers to the use of best evidence derived from methodologically rigorous, valid research.

Expressive communication: Sending information or messages to other people. This could involve use of speech or augmentative communication.

Fine motor skills: Activities which require the co-ordination of smaller body muscles eg writing.

Functional analysis: Process of carefully observing behaviour to determine what sets off the chain of events that leads to a problem behaviour, such as tantrums or aggression.

Gluten-free, casein-free (GFCF) diet: A diet believed by some to help improve the symptoms of autism. It involves elimination from the diet of gluten (a protein found in wheat and other grains) and casein (a protein found in dairy products).

Griffiths Scales of Mental Development: A developmental assessment.

Gross motor skills: Body movements which utilise larger muscle groups such as sitting, kicking and jumping.

High functioning autism (HFA): Autism in individuals with normal/ near-normal IQ.

Individual education plan (IEP): A document that delineates special education services for special needs students.

Intellectual disability: An impaired ability to learn, as measured by IQ score (<70) and associated difficulties in adaptive functioning. It is a condition which presents before the age of eighteen.

Intelligence quotient (IQ): The ratio of tested mental age to chronological age, usually expressed as a quotient multiplied by 100.

Intensive behavioural intervention (IBI): An individualised, intensive intervention program which involves the systematic use of ABA techniques.

International Statistical Classification of Diseases and Related Health Problems (ICD 10): Manual produced by the World Health Organisation, which provides codes to classify diseases and disorders. The latest version is known as ICD 10. The definition of autistic disorder in the ICD 10 is almost identical to that in the DSM-IV.

Joint attention: Ability to follow someone else's gaze and share the experience of looking at an object or activity

Low functioning autism (LFA): Autism associated with an intellectual disability.

Mainstreaming: The concept that students with special needs should, when appropriate, be integrated with their non-disabled peers to the maximum extent possible.

Makaton®: A manual signing system sometimes used to augment verbal communication for individuals with ASD.

Modified Checklist for Autism in Children (M-CHAT): An ASD screening tool.

Motor planning: The brain's ability to conceive, organise and execute a sequence of complex physical actions.

Neurobehavioural: Relating to the relationship between the action of the nervous system and behaviour.

Neurological: Having to do with the nerves or the nervous system.

Neurology: The medical science that deals with the nervous system and disorders affecting it.

Neurotransmitter: A chemical messenger released from one nerve cell which makes its way to another nerve cell where it influences a particular chemical reaction to occur.

Neurotypical: A term sometimes used to describe people without an ASD.

Observational Study: A study in which the investigators do not seek to intervene, and simply observe the course of events.

Obsessive compulsive disorder (OCD): Disorder where a person has recurrent unwanted ideas (obsessions) and an urge (compulsion) to do something to relieve the obsession

Open Trial: A clinical trial in which the investigator and participant are aware which intervention is being used for which participant (ie not blinded).

Opioid: A substance with pharmacological action like that of opium or its derivatives (eg morphine).

Outcome measure: The measure of an effect or impact of an intervention on the participants.

Parkinsonism: Condition that causes movement abnormalities like those seen in Parkinson's disease eg tremors, slow movement, or muscle rigidity.

Peer-review: A refereeing process for checking the quality and importance of reports of research. An article submitted for publication in a peer-reviewed journal is reviewed by other experts in the area.

Pervasive developmental disorder - not otherwise specified (PDD-NOS): An ASD where a child presents with impairments in social interaction, communication and behaviour but symptoms are not severe enough or of sufficient number to qualify for a diagnosis of autistic disorder.

Phenotype: The appearance of an individual, which results from the interaction of the person's genetic makeup and his or her environment.

Pica: Ingestion of non-food items.

Picture Exchange Communication System (PECS): A visual augmentative communication system.

Pivotal Response Training: A contemporary ABA intervention.

Placebo effect: Psychological benefit to the participant through a belief that they are receiving treatment

Placebo: An inactive intervention, received by the participants in the control group in a clinical trial, which is indistinguishable from the active intervention received by patients in the experimental group.

Pragmatics: Use of language in the social contexts.

Prevalence: A measure of the number of cases of a disorder in a defined population at a particular point in time. It differs from incidence, the rate at which new cases occur in a population during a specific time period.

Prolactin: A hormone which stimulates breast development and milk production.

Proprioception: A sense that informs us the position of our body parts.

Randomised controlled trial (RCT): Study design in which enrolment into a study is done by random allocation, that is, the patient has no greater likelihood of receiving the treatment or placebo (or the comparison treatment) than could be expected by chance alone.

Receptive communication: Receiving and understanding messages from others.

Relationship Development Intervention (RDI®): A developmental intervention model.

Rett's disorder: A rare genetic disorder, usually only found in females, in which a child appears to develop normally for a period and then regresses.

Risk factor: An aspect of a person's condition, lifestyle or environment that increases the probability of occurrence of a disease or condition.

Rubella: German measles.

Selective serotonin reuptake inhibitors (SSRI): A class of antidepressant medicines sometimes prescribed to help manage anxiety and repetitive behaviours associated with ASD.

Self-stimulatory behavior: Commonly referred to as a 'stim'. Any kind of repetitive or stereotypic behavior (e.g. staring at lights, flapping hands, rocking etc.), which is believed to provide some form of sensory stimulation.

Sensory integration therapy: Therapy which aims to improve the way the brain processes and organises the senses.

Sensory processing disorder: Disorder which makes people misinterpret everyday sensory information, such as touch, sound and movement.

Sensory profile: Questionnaire that describes responses to sensory events in daily life.

Social Communication Emotional Regulation Transactional Supports Model (SCERTS®): An early intervention model combining elements of contemporary ABA and developmental methods.

Social pragmatics: see Pragmatics.

Stereotypy: Persistent repetition of body movements, ideas, or words.

Stimming: Engaging in self-stimulatory behavior.

Stimulant medications: Class of drugs used to treat ADHD.

Theory of mind: Ability to attribute mental states to oneself and others and to understand what another person thinks, feels, desires, intends or believes.

Treatment and Education of Autistic and related Communication-handicapped CHildren (TEACCH): An early intervention model which emphasises structured teaching.

Vestibular: Pertaining to the sensory system in the inner ear that governs posture and balance.

Vineland Adaptive Behaviour Scales: Measures designed to assess adaptive living skills.

Visual supports: The presentation of information in a visually structured manner to make it easier to understand eg a daily schedule may be shown by photographs or cartoons.

Wechsler Intelligence Scale for Children (WISC): An IQ test.

Wechsler Preschool and Primary Scale of Intelligence (WPPSI): An IQ test.

Acknowledgements

Firstly, we would like to acknowledge the contribution of a range of Australian experts in the field of ASD, who have willingly offered us their time and expertise. Dr Richard Couper, Associate Professor Deb Keen, Dr Antony Underwood and Associate Professor Robyn Young have most generously shared their specialist knowledge with us and we are thrilled to include their contributions in this book. Justine Watson, counsellor and parent of a child with ASD, has written 'Through Grief to Self Care' perhaps one of our most important chapters. Another fellow parent and champion of the rights of people with ASD, Bob Buckley, penned the very helpful Advocacy appendix.

Behind the scenes many other eminent specialists provided us with expert guidance. These include the leading developmental paediatricians Dr Natalie Silove of the Children's Hospital at Westmead (Sydney) and Dr John Wray of the Women's and Children's Health Service in Perth. Associate Professor Katrina Williams, paediatric epidemiologist at the Sydney Children's Hospital and the University of NSW provided advice for 'How Did It Happen?' Psychologist Anne Chalfant from Annie's Centre gave us her unique insights into diagnosis and the social impacts of ASDs. Occupational therapist Kim Bulkeley and paediatrician Dr Joanne Leal also offered advice willingly and most helpfully. Special thanks must go to Dr Jacqueline Roberts, co-author of the 2006 federal government-sponsored *Review of the Research to Identify the Most Effective Models of Practice in Early Intervention for Children with Autism Spectrum Disorders*, who kindly reviewed three chapters in total — a considerable chunk of the book.

We'd also like to express our appreciation to our other contributors: the many parents who provided the quotes (some anonymous; some attributed) and personal stories which give this book its heart and illustrate the impact of ASDs in a way that science and statistics could never do. Many are acknowledged throughout the pages of the book but we need also to express thanks to the following people: Julie Allen, Jenny Badger, Elena Barnes, Michelle Barrett, Susan Bowman, Alison Cornish, Ruth Evatt, Valerie Foley, Sandy Gray, Jenny Grindell, Marion Redmond, Elizabeth Sheedy and Audrey Uren.

The writers of our 'Where Are They Now?' chapter deserve a special mention for their bravery and honesty. Grateful thanks to Elena Barnes, Jennifer Couper, Kate Hurley, Dorothy Macrae-McMahon, Caroline McCallum, Therese Potma, Wendy Rafferty, Nicole Rogerson and Kim Stockton.

Many thanks to all the people who responded so positively to requests for information for the Resource Guide. There is great goodwill in the ASD community and the support for this project was tremendously encouraging.

We would like to thank the publisher of this book, Jane Curry, who has known for a long time that this book really needed to be written and has been unfailingly generous in her efforts. Our editor, Sarah Plant, has taken the writing of two different authors and expertly merged them into a coherent whole. The book is so much better as a result of her efforts.

On a personal note Seana would like to thank Kathryn Eardley-Wilmot, Ruth Evatt, Susanne Fraser, Kelly Hargreaves, Liz Heath, Maria Mitsios, Elizabeth Sheedy and Desley Stewart for their longstanding practical and emotional support. Benison would particularly like to acknowledge the following people: Dr Greg Rowell, Donna White, Micaela Middleton, Susan Hollar, Debbie Evans, Karin Raynal, Emily Pidcock, Joe's longest-serving therapists, Bianca Circosta and Vedran Vulovic, and all her friends who have provided wise counsel and laughter over the years. To all those other therapists and teachers who have worked with our boys and helped them to get to where they are today, unfortunately we can't single you all out, but you know who you are! Sincere thanks from us both.

Finally we would like thank our extended families and particularly our long-suffering husbands, Paul (Seana) and James (Benison) for their patient and loving support and — last but not least — Seana's children Dexter, Jamie and Iona, and Benison's big boys Matthew and Nicholas for putting up with distracted and occasionally cranky mothers in the months leading up to publication.

But of course, our biggest debt of gratitude must go to our brave and clever boys, Tom and Joe, without whom this book would never have been written.

INDEX